ATLAS OF
Clinical Gynecology

ATLAS OF

Clinical Gynecology

SERIES EDITOR

Morton A. Stenchever, MD

Professor, Chairman Emeritus
Department of Obstetrics and Gynecology
University of Washington Medical Center
Seattle, Washington

Volume V

Urogynecology and Reconstructive Pelvic Surgery

VOLUME EDITOR

J. Thomas Benson, MD

Clinical Professor of Gynecology
Director of Urogynecology and Reconstructive Pelvic Surgery
Indiana University School of Medicine
Indianapolis, Indiana

With 14 contributors

Developed by Current Medicine, Inc.
Philadelphia

McGraw-Hill
Health Professions Division

New York St. Louis San Francisco Auckland Bogotá Caracas Lisbon London
Madrid Mexico City Milan Montreal New Delhi San Juan
Singapore Sydney Tokyo Toronto

McGraw-Hill
A Division of The McGraw-Hill Companies

Current Medicine, Inc.
400 Market Street
Suite 700
Philadelphia, PA 19106

Managing Editor	*Mary Kinsella*
Development Editor	*Susan L. Hunsberger*
Editorial Assistant	*Lisa M. Janda*
Design	*Robert LeBrun*
Layout	*Rachel Berlin, Christoper Allan*
Illustrators	*Nicole Mock, Paul Schiffmacher, Anne Rains, Wieslawa Langenfeld, Debra Wertz, Sharon Harris, Joel Harris, Becky Slemmons, Larry Ward, Andra Ross, Terri Mulley, Chris Peterson*
Art Director	*Jerilyn Kauffman*
Illustration Director	*Debra Wertz*
Production Manager	*Lori Holland*
Production Associate	*Constance Copeland*
Index	*Dorothy DiRienzi*

Urogynecology and pelvic reparative surgery / volume editor, J. Thomas
Benson ; with 37 contributors.
p. cm. —(Atlas of clinical gynecology ; v. 5)
Includes bibliographical references and index.
ISBN 0-8385-0320-9 (alk. paper)
1. Urogynecology—Atlases. 2. Generative organs, Female—Surgery
Atlases. 3. Urinary incontinence—Atlases. 4. Fecal incontinence
Atlases. 5. Pelvis—Diseases—Surgery Atlases I. Benson, J.
Thomas. II. Series.
[DNLM: 1. Gonadal Diseases, Female Atlases. 2. Fecal
Incontinece—surgery Atlases. 3. Rectal Prolapse—surgery Atlases.
4. Urinary Incontinence—surgery Atlases.WP 17 A8806 1998 v.5]
RG484.U755 1999
618.1—dc21
DNLM/DLC
for Library of Congress 99-33745
CIP

Printed in Singapore by Imago Productions (FE) Pte Ltd.

10 9 8 7 6 5 4 3 2 1

Series Preface

The *Atlas of Clinical Gynecology* is an ambitious 5-volume series covering the field of gynecology. Volume topics include pediatric and adolescent gynecology, oncology, pathology, reproductive endocrinology, urogynecology, and reparative surgery. Each volume contains more than 500 images. The images in this collection include not only traditional photographs, but also charts, tables, algorithms, and diagrams, making this collection much more than an atlas in the conventional sense.

The atlas series serves as an excellent teaching tool and resource. In the past few decades, individual learning styles have changed dramatically. In the past, the printed work in book and journal was the primary way in which information was transferred and learning accomplished. In recent decades, however, education has been greatly enhanced by the addition of audio and visual technology. More recently, the advent of personal computers has further enriched the types of learning modalities available.

The *Atlas of Clinical Gynecology* series is designed to use the printed word and visual modalities. The information can be used by individual students and by those who teach physicians, medical students, and other health care professionals. The atlas may also serve as a valuable patient education tool.

The series is comprehensive and includes topics that may neglected in the literature or absent from some training programs. Often practitioners do not see enough patients with a given condition to develop expertise in diagnosis and management. The series is designed to expose the clinician to the unfamiliar as well as to update information on more common gynecologic problems.

I wish to thank the volume editors for their expertise and dedication-Alvin Goldfarb, Barbara Goff, Daniel Mishell, Benjamin Greer, F. J. Montz, and J. Thomas Benson. We hope that physicians, health care professionals, and the educators who train them find the quality and format of this series useful in the diagnosis and treatment of women of all ages. They deserve the best care available.

Morton A. Stenchever, MD

Volume Preface

Pelvic floor disorders have plagued women since their evolution into upright, two-legged, live-bearing creatures. With the aging of the population and the increased quality-of-life expectations, patients with these disorders represent a rapidly growing segment requiring rapidly improving therapies.

Pelvic floor disorders include pelvic organ prolapse, urinary voiding dysfunction and incontinence, colorectal constipation and incontinence, sexual difficulties, and pelvic pain problems. For years specialists have compartmentalized the therapies into piecemeal treatments with limited specific training in either the anterior, middle, or posterior compartments of the pelvic floor. During the past five years, a subspeciality dealing specifically and totally with these disorders has advanced from a special interest group to the fourth subspecialty accredited by the American Board of Obstetrics and Gynecology. This subspeciality is Urogynecology and Reconstructive Pelvic Surgery. Its accreditation has created multimodality training leading to comprehensive care for women with pelvic floor disorders.

This volume is intended to provide, in an interesting visual format, current material covering the basic aspects of urogynecology and reconstructive pelvic surgery for teachers, practitioners, and students.

J. T. Benson

Contributors

J. Thomas Benson, MD
Clinical Professor of Gynecology
Director of Urogynecology and Reconstructive Pelvic Surgery
Indiana University School of Medicine
Indianapolis, Indiana

Alfred E. Bent, MD
Division of Urogynecology and Reconstructive Pelvic Surgery
Department of Gynecology
Greater Baltimore Medical Center
Baltimore, Maryland

Mark I. Brand, MD
Assistant Professor
Department of Surgery
Rush Medical College
Chicago, Illinois

Linda Brubaker, MD
Associate Professor
Department of Obstetrics and Gynecology
Director
Section of Urogynecology and Reconstructive Pelvic Surgery
Rush Presbyterian St. Luke's Medical Center
Chicago, Illinois

Jeffrey L. Cornella, MD
Assistant Professor
Department of Gynecologic Surgery
Mayo Medical School
Head
Division of Urogynecology
Mayo Clinic Scottsdale
Scottsdale, Arizona

John O.L. DeLancey, MD
Associate Professor
Director, Division of Gynecology
University of Michigan Medical School
Ann Arbor, Michigan

Dee E. Fenner, MD
Associate Professor
Department of Obstetrics and Gynecology
Rush Medical College
Chicago, Illinois

Douglass S. Hale, MD
Associate Director
Urogynecology and Reconstructive Pelvic Surgery Fellowship
Methodist/Indiana University Hospital
Indianapolis, Indiana

W. Glenn Hurt, MD
Professor
Department of Obstetrics and Gynecology
Medical College of Virginia
Virginia Commonwealth University
Richmond, Virginia

Mary T. McLennan, MD
Assistant Professor
Department of Obstetrics and Gynecology
St. Louis University
St. Louis, Missouri

J. Scott Pittman, MD
Midwest Colon and Rectal Surgery, P.C.
Carmel
St. Vincent Hospital
Indianapolis, Indiana

Jack R. Robertson, MD
Professor Emeritus
Department of Urogynecology
University of Nevada at Las Vegas
Las Vegas, Nevada

Theodore J. Saclarides, MD
Professor
Department of Surgery
Rush Medical College
Chicago, Illinois

Stephen B. Young, MD
Associate Professor
Department of Obstetrics and Gynecology
Chair
Division of Urogynecology and Vaginal Surgery
University of Massachusetts
Worcester, Massachusetts

Contents

CHAPTER 1

Anatomy

John O. L. DeLancey

Muscles and connective tissues support the pelvic organs by attaching them to the bony pelvis. In women with pelvic organ prolapse and incontinence, damage to these muscles and fibrous structures result in descent of the vaginal walls and pelvic organs through the urogenital hiatus in the levator ani muscles. Different types of prolapse exist in different women. One woman may have a cystocele, while another may have a cystocele and rectocele. The site at which a muscle or fascia is damaged determines the type of prolapse present. Of course, understanding the nature of these different clinical problems must be based on an accurate understanding of the site and type of defect present.

The supportive apparatus that holds the pelvic organs in place was designed to operate in the standing position. This is the orientation in which the pelvic organ supports must be studied and understood. Physicians learn about pelvic anatomy from observing supine cadavers and by examining women in the clinic and operating room who are recumbent. This is somewhat like trying to understand how a parachute works while observing it lying crumpled on the ground. In considering the following anatomy, the reader should keep in mind the anatomical and topographical relationships as they exist under the effects of gravity in the standing individual.

Anatomy is the basic science of reconstructive pelvic surgery. This chapter is intended to provide a view of pelvic anatomy useful to clinicians that wish to understand the nature of pelvic organ prolapse. It is based on illustrative material taken directly from dissections of female cadavers supplemented with macroscopic and microscopic examination of serial sections containing the whole pelvis. Special techniques have been used to minimize embalming artifacts.

Careful attention to the illustrations should provide a framework for understanding the clinical topics that follow.

THE BONY PELVIS AND BORDERS OF THE PELVIC FLOOR

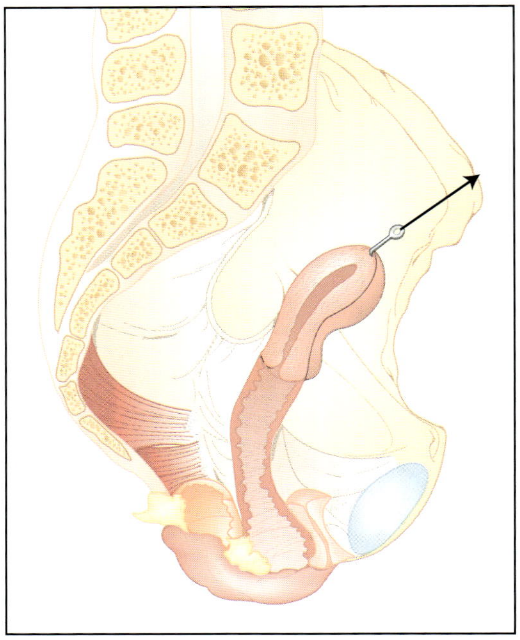

FIGURE 1-1.

Compartments of the pelvis. The pelvis is divided into an anterior and posterior compartment by the vagina and its attachments to the pelvic wall. The walls of the posterior compartment are formed by the sacrum, levator ani muscles. The pubic bones, internal obturator muscles, and the anterior projection of the levator ani muscles form the walls of the anterior compartment. The walls of the vagina are attached to the pelvic walls by the endopelvic fascia and form the separating wall that divides the anterior and posterior compartments.

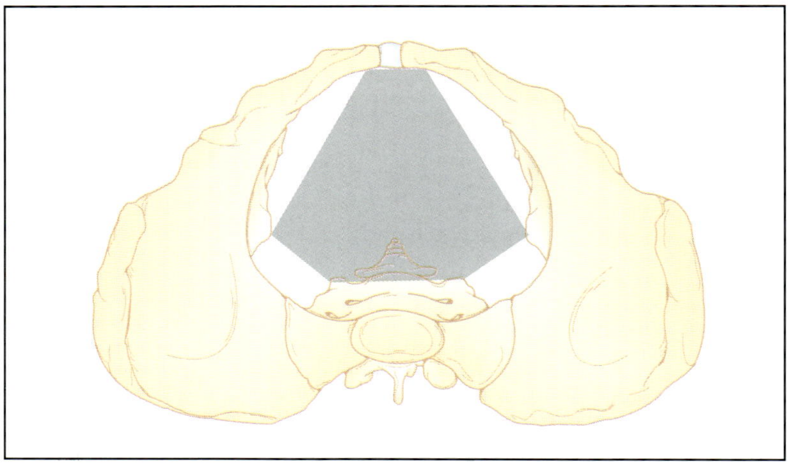

FIGURE 1-2.

Space occupied by the pelvic floor. The boundaries of the pelvic floor are hexagonal. The ventral bounds are the pubic bones anteriorly, the arcus tendinei laterally, and the sacrum and sacrospinous ligaments dorsally. The ischial spines form the lateral points of attachment for both the sacrospinous ligament and the arcus tendinei.

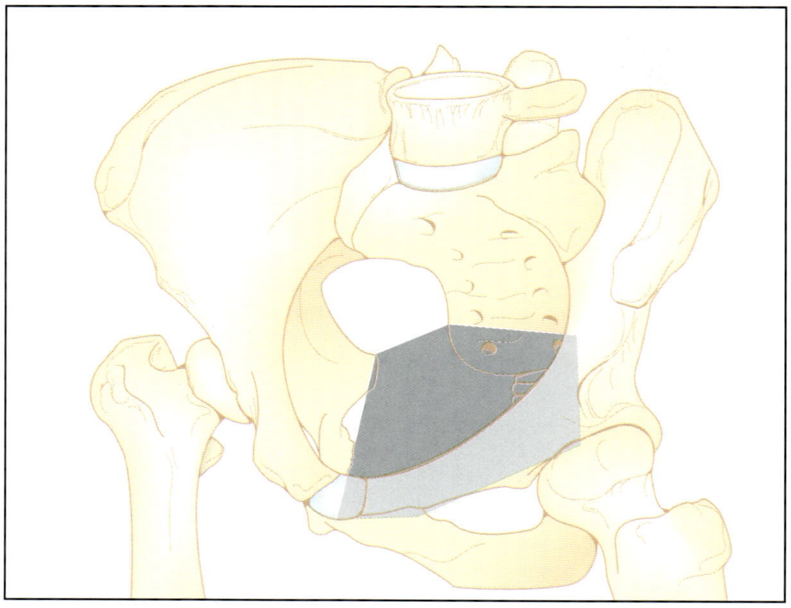

FIGURE 1-3.

Pelvic plane. The plane of the pelvic floor lies oblique to the horizontal plane in the standing position.

LEVATOR ANI MUSCLES AND ENDOPELVIC FASCIA

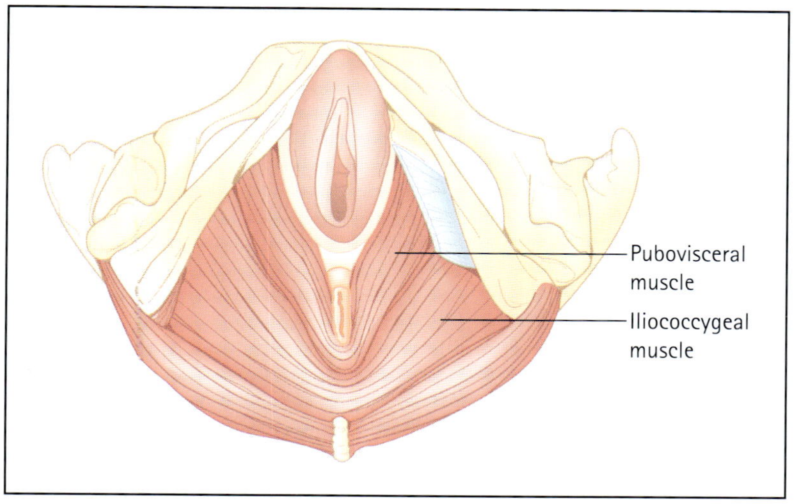

FIGURE 1-4
Levator ani muscles from below. This illustration shows the muscles of the pelvic floor from below, after the anal sphincters and the perineal membrane (urogenital diaphragm) have been removed. The cut edge of the left portion of the perineal membrane can be seen still attached to the ischiopubic ramus. The levator ani muscles span the opening in the pelvic bones. Note the thick portions adjacent to the vaginal wall. These are the puborectalis, pubococcygeus portion of the levator ani muscle, and they pull the pelvic opening closed constricting the genital hiatus in the levator ani muscles. The constant action of the muscles holds the perineal body, anus, and rectum anteriorly against the pubic bones closing the urogenital hiatus and vagina. The connective tissue of the perineal body helps to unite the levator ani muscles in the midline.

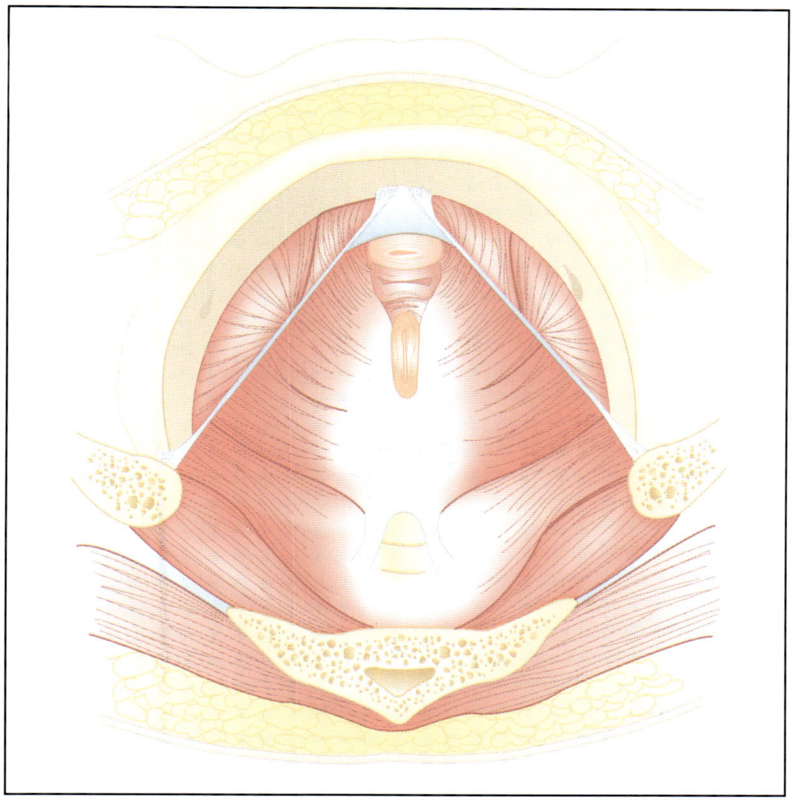

FIGURE 1-5.
Levator ani muscles from above. This figure shows the anatomy of the levator ani muscles seen from above. Note the ventral fibers of the levator ani muscle pass lateral to the tendinous arch of the pelvic fascia to arise from the pubic bones while the iliococcygeal fibers that arise closer to the ischial spine terminate at the level of the arcus.

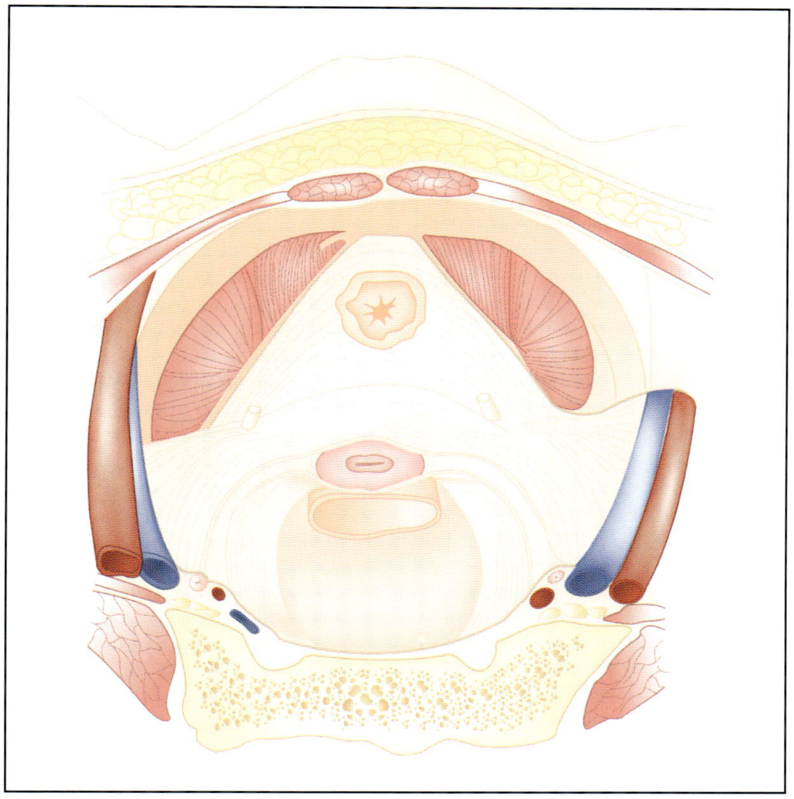

FIGURE 1-6.
Fascial tissues of the pelvis. The fascial tissues that attach the cervix to the pelvic wall are shown from above after the removal of the uterine corpus. Note how the uterosacral ligaments are simply the medial margin of these tissues. Also note the lateral boundary of the pelvic floor formed by the tendinous arch of the pelvic fascia.

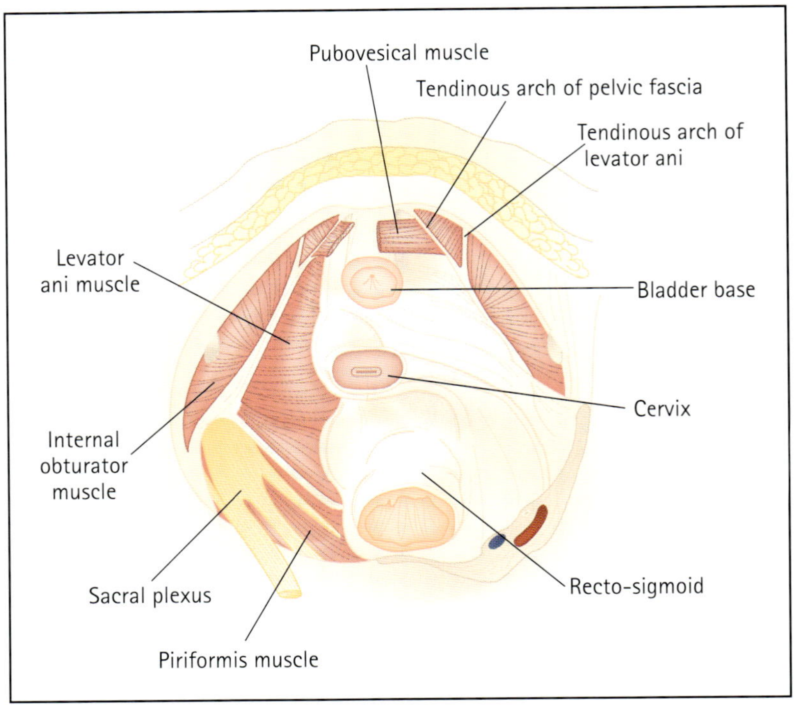

FIGURE 1-7.
The right side of this dissection shows the endopelvic fascia's attachment to the pelvic walls. The other side reveals the position of the levator ani muscles below this level as well as the nerves of the sacral plexus. Note the close proximity of the sacral plexus of nerves to the sacrospinous ligament as they exit the pelvis through the greater sciatic foramen on the inner surface of the piriformis muscle. The boundaries of the pelvic floor, the arcus tendineus, and coccygeus muscle/sacrospinous ligament complex is visible on the cadaver's left side.

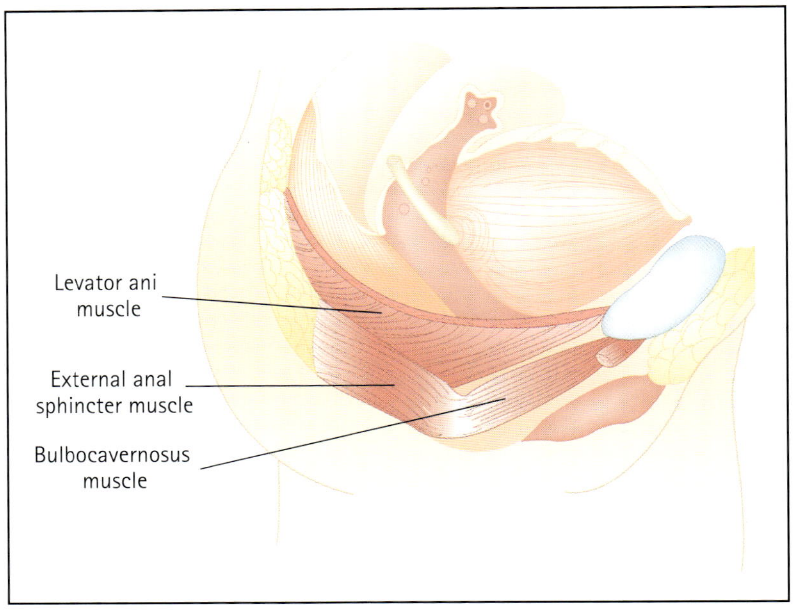

FIGURE 1-8.
Lateral view of the pelvis. This illustrates the relationship between the pelvic organs and the levator ani muscles. A portion of each organ system (urinary, genital, and intestinal) lies above the levator ani muscles. Each system has an orifice below the muscles. As the viscera pass through the pelvic musculature, they are influenced in two ways. First, the sling of the levator ani muscles pulls them toward the pubic bones constricting their lumens and preventing their downward descent through the attachment of the visceral walls and the muscles. Second, distal sphincters help occlude the lumens of each organ systems.

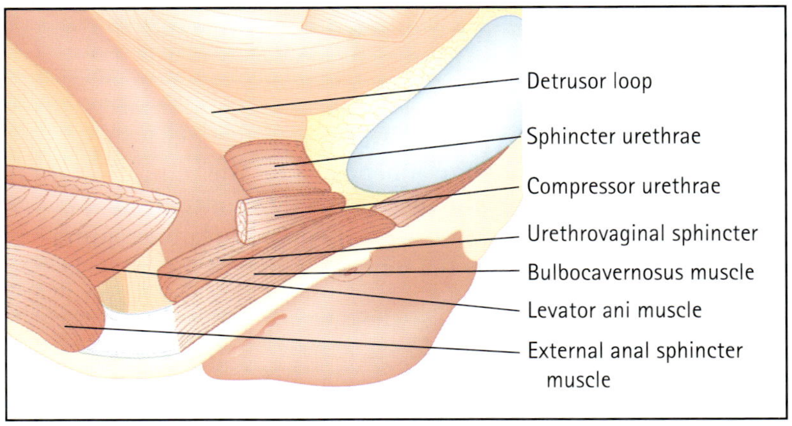

FIGURE 1-9.
In this illustration, the anterior portion of the levator ani muscle has been removed to show the urogenital sphincter muscles. The striated urogenital sphincter muscle has two regions. Just below the vesical neck, the muscle encircles the urethra. Nearer the external meatus, two bands of muscle arch over the dorsal urethral wall. One band, the urethrovaginal sphincter muscle, encircles both the vagina and urethra while the other, the compressor urethra, passes laterally along the ischiopubic rami just cephalad to the perineal membrane (urogenital diaphragm).

LEVELS OF FASCIAL SUPPORT

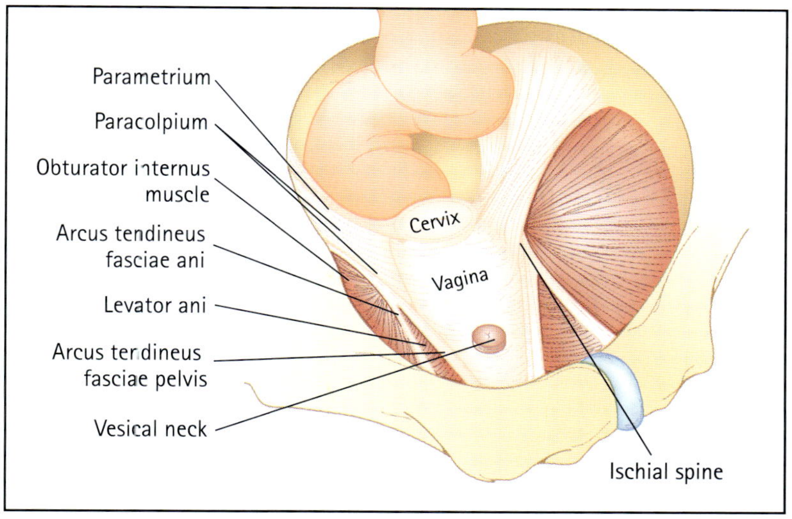

FIGURE 1-10.
Fascial supports of the vaginal apex and anterior vaginal wall. This illustration demonstrates the regional differences in the fascial attachments of the vagina and cervix to the pelvic walls. The bladder and corpus of the uterus have been removed so only the vesical neck and cervix remain. Note fascial fibers near the cervix and upper vagina are vertical in orientation while those attaching to the mid vagina are transverse, spanning the space between the fascial arches. It is also possible to see divergence between the two fascial arches. The tendinous arch of the levator ani from which the levator ani muscle arises attaches higher on the pubic bone than the tendinous arch of the pelvic fascia which is the structure to which the endopelvic fascia is attached.

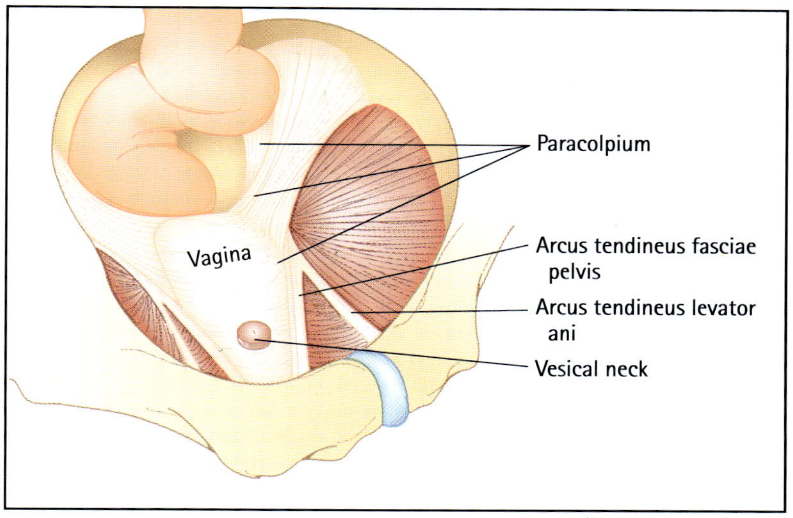

FIGURE 1-11.
Attachments to pelvic wall after hysterectomy. This figure reveals the situation present after hysterectomy. The upper vaginal supports differ from the mid-vaginal supports.

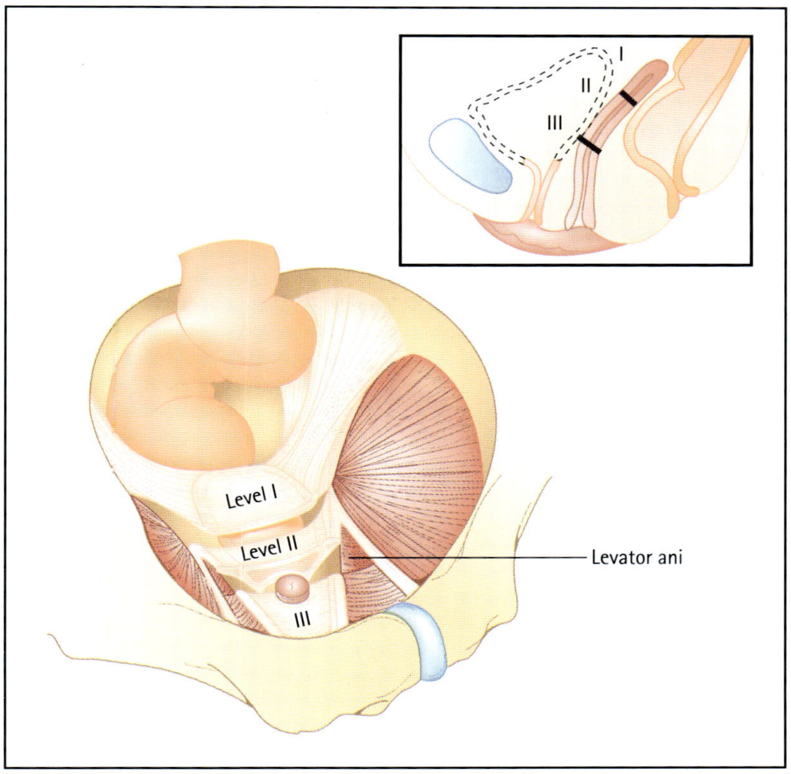

FIGURE 1-12.
The attachments of the vagina to the pelvic walls can be divided into three regions. Note that despite the removal of the cervix, the fibers in Level I, the long suspensory fibers of the paracolpium, suspend the upper vagina. In the mid vagina, Level II, the vagina is attached laterally to the tendinous arch of the pelvic fascia. Level III is characterized by fusion of the vagina to surrounding structures.

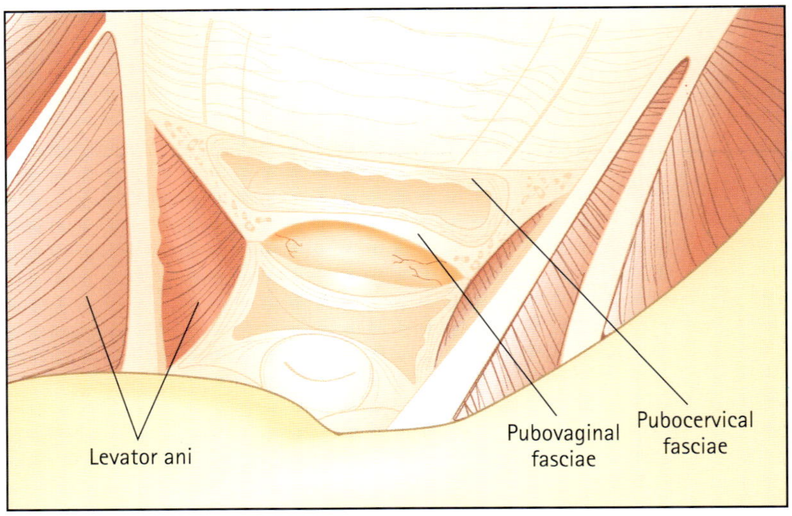

FIGURE 1-13.
Nature of level II. This view shows the caudal margin of Level II after a triangular wedge of the vagina wall has been removed. This exposes the distal urethra and the anterior surface of the rectum. The fascial attachment between the anterior vaginal wall and the tendinous arch of the pelvic fascia is visible. The structural layer on which the bladder rests is comprised of the vaginal wall and its connections through the pubocervical fascia to the arcus. At this level of the vagina, there is no separate layer that separates the vagina from the bladder. It is the wall of the vagina itself that is responsible for bladder base support.

ANATOMY OF THE URINARY CONTINENCE MECHANISM

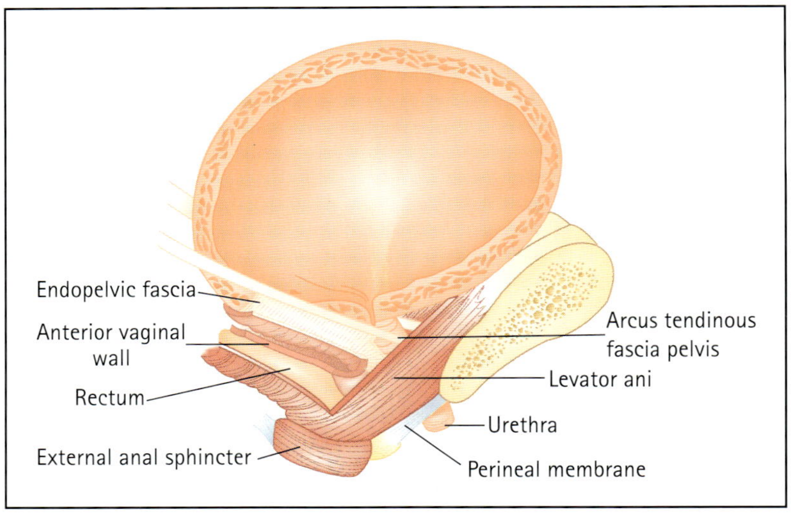

FIGURE 1-14.
Lateral view of the pelvic floor structures related to urethral support seen from the side in the standing position, cut just lateral to the midline. Note that windows have been cut in the levator ani muscles, vagina, and endopelvic fascia so that the urethra and anterior vaginal walls can be seen. Note the tendinous arch of the pelvic fascia stretched from the pubic bone to its eventual attachment to the ischium. The anterior vaginal wall is attached to the arcus by the endopelvic fascia and forms a supportive layer for the bladder and urethra. The levator ani muscle attaches to the endopelvic fascia so that contraction of the levator muscle can elevate the urethra.

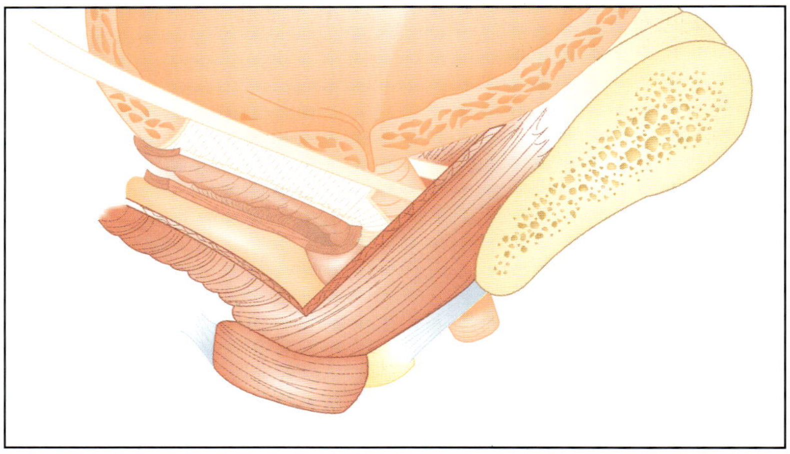

FIGURE 1-15.
Closeup of the urethral support structures shown in Figure 1-14.

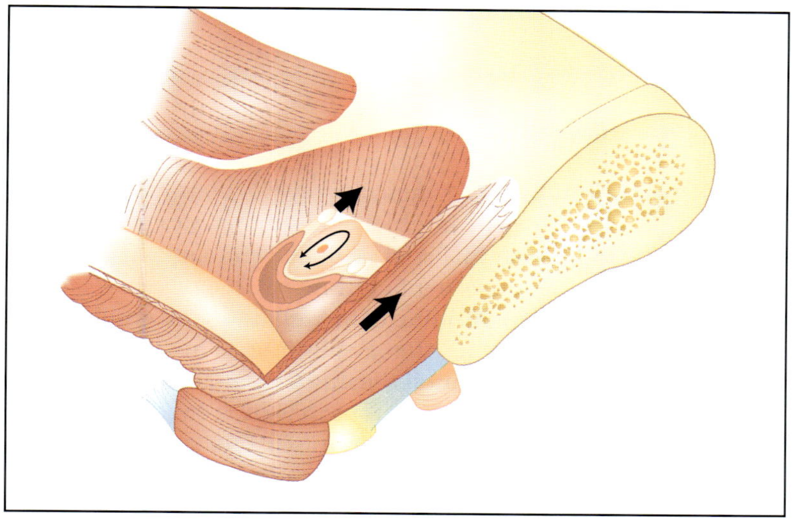

FIGURE 1-16.

There are two ways in which the striated muscles of the pelvic floor can affect urinary continence. The constrictive effects of the striated urogenital sphincter muscle within the wall of the urethra can increase urethral closure pressure during times of increased need and during increases in abdominal pressure. The levator ani muscles can also stiffen the supports of the urethra. As abdominal pressure pushes the urethra downward, this stiffened support system provides a firm and unyielding backboard against which the urethra can be compressed closed.

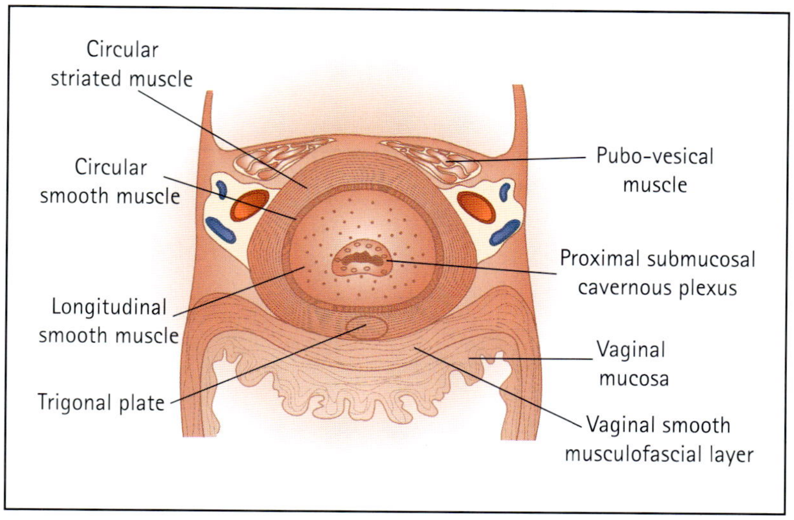

FIGURE 1-17.

This illustration depicts the structures seen in the mid-urethra. Here the striated muscle of the urethra can be seen to surround the circular and longitudinal smooth muscle layers. The submucosal vaginal musculofascial layer is the layer that provides support for the urethra. Note also the prominent vascular plexus that surrounds the mucosal lining of the urethra. This probably provides a flexible filling between the mucosa and muscular layers. The trigonal plate bridges the gap between the ends of the striated urogenital sphincter muscle. This gap does not impede its ability to constrict the lumen because the trigonal plate spans the separation between the muscles, forming a tendon-like union of the two sides mechanically connecting them.

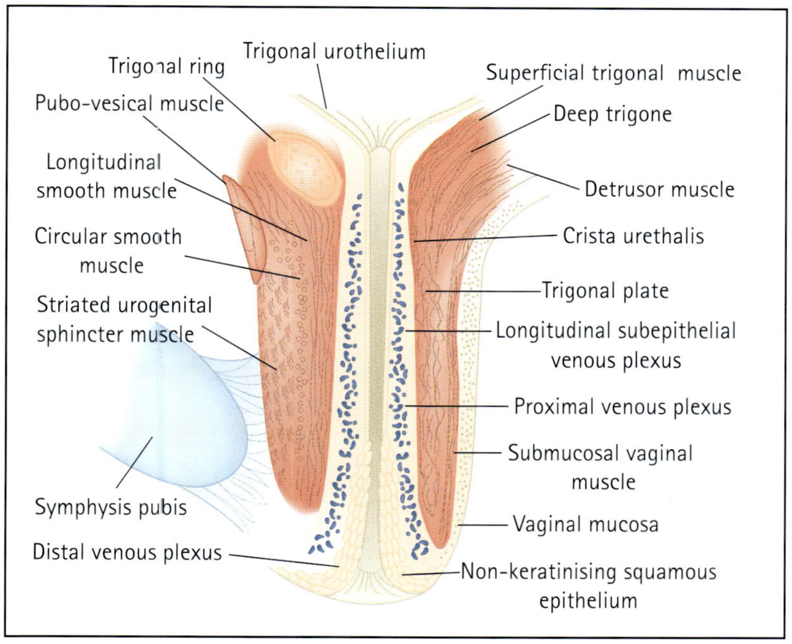

FIGURE 1-18.

The layered structure of the urethral wall can be seen in sagittal section. Just below the internal urinary meatus, the urethral lumen is surrounded by muscle that forms the bladder. The trigonal ring anteriorly marks the most caudal extent of the bladder. Inserting into the vesical neck in the dorsal wall of the urethra are fibers of the detrusor muscle that probably act to help open the vesical neck when the detrusor muscle contracts. The striated urogenital sphincter muscle begins below the vesical neck and extends along the mid-urethra. The pubovesical muscle is an extension of the detrusor muscle that passes laterally to attach the bladder muscle to the tendinous arch of the pelvic fascia and may also be involved in vesical neck opening at the beginning of micturition.

THE ANAL SPHINCTERS

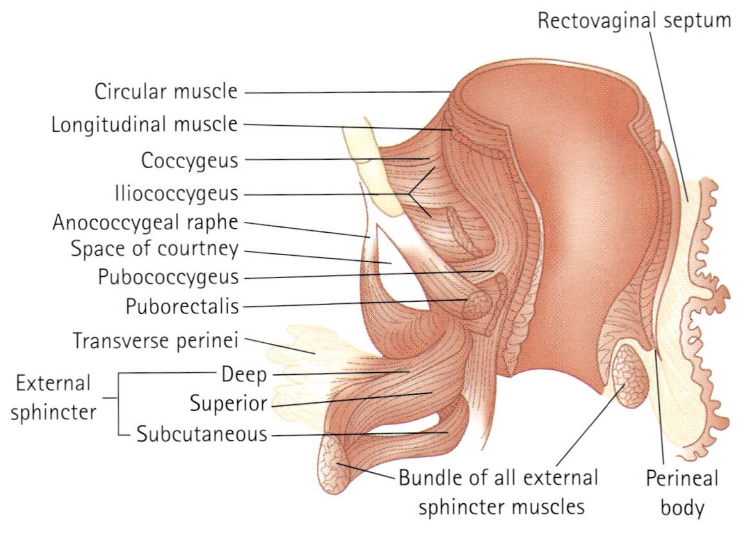

FIGURE 1-19.

This lateral view of the anal sphincters reveals their important relationships. Note that the internal anal sphincter extends down to overlap the external anal sphincter so that a 4th degree laceration of the perineum during vaginal delivery must transect the internal sphincter as well as the external sphincter. Note also that the puborectalis muscle lies cephalic to the external sphincter behind the anorectum at the anorectal angle. Note that the pubococcygeus muscle lies cephalic to the puborectalis and to the iliococcygeus muscle. The anal sphincter complex is attached to the coccyx by the anococcygeal raphe.

SUGGESTED BIBLIOGRAPHY

Berglas B, Rubin IC: Histologic study of the pelvic connective tissue. *Surg Gynecol Obstet* 1957;97:227–89.

Berglas B, Rubin IC: Study of the supportive structures of the uterus by levator myography. *Surg Gynecol Obstet* 1953;97:677–92.

Campbell RM: The anatomy and histology of the sacrouterine ligaments. *Am J Obstet Gynecol* 1950;59:1–12

DeLancey JOL: Anatomic aspects of vaginal eversion after hysterectomy. *Am J Obstet Gynecol* 1992;166:1717–28

DeLancey JOL: Anatomy and biomechanics of genital prolapse. *Clin Obstet Gynecol* 1994;36:897–909.

DeLancey JOL: Structural anatomy of the posterior pelvic compartment as it relates to rectocele. *Am J Obstet Gynecol* 1999;180: in press.

DeLancey JOL: Structural support of the urethra as it relates to stress urinary incontinence: the hammock hypothesis. *Am J Obstet Gynecol* 1994;170:1713–20.

Halban J, Tandler J: *Anatomie und Aetiologie der Genitalprolapse beim Weibe*. Vienna and Leipzig, Wilhelm Braumuller, 1907.

Lawson JO: Pelvic anatomy. II. Anal canal and associated sphincters. *Ann R Coll Surg Engl* 1974;54:288–300.

Lawson JO: Pelvic anatomy. I. Pelvic floor muscles. *Ann R Coll Surg Engl* 1974;54:244–52.

Oelrich TM: The striated urogenital sphincter muscle in the female. *Anat Rec* 1983;205:223–32.

Oh C, Kark AE: Anatomy of the perineal body. *Dis Colon Rectum* 1973;16:444–54.

Paramore RH: The statics of the female pelvic viscera. Vol. 1, Chapter 2. In *The Uterus as a Floating Organ*. 1918 London, England; H.K.Lewis & Co. Ltd, 12–15.

Paramore RH: The supports-in-chief of the female pelvic viscera. *J Obstet Gynaecol Br Emp* 1908;13:391–409.

Range RL, Woodburne RT: The gross and microscopic anatomy of the transverse cervical ligaments. Am J Obstet Gynecol 1964;90:460–67.

Ricci JV, Lisa JR, Thom CH, Kron WL: The relationship of the vagina to adjacent organs in reconstructive surgery. Am J Surg 1947;74:387–410.

CHAPTER 2

Neurophysiology

J. Thomas Benson

The complexity of the neural networks involved in pelvic organ activity deserves attention by the clinician treating patients with dysfunction. Such attention leads to understanding the myriad pathologic processes that have potential for producing abnormality. Therapeutically, the understanding of the neurophysiology leads to possible treatment. Neurotransmitters may be modulated, receptors can be effected, protein channels can be blocked or opened, nerve growth factors and gene therapy may affect neuroplasticity, and electrical stimulation may affect reflex activity. As more advances in the neurophysiologic sciences meet collaboration with clinicians, the benefit to patients and society will escalate.

In this chapter, we consider the nerve cell as it functions in the peripheral nervous system to innervate skeletal and smooth muscle (the somatic and autonomic systems) and as it functions in the central nervous system to modulate activity. Pathways of central and spinal reflex circuits as they relate to pelvic viscera are demonstrated, including currently understood neurotransmitters, channels, and receptors. The recently appreciated development of "pathologic reflexes" in spinal cord injury and bladder outlet obstruction are described, including treatment modalities that affect them. The advances in basic science in this field are occurring rapidly and clinical usefulness is prompted by understanding these advances.

COLLABORATION OF BASIC SCIENCE AND THE CLINICIAN

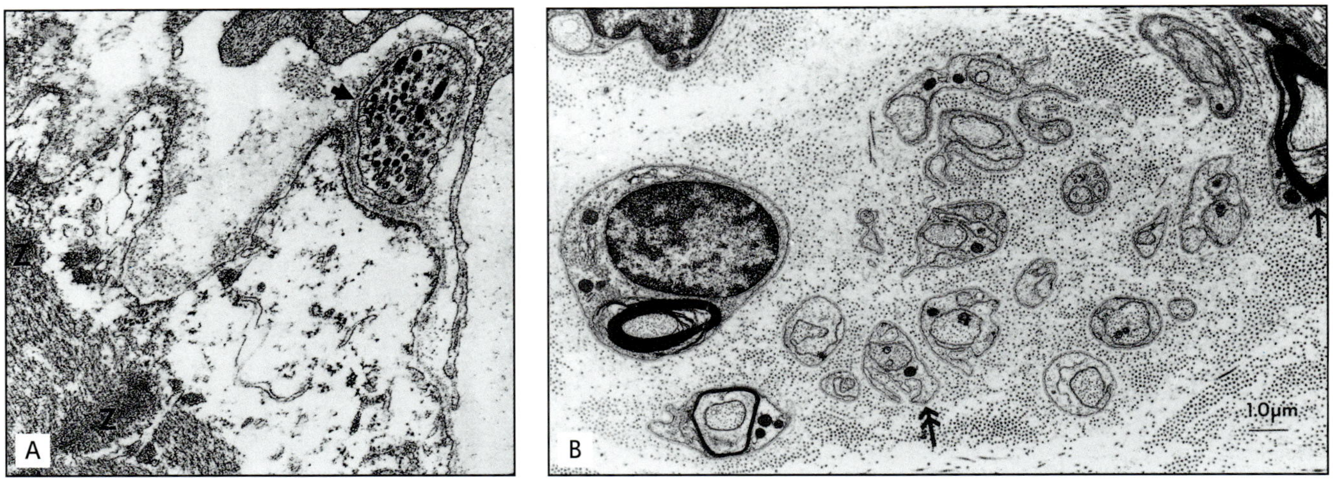

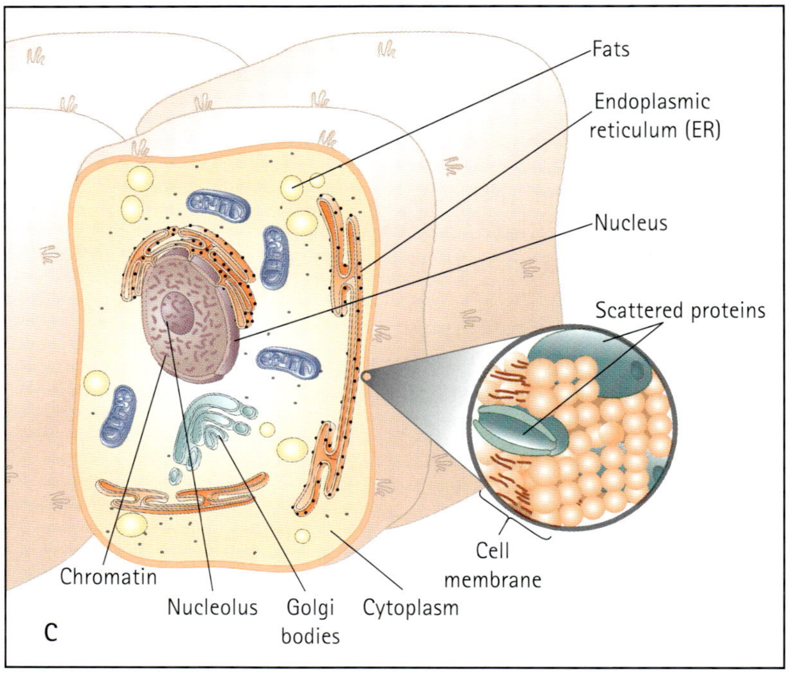

FIGURE 2-1.

A, Basic scientific study. The cat urethral electron microscopic study shows the adrenergic axon terminal (*arrow*) with synaptic vesicles containing neurotransmitter. Z—myofibril. **B**, Clinical study, electron microscopic evaluation of human urethral biopsy; axon terminal with vesicles containing neurotransmitter in myelinated (*arrow*) and unmyelinated (*double arrow*) nerves.

Urinary and fecal storage and elimination processes are complex and involve the entire nervous system. The processes involve simultaneous smooth muscle (detrusor, rectal, internal anal, and urethral sphincters) and skeletal muscle (external anal sphincter, urethral sphincter, pelvic floor muscles) activity. These activities depend on autonomic (to smooth) and somatic (to skeletal) efferent neural mechanisms that are integrated within the lumbosacral spinal cord with an element of supraspinal control. The control mechanisms are both excitatory and inhibitory. The nervous control consists of neural circuits located in the brain, spinal cord, and peripheral ganglia. Many of these neural circuits exhibit phasic, rather than tonic, patterns of activity, which operate to turn "on" or turn "off" mechanisms involved in storage and elimination. The effect of such switchlike activity is to allow voluntary control over the storage and elimination processes. Some visceral functions (*e.g.*, the gastrointestinal tract and the cardiovascular system) have tonic patterns of autonomic pathway activity and maintain an involuntary level of function even after elimination of extrinsic neural input. The urinary and fecal storage and elimination differ from tonic, involuntary viscera in their dependence on central nervous control.

The basic unit of the nervous system is the nerve cell. The nerve cell is intended to last the lifetime of the organism and is able to do so by its plasticity, the ability to be dynamic and constantly reorganizing, restructuring, and regrowing to retain function. The nerve cell transmits "signals," referred to as action potentials, to an effector organ (*e.g.*, muscle fiber) or to another neural structure. The transmission within the nerve cell process is ionic (electrical), using protein channels in the bilayered axon membrane (**C**) that allow passage of sodium, potassium, and chloride ions. At the neuro-effector site or synapse, the transmission is chemical, depending on neurotransmitters acting on receptors. The neurotransmitters include proteins, made on ribosomes, under nuclear direction. Once neurotransmitters reach the effector organ, an electrical process again occurs to effect organ activity. (Part A *from* Elbadawi [1], with permission; part B *from* Hale and Benson [2] with permission; part C *from* Merrill Life Science [3].)

NEURONS OF THE CENTRAL AND PERIPHERAL NERVOUS SYSTEMS

UPPER AND LOWER MOTOR NEURONS AND INTERNEURONS

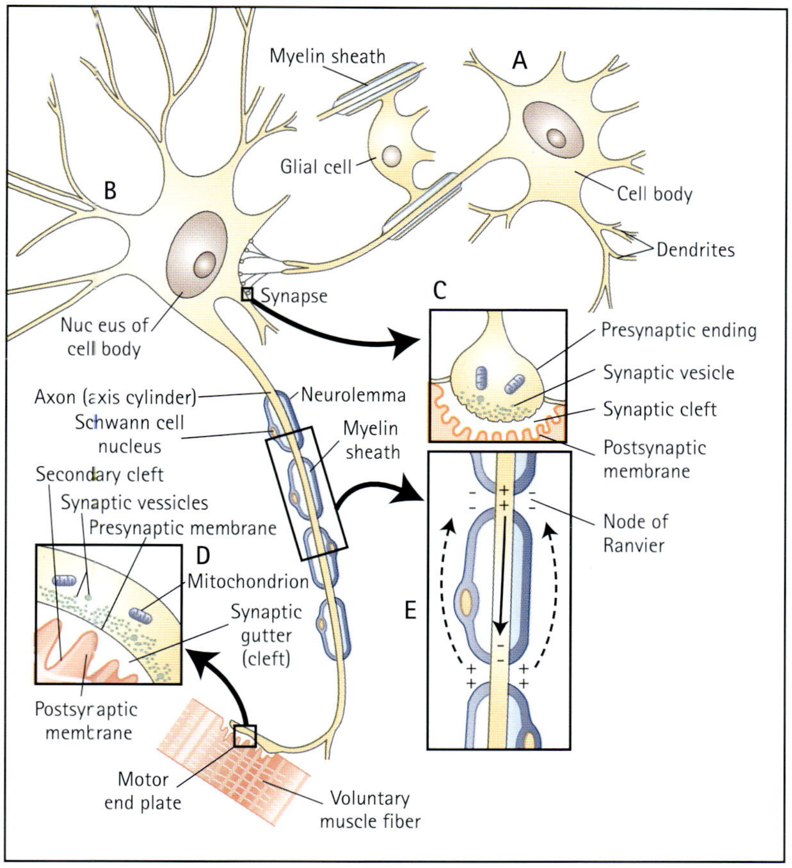

FIGURE 2-2.

Development of the upper and lower motor neurons. The brain and spinal cord develop from the neural tube. Neuron **A** is confined to the central nervous system (CNS), its cell body frequently supraspinal, dendrites communicating with other neurons. Its axon travels in tracts, supported by glial cells, myelinated by oligodendrocytes. It joins neuron **B** at a chemical junction, the synapse (**C**). Many single neurons of the CNS receive thousands of connections from other neurons. The presynaptic nerve terminal contains synaptic vesicles with chemical neurotransmitters and the postsynaptic membrane has specialized receptors for the neurotransmitters. These chemical synapses can be excitatory or inhibitory. Neurotransmitter release is effected by an action potential entering the axon terminal and opening voltage-dependent calcium channels. When the neurotransmitter binds to receptor, ion channels open in the postsynaptic neuron. If excitatory, Na^+ channels allow sodium influx and depolarization will generate an action potential. If inhibitory, Cl^- channels allow influx, K^+ channels allow egress, and hyperpolarization develops, preventing action potential development. Acetylcholine, the primary neurotransmitter in the body, acts in limited areas of the CNS. The chief excitatory neurotransmitter in the CNS is glutamate, the most plentiful amino acid neurotransmitter in the adult CNS. Sites of action include the cerebral cortex, hippocampus, subthalamic nucleus, and cerebellum. Although excitation of synapses is essential for neuronal function, overstimulation may be toxic to the neuron. Glutamate, acting on *N*-methyl-D-aspartate (NMDA) receptors, opens calcium channels. If the effect is too prolonged, cell death may occur. Clinical therapies related to blocking NMDA receptors are now available. The chief inhibitory neurotransmitters are gamma-aminobutyric acid (GABA) and glycine, and clinical application of agents acting on GABA transmission is being developed.

Neuron **B** is a motor neuron, its cell body is within the CNS system and its axon extends to a peripheral nerve and innervates a striated muscle. The axon is surrounded by myelin, produced by Schwann cells, and interrupted segmentally at the node of Ranvier, an area rich in sodium channels. Action currents flow from node to node ("saltatory" conduction, **E**), a much more effective propagation than is present in unmyelinated nerves. Each functioning skeletal muscle fiber is innervated by an axon (**D**), connecting to the muscle fiber through a neuromuscular junction. (*From* Gilman and Newman [4].)

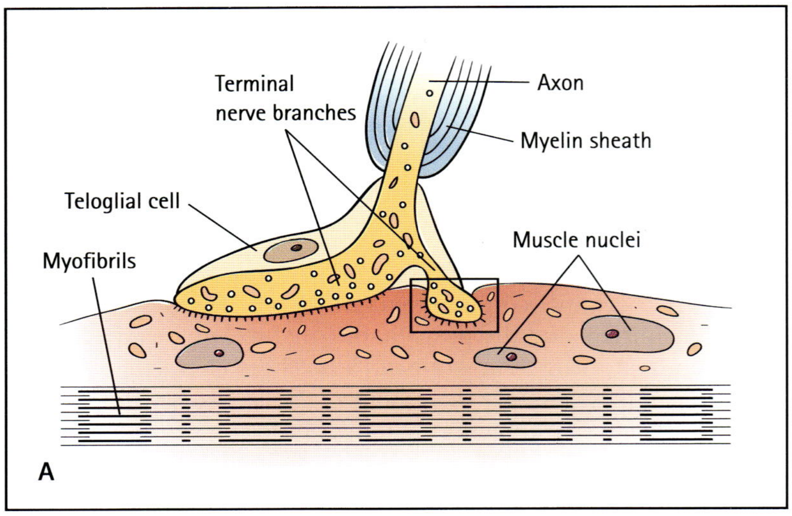

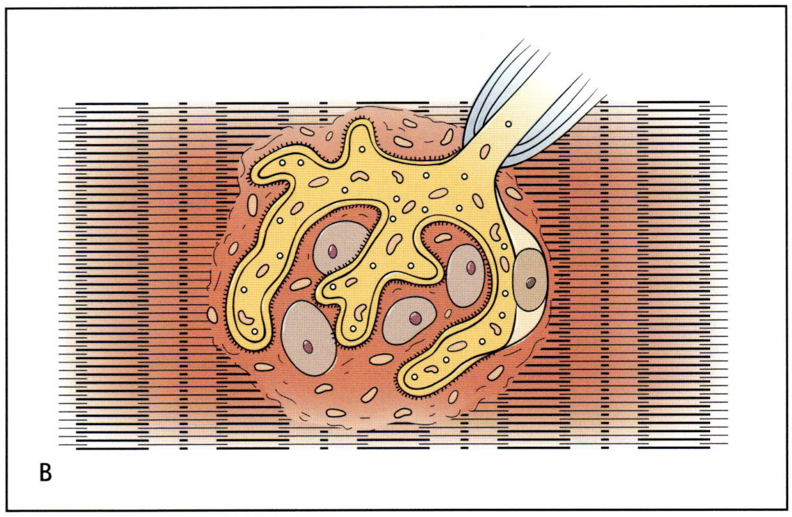

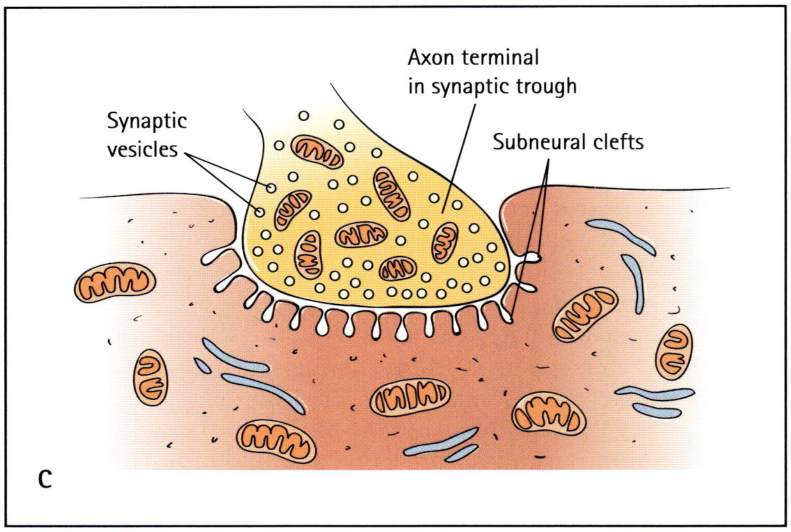

FIGURE 2-3.

The neuromuscular junction. The motor end plate is seen in histologic sections in the long axis of the muscle fiber (**A**) and in a surface view (**B**) under the light microscope. The area in the rectangle in (**A**) is depicted under the electron microscope in (**C**). The neuromuscular junction is composed of the nerve terminal, a synaptic cleft, and a postsynaptic portion of the muscle fiber containing synaptic "folds." The nerve terminal contains vesicles with acetylcholine, which are released with invasion of an action potential, a calcium-dependent process. The postsynaptic membrane has acetylcholine receptors (nicotinic) and when sufficient acetyl-chloline is received, an end-plate potential is formed, causing depolarization of the muscle fiber membrane. Acetylcholine neurotransmitter, acting on nicotinic receptors, is the activity present in all alpha, beta, and gamma motoneurons and spinal Renshaw interneurons, controlling the rate of lower motor neuron firings. (*From* Kimura [5].)

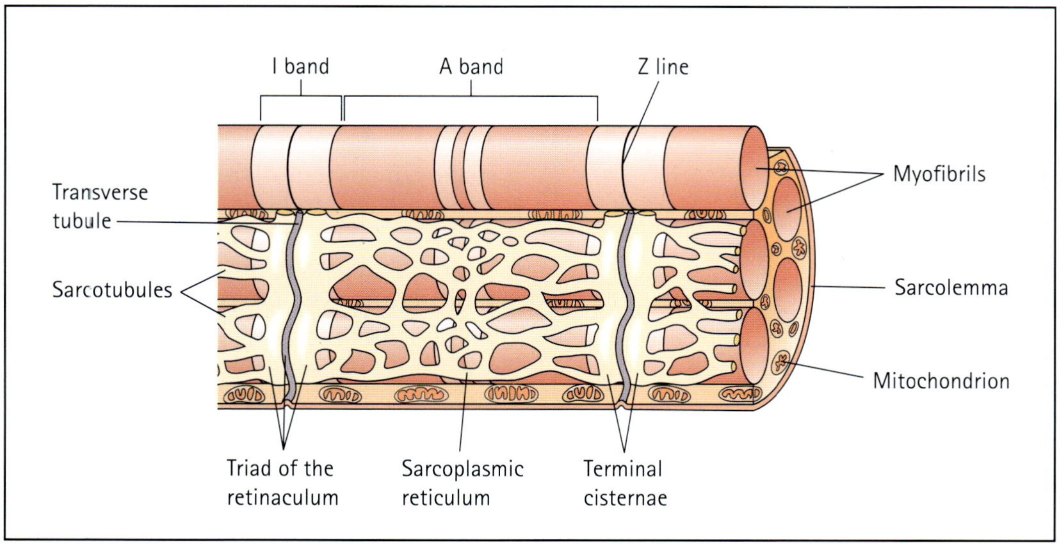

FIGURE 2-4.

Muscle fibril contraction. The action potential spreads in the muscle and electromechanical coupling at the triad of the reticulum occurs. The triad consists of two terminal cisterns of the longitudinal tubules and one transverse tubule between them. The calcium is released from the longitudinal tubules into the sarcoplasm surrounding the myofilaments and a chemical interaction bridges thin and thick filaments causing contraction of the muscle fibril. (*From* Kimura [5].)

Sensory Neurons

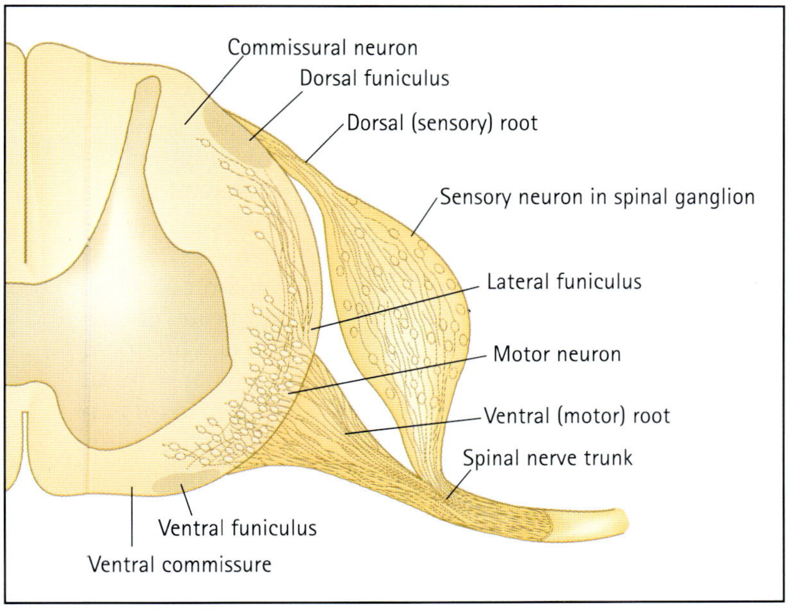

FIGURE 2-5.

Sensory neurons. The sensory neurons develop from a proliferation of the neural crest resulting in cellular aggregations *lateral* to the neural tube. The nerve cell body has two primary axon processes that fuse into one, dividing like a "T". The cell body is located in the dorsal root ganglion and the peripheral process goes to the peripheral sensory site and the central process enters the spinal cord through the dorsal root. The action potentials generated at the sensory organ travel to the cord through this single neuron because there are no synapses in the dorsal root ganglion. Sensory small fiber naked terminals may be excited by a variety of substances including histamine, bradykinin, serotonin, acetylcholine, and substance P ,whereas various types of touch or pressure sensations are perceived by encapsulated receptors such as muscle spindles, Golgi tendon organs, Pacinian corpuscles, Meissner's corpuscles, and others.

Neurotransmitters at the central processes include neuropeptides. Unlike neurons that produce acetylcholine and monoamines by alteration of ubiquitous molecules delivered to the cell, peptides are produced *de novo* in the cell. A number of peptides, many first identified in the gut then later found in neural tissue, are involved in sensory nerve neurotransmission. Peptides so involved include vasointestinal peptide (VIP), substance P, cholecystokinin, calcitonin gene-related peptide (CGRP), and enkephalin. After significant axonal injury, tonic firing of sensory neurons may occur, a process involving nitric oxide neurotransmission [6] in dorsal root ganglion cells. This process is important in chronic pain syndromes and offers a pathway of possible therapy. (*From* Clemente [7].)

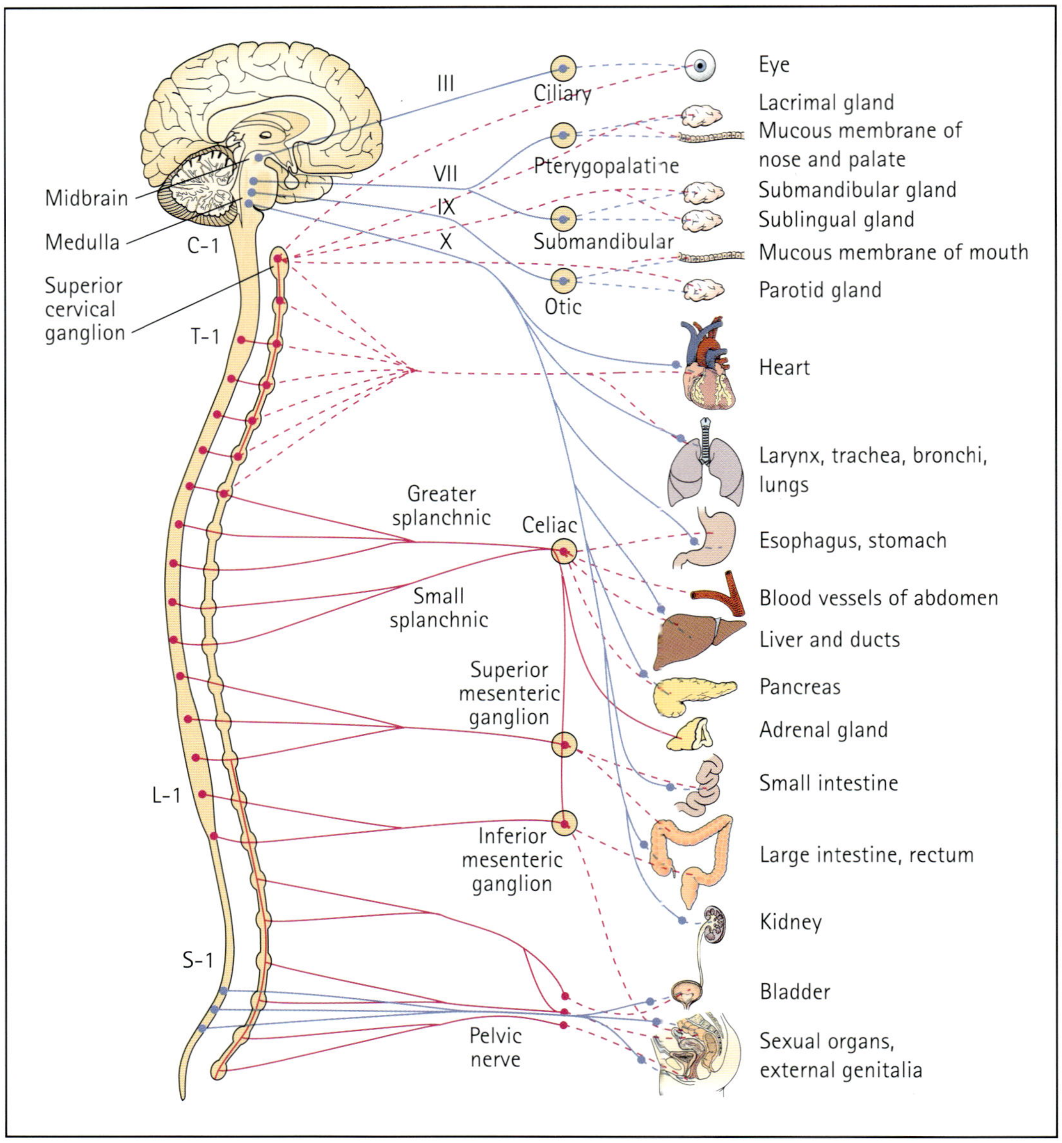

FIGURE 2-6.

Diagram of efferent autonomic nervous system; sympathetic division in red and parasympathetic in blue. The autonomic nerves are composed of at least two neurons, a preganglionic and a postganglionic neuron. The preganglionic neuron bodies are located in the lateral gray matter of the spinal cord, the sympathetic division in a column extending from the first thoracic through the second lumbar segments and the sacral portion of the parasympathetic system in a similar column in the second, third, and fourth sacral segments. The cranial portion of the parasympathetic division's preganglionic neurons arise in the visceral efferent nuclei of the brainstem.

The postganglionic neurons of the sympathetic and sacral parasympathetic system arise, like the sensory neurons, from the neural crest. The sympathetic ganglia neurons form paravertebral chains and outlying collateral ganglia located adjacent to branches of the abdominal aorta. The sacral parasympathetic ganglionic neurons are located adjacent to the organ innervated.

Sympathetic preganglionic axons exit the cord through ventral root, course to the sympathetic chain via white rami communicantes. Some synapse in the chain and the postganglion axon joins the spinal nerves via gray rami communicantes (the paravertebral sympathetic system), whereas others course through the chain to synapse with ganglion cells in the outlying collateral ganglia (prevertebral sympathetic system). Sacral preganglionic axons exit the cord via the ventral roots to the pelvic splanchnic nerves (nerve erigens) and traverse the pelvic plexus to synapse with the ganglion cell at the organ. (*From* Clemente [7].)

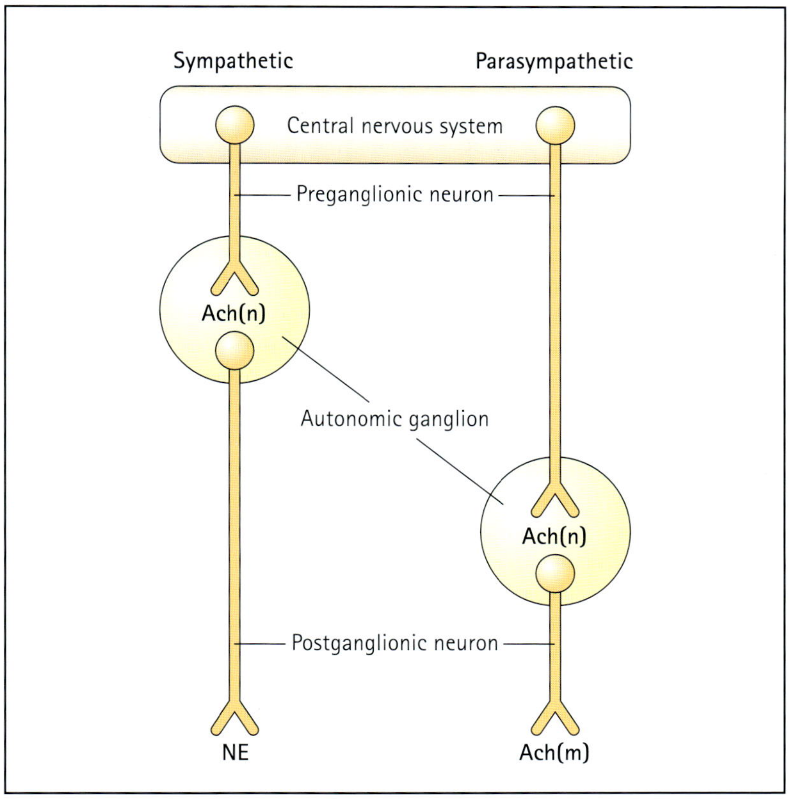

FIGURE 2-7.

Preganglionic autonomic neurons. The preganglionic autonomic neurons use acetylcholine as a primary neurotransmitter and synthesize nitric oxide; some sympathetic preganglionic neurons release enkephalin or neurotensin. Acetylcholine acts on nicotinic receptors (*ACh[n]*) for excitation and on muscarinic receptors (*ACh[m]*) for excitation and inhibition. The autonomic ganglion neurons are not just relay stations but are the site of complex interactions.

At the neuroeffector junctions, sympathetic terminals release norepinephrine (*NE*), neuropeptide Y, and adenosine triphosphate (ATP) except at sweat glands where acetylcholine is used. Norepinephrine acts on different types of adrenergic receptors. Norepinephrine is mainly inactivated by *reuptake* by prejunctional terminals. The limiting of norepinephrine activity by its reuptake is a process that can be clinically modulated by the use of norepinephrine reuptake inhibitors.

Parasympathetic terminals release acetylcholine, vasointestinal protein (VIP), ATP, and nitric oxide. Acetylcholine acts on different subtypes of muscarinic receptors. Cotransmitters such as purine (ATP, adenosine), local factors (histamine, serotonin, prostaglandins), and circulating influences (epinephrine, steroids, cytokines) modulate autonomic neurotransmission.

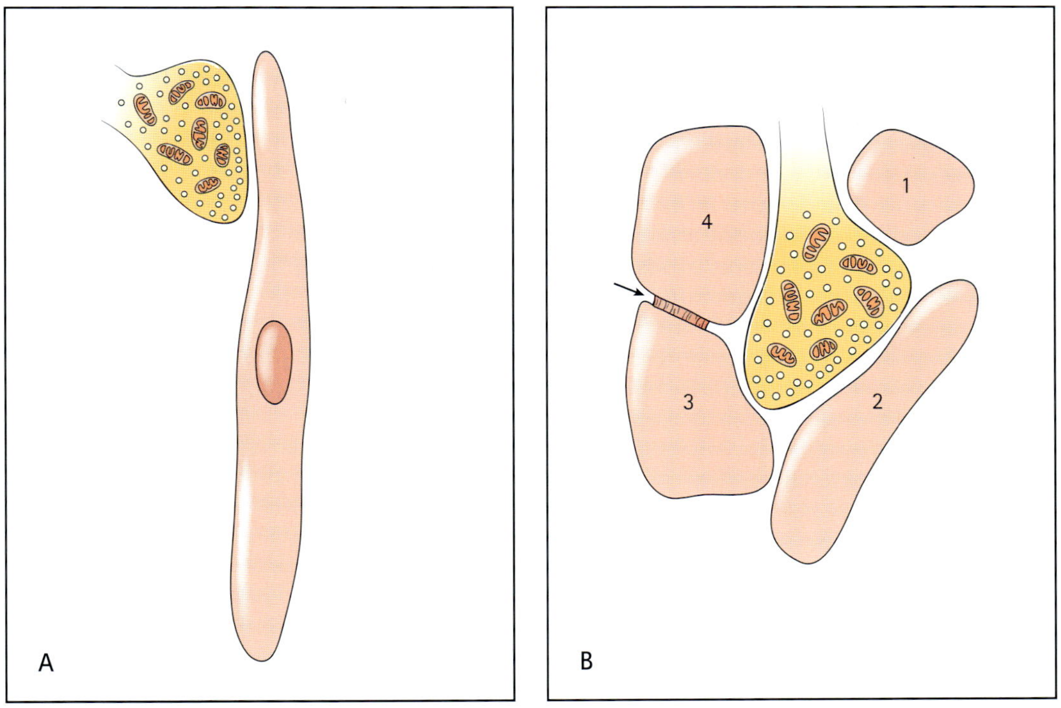

FIGURE 2-8.

The neuroeffector junctions in the autonomic nervous system are much more complex than with the somatic motor system to skeletal muscle. There are many varieties of neuroeffector junctions: **A**, chloinergic neuroeffector junction; **B**, adrenergic multieffector junction (with four muscle cells);

(*Continued on next page*)

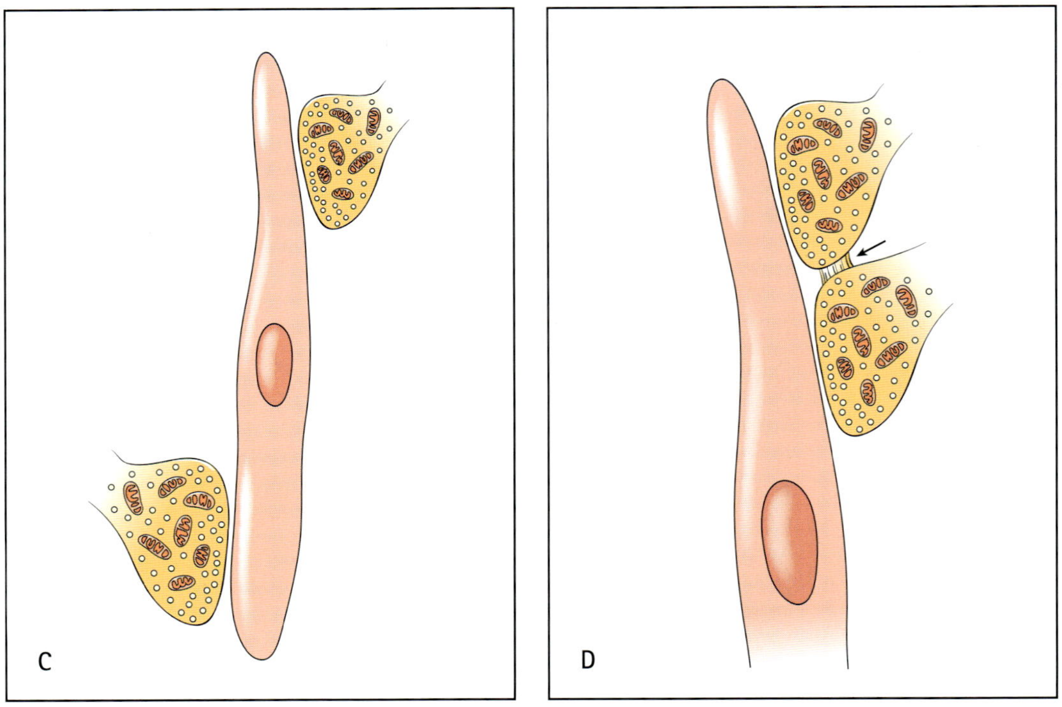

FIGURE 2-8. *(Continued)*
C cholinergic multiaxonal junction; **D**, diautonomic junction with axono-axonal synapse *(arrow)*. There is variation of neurotransmission with signal frequency, with intramural cholinergic ganglia acting as "high-pass" filters. (*From* Krane and Siroky [8].)

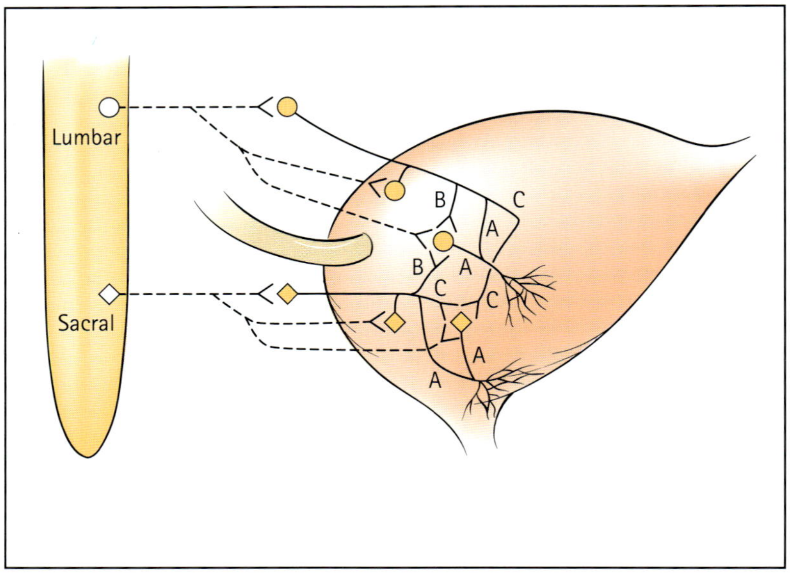

FIGURE 2-9.
Concept of postganglionic synapses in vesicourethral peripheral neural pathways. Sympathetic pathway *(top)*. *Open circle* is preganglionic and *solid circles* are postganglionic. Parasympathetic pathway *(bottom)*. *Open square* is preganglionic and *solid squares* are postganglionic with synapses as shown (**A, B**,and **C**). Visceral effectors are characterized by *automatic activity*, the ability to sustain rhythmic contractions in the absence of innervation, *intramural conduction*, transmission of electric inputs between synctial fibers, and *denervation supersensitivity*. Whereas the main consequence of denervation in striated muscle is paralysis and atrophy, most autonomic effectors develop no atrophy and an exaggerated response to the specific neurotransmitter, secondary to up-regulation of postjunctional receptors. This property allows clinical testing for postganglionic bladder denervation by measuring the bladder response to bethanechol injection. (*From* Elbadawi and Schenk [9].)

*N*EURONAL NEUROPLASTICITY

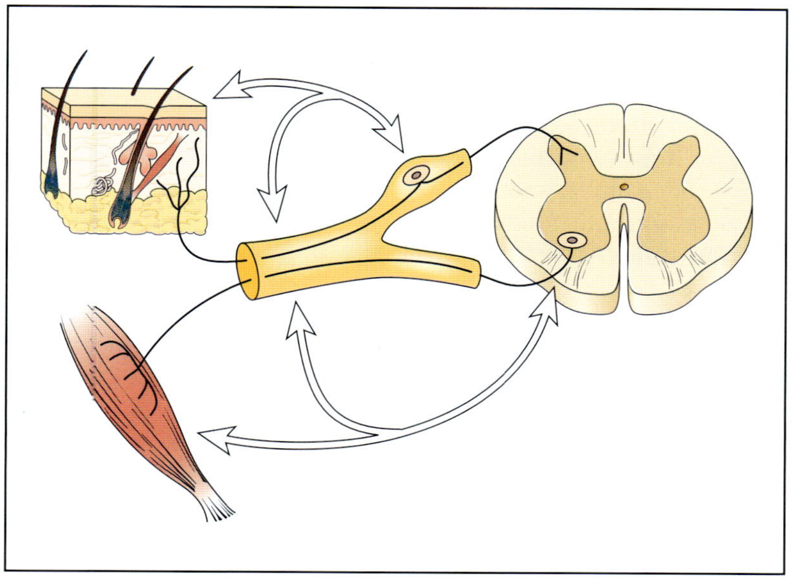

FIGURE 2-10.

Neuroplasticity. A very important concept for the clinician to realize is that neurons in the adult are dynamic and capable of marked morphologic and physiologic changes in response to a target organ change. Understanding this concept paves the way to comprehension of the evolving processes being discovered, which affect pelvic organ function and therapies (*eg*, see Figure 2-39). There is interaction between neuronal cell bodies and peripheral target organs. The end organs are under trophic influence from the neuronal cell bodies, and the cell bodies are dependent on a constant supply of neuronotrophic factors synthesized by the end organs. (*From* Lundborg [10].)

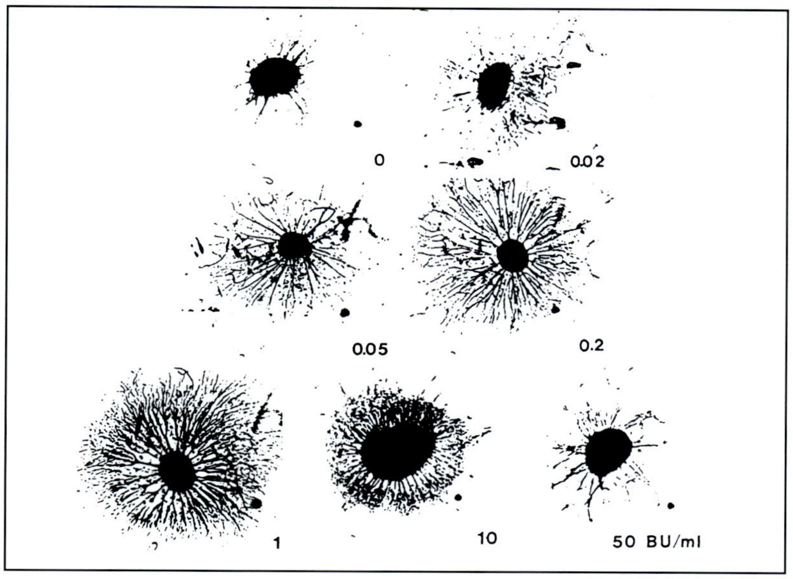

FIGURE 2-11.

Nerve growth factor. A protein found to enhance the outgrowth of neurites from neurons of sympathetic and dorsal root ganglia has been termed nerve growth factor (NGF). The effects are dose related as shown in this 8-day chick dorsal root ganglia explant. Indicated are levels of biologic units of NGF/mL of culture. (*From* Lundborg [10]; with permission.)

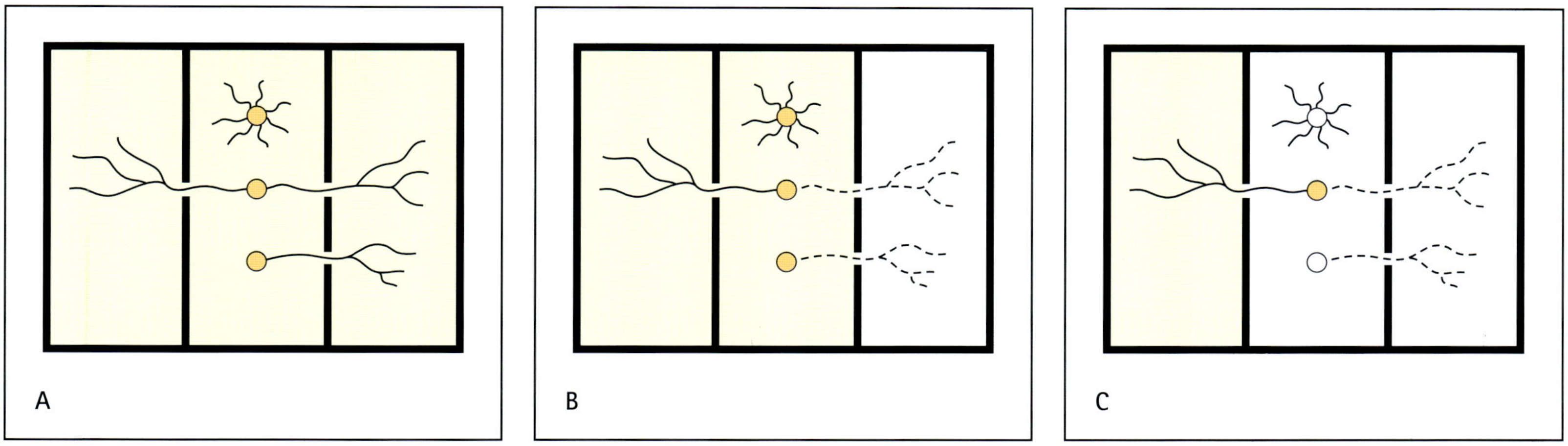

FIGURE 2-12.

Campenot's experiment [11]. Dissociated sympathetic neurons can, in the presence of nerve growth factor (NGF), extend processes from the central compartment of a specially designed culture dish into the side compartments with the NGF. **A**, NGF in both side compartments; **B**, NGF removed from the right compartment; **C**, NGF removed from middle and right compartment. If NGF is available to some of the processes of the parent cell, the cell can survive. (*From* Lundborg [10].)

THE PERIPHERAL NERVE

FORMATION

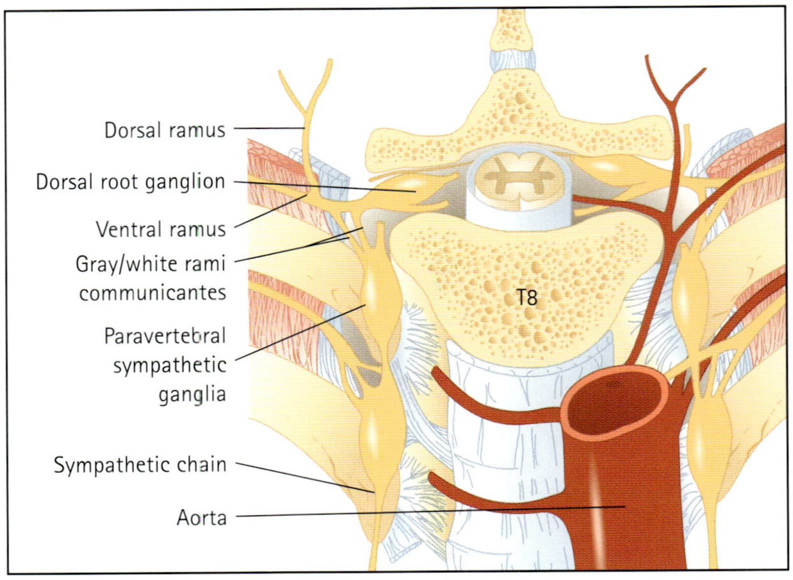

FIGURE 2-13.
Formation of a peripheral nerve. The motor neurons from the anterior horn cells, the sensory neurons with cell bodies in the dorsal root ganglia, and the preganglionic parasympathetic (in cranial and sacral cord levels) and postganglionic sympathetic neurons (from paravertebral sympathetic ganglia at all spinal cord levels) constitute a peripheral nerve. In this section from the T8-9 cord level, the gray rami communicantes are also depicted, conveying preganglionic sympathetic neurons to the sympathetic chain. (*From* Low [12].)

ANATOMY

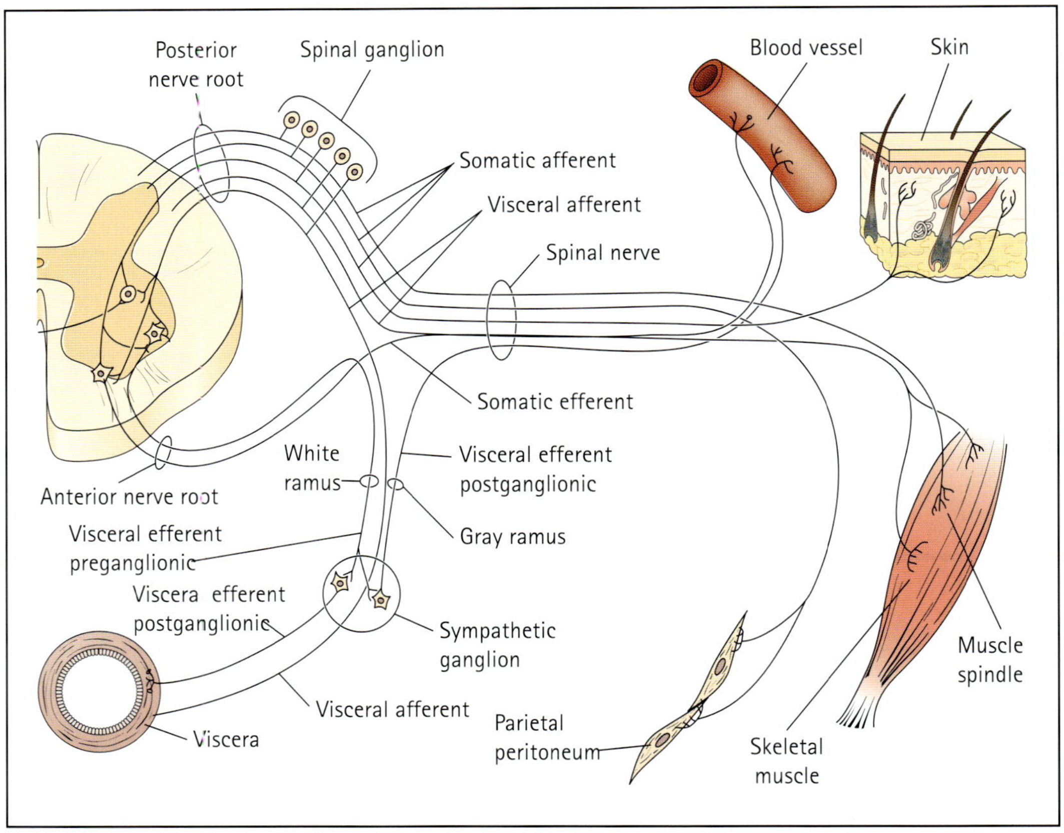

FIGURE 2-14.
Schema showing structure of a typical spinal nerve. (*From* Clemente [7].)

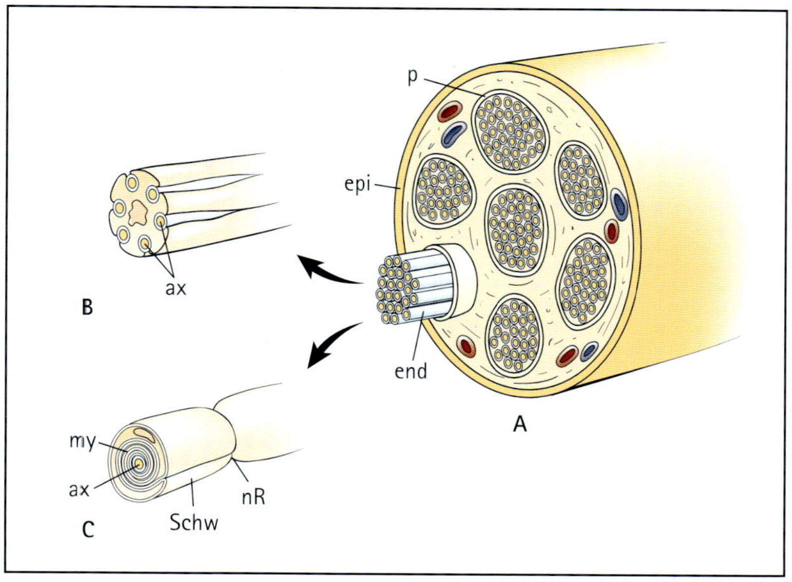

FIGURE 2-15.

Microanatomy of peripheral nerve. **A**, Fascicle is surrounded by multilaminated perineurim (*p*), embedded in loose connective tissue. The epineurium (*epi*) is the outside lining of the nerve. Within the fascicals is the endoneurium (*end*). The outer layers of the endoneurium are condensed into a sheath (**B** and **C**) containing myelinated and unmyelinated nerves. The portion of the intraneural vascular system going through the perineurium is at an angle that is subject to "kinking" in the event of stretch and pressure, affecting blood flow. Mercury pressure of 80 mm can stop the blood flow. Periods as long as 6 hours of complete blood flow obstruction can be followed by resumption of flow without coagulation, but 8 hours will lead to no reflow with thromboses. Stretching the nerve 15% of its length can also lead to complete obstruction. ax— axon; my—myelin sheath; nR—node of Ranvier; Schw—Schwann cell. (*From* Lundborg [10].)

CLASSIFICATION OF NERVE FIBERS

Sensory and Motor Fibers	Sensory Fibers	Largest Fiber Diameter	Fastest Conduction Velocity (m/s)	General Comments
A-α	Ia	22	120	Motor: The large alpha motoneurons of lamina IX, innervating extrafusal muscle fibers
				Sensory: The primary afferents of muscle spindles
A-α	Ib	22	120	Sensory: Golgi tendon organs, touch and pressure receptors
A-β	II	13	70	Motor: The motoneurons innervating both extrafusal and intrafusal (muscle spindle) muscle fibers
				Sensory: The secondary afferents of muscle spindles, touch and pressure receptors, and pacinian corpuscles (vibratory sensors)
A-γ		8	40	Motor: The small gamma motoneurons of lamina IX, innervating intrafusal fibers (muscle spindles)
A-δ	III	5	15	Sensory: Small, lightly myelinated fibers; touch, pressure, pain, and temperature
B		3	14	Motor: Small, lightly myelinated preganglionic autonomic fibers
C	IV	1	2	Motor: All postganglionic autonomic fibers (all are unmyelinated)
				Sensory: Unmyelinated pain and temperature fibers

FIGURE 2-16.
Classification of nerve fibers. (*From* Erlanger [13].)

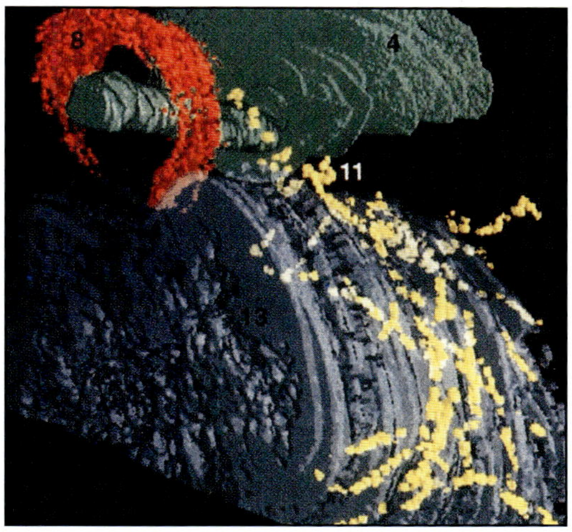

FIGURE 2-17.

Three-dimensional reconstruction of nerve supply to cranial portion of urethra and bladder neck. The majority of neural supply to the bladder neck and urethra course alongside the lateral vaginal walls as indicated in this three-dimensional reconstruction of nerve supply from digitized histologic sections [14]. In vaginal deliveries, average pressures on the lateral pelvis during the second stage of labor are 100 mm Hg during contractions and maximum pressures usually reach 240 mm Hg. The pudendal nerve, supplying the external urethral sphincter, courses through Alcock's canal in the obturator fascia where it is relatively bound. Movement of the pelvic floor, such as with Valsalva maneuvers during vaginal delivery, can place significant stretch on the pudendal nerve fibers. With the pudendal nerve supported firmly in Alcock's canal, movement of the perineum 1.35 cm can produce cessation of blood flow in the vessels supplying the nerve. Thus, stretch and pressure during vaginal delivery can produce profound nerve effects proportional to amount and temporal duration. (*From* Colleselli [14]; with permission.

SPINAL PATHWAYS

EFFERENT SPINAL NEURONS

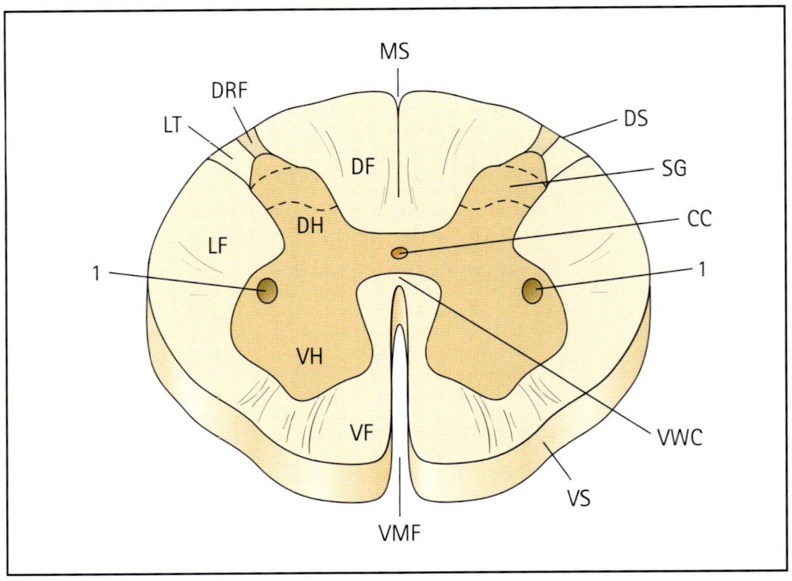

FIGURE 2-18.

Efferent autonomic spinal neurons (*1*). Parasympathetic: Preganglionic neurons in the sacral cord segments. Dendrites of these neurons go to the lateral and dorsolateral funiculus, receiving glutaminergic neurons from the pontine micturition center, the "M" region of the pons. These terminals are excitatory and responsible for bladder contraction during micturition. Other dendrites go to the lateral edge of dorsal horn, dorsal gray commissure, which also has excitatory connection to pons "M" region, and to the ventral gray matter. The sacral parasympathetic outflow is critical for defecation, micturition, and erection, mediated chiefly by muscarinic cholinergic receptors.

Sympathetic: The lumbar intermediolateral gray matter (T11-L2) gives origin to sympathetic preganglionic neurons involved with pelvic structures. Lumbar sympathetic neurons mediate inhibitory viscerosympathetic reflexes, activated by low bladder pressure afferent activation, which ascends to the lumbar cord to reflexly activate sympathetic continence reflex. This reflex pathway is facilitated by norepinephrine and serotonin. The efferent limb of this reflex has an inhibitory effect on parasympathetic ganglionic transmission, increases outlet resistance by alpha-adrenergic receptors in the bladder neck, and may cause bladder contractility decrease by beta-adrenergic receptors in the body of the bladder. CC—central canal; DF—dorsal funiculus; DH—dorsal horn; DRF—dorsal root fibers; DS—dorsolateral sulcus; LF—lateral funiculus; LT—Lissauer's tract; MS—dorsal median sulcus; SG—substancia gelatinosa; VF—ventral funiculus; VH—ventral horn; VMF—ventral median fissure; VS—ventrolateral sulcus; VWC—ventral white commissure; 1—intermediolateral gray matter.

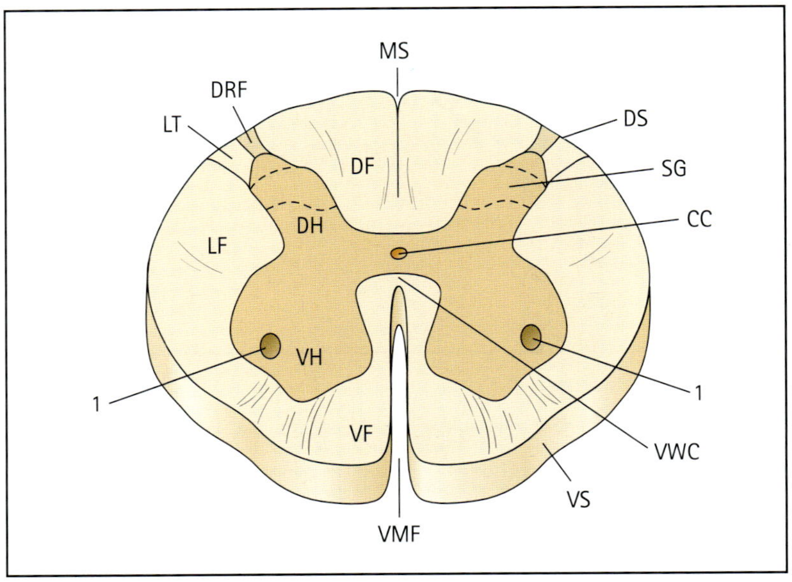

FIGURE 2-19.

Motor neurons. Sphincter motor neurons, Onuf's nucleus (*1*). In the sacral cord, these anterior horn cells differ from other somatic anterior horn cells in many respects; they are structurally smaller, have resistance to anterior horn cell disease (amyotrophic lateral sclerosis, polio), and have supraspinal connection similar to autonomic preganglionic neurons. The dendritic projections are similar to the distribution of the sacral preganglionic neurons. Onuf's nucleus activity is controlled by another group of neurons in the pons, the "L" region. The terminals from the pons micturition center are excitatory to the dorsal commissural gray, where they make contact with inhibitory gamma-aminobutyric acid (GABA) neurons that, in turn, inhibit the Onuf motoneurons. During storage, this inhibition is not present, allowing the sphincter to contract. Again, norepinephrine and serotonin input to the Onuf's nucleus motoneurons tends to facilitate storage. Abbreviations as defined in Figure 2-18.

Afferent Projections to Spinal Cord

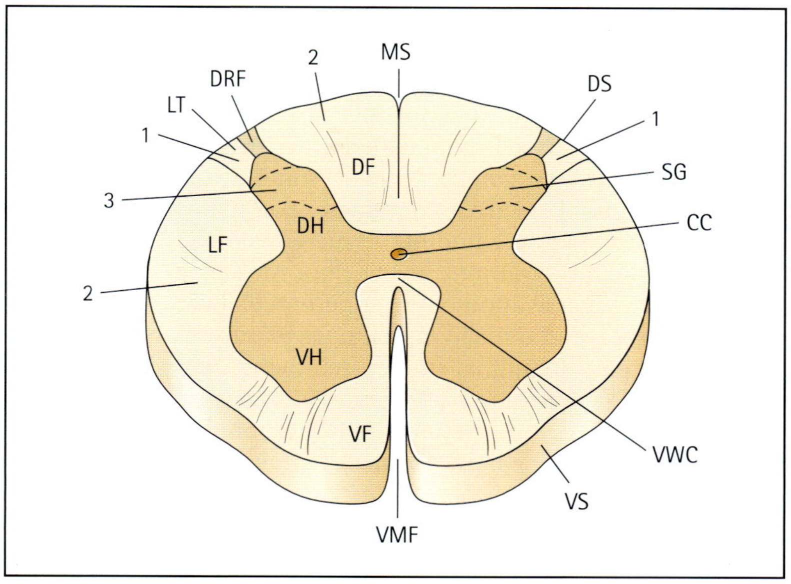

FIGURE 2-20.
Afferent spinal cord projections. Afferent activity in the bladder is transmitted to the central nervous system over both sets of autonomic nerves, the ones initiating micturition passing through pelvic nerves to the sacral cord. The majority of the afferents are alpha-delta neurons although C fibers can be activated by chemical irritation or cold temperature. The C-fiber pathway bladder overactivity induced by noxious stimuli can be blocked by capsaicin, a neurotoxin that desensitizes C-fiber afferents. The C-fiber reflex pathway is weak in animals with an intact nervous system but emerges in chronic spinal animals (see Figure 2-38). Pelvic nerve afferent pathways (*1*) from the lower urinary tract project into Lissauer's tract and pass rostrocaudally, giving off collaterals passing to base of dorsal horn. The synaptic connections in the dorsal horn involving alpha-delta and C-fiber transmission use substance P, which has an excitatory effect of long duration. Vasointestinal peptide is the most common peptide involved with sensory afferent activity from the pelvis and is only released from myelinated neurons. Other involved peptides are calcitonin gene-related peptide, enkephalin, and cholecystokinin. Terminations are made in the region of the sacral parasympathetic nucleus and dorsal commissure. Pudendal afferents from the urethra follow a similar pattern.

Some interneurons, synapsing with the afferent projections to the cord, send long projections to supraspinal areas, whereas others make local connections to participate in segmental spinal reflexes. Ascending pathways are in the lateral and dorsal funiculus (*2*). Neurons in the lateral dorsal horn (*3*) project via ascending pathways to the periacqueductal gray where they are relayed to the pontine micturition center where they initiate the micturition reflex. Interneurons located near the parasympathetic nucleus have both excitatory glutamatergic and inhibitory gamma-aminobutyric acid (GABAergic) actions on the preganglionic neurons. Descending serotonergic pathways tonically suppress afferent activity at the spinal level, inhibiting the micturition reflex. With increased stretching of the smooth muscle of the bladder, proprioceptive information (bladder "fullness") is carried to pontine and sacral reflex centers, the former resulting in excitation of parasympathetic sacral neurons and inhibition of sacral motoneurons to produce coordinated bladder contraction and urethral relaxation. Interruption of the pontine and sacral connections leads to incoordinated activity, detrusor-sphincter dyssynergia.

Brain Pathways

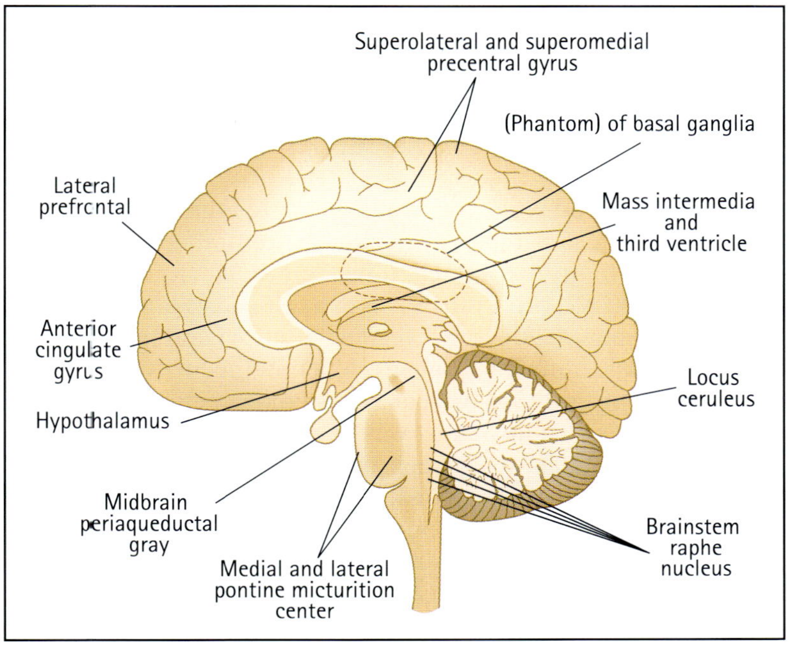

FIGURE 2-21.
Areas of the brain known to be associated with pelvic organ (especially bladder) activity. Newer methodologies for mapping pathways include (1) positive emission tomography scans, which demonstrate increased activity in the central nervous system (CNS) associated with a given activity such as micturition; (2) transneuronal virus tracing (pseudorabies viruses pass by retrograde axonal transport from a target organ to the CNS where they infect second- and third-order neurons across synapses) [15]; and (3) measurements of gene expression (irritation of target organ increases level of immediate early gene, c-*fos*, in spinal neurons involved in processing afferent input. Areas of involvement for lower urinary tract activity include precentral gyrus, lateral prefrontal cortex, and anterior cingulate gyrus of the cortex, basal ganglia, brainstem raphe nuclei, locus ceruleus, hypothalamus, the midbrain periacqueductal gray, and medial and lateral pons.

Cortical Pathways

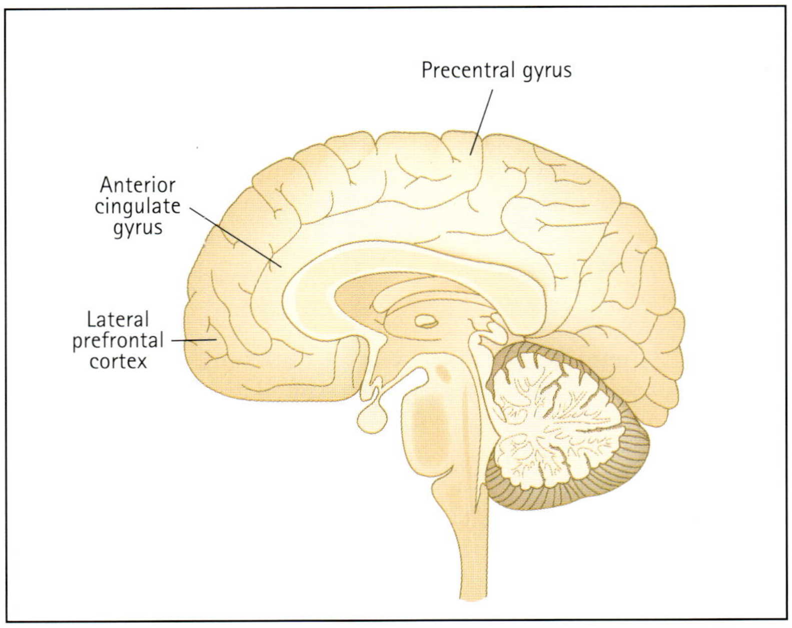

FIGURE 2–22.

Precentral gyrus. The prefrontal cortical areas are involved in high-order processing of visceral information. Positron emission tomography experiments demonstrate that the anterior cingulate gyrus and the lateral prefrontal cortex are activated during attempted micturition, whether micturition is actually achieved or not. The active areas are predominately on the right side of the brain, consistent with the findings of increased urge incontinence with right hemisphere lesions. Pelvic floor muscular contraction is associated with activation of the superomedial part of the precentral gyrus, and the abdominal musculature with the superolateral part. In animal studies, removing these cortical areas reduces bladder capacity by removing the cortical *tonic inhibition*. The effect can be eliminated by administration of *N*-methyl-D-aspartate glutaminergic receptor antagonist.

Subcortical Pathways

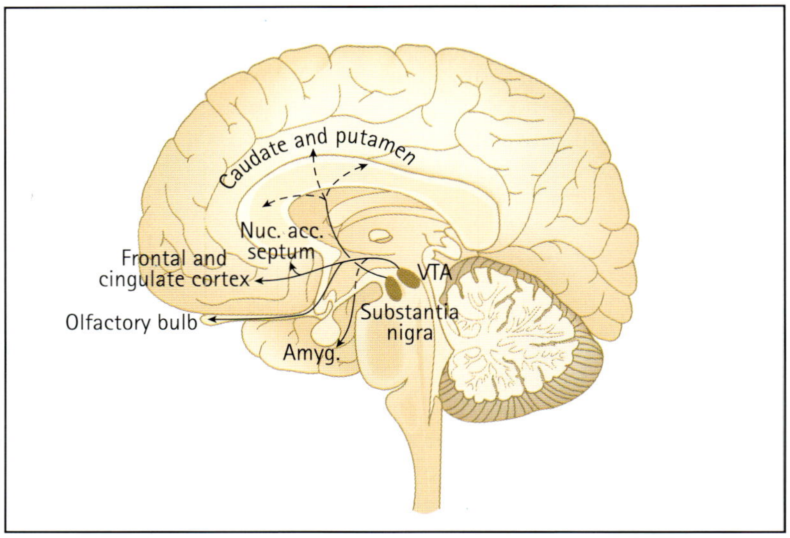

FIGURE 2–23.

Basal ganglia and dopamine. Patients with Parkinson's disease often (75%) have bladder overactivity. Animal studies indicate the overactivity is due to loss of dopaminergic inhibition. Dopamine is one of the catecholamine neurotransmitters. Catecholamine is produced in the brain (and sympathetic ganglia) from the amino acid precursor tyrosine. The production is by a series of enzymatic steps in which dopamine appears first, can be converted to norepinephrine, which, in turn, can be converted to epinephrine. AMYG—amygdaloid body; NUC ACC— nucleus accumbens; VTA—ventral tegmental area. (*From* Manter and Gatz [4]; with permission.)

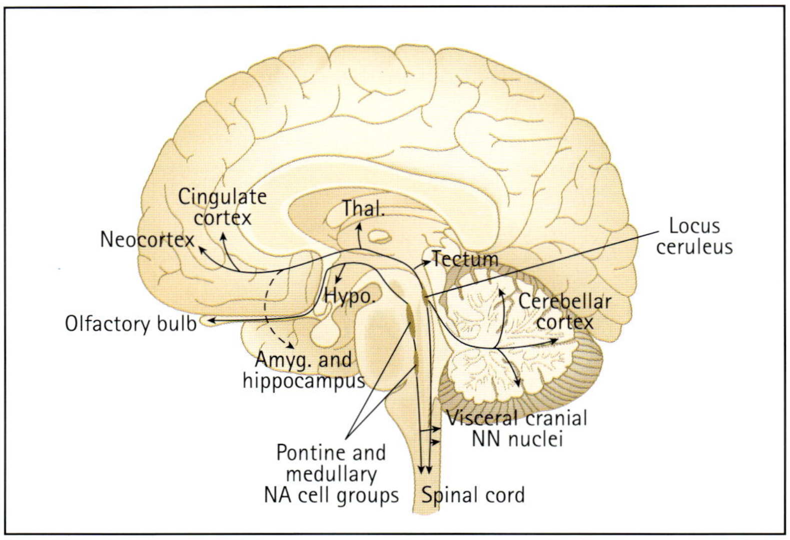

FIGURE 2–24.

Locus ceruleus. Norepinephrine cell bodies are found in the sympathetic ganglia peripherally, but in the central nervous system (CNS), they are confined to the brainstem, although their axons extend to all parts of the CNS. The cell bodies are found in a group of noradrenaline lateral tegmental nuclei and in the locus ceruleus. In cats, norepinephrine depletion in the locus ceruleus abolishes micturition. Alpha-1 blockers suppress pelvic nerve stimulation-evoked reflex discharges on the hypogastric and pudendal nerves, indicating that norepinephrine tonically facilitates continence-related reflexes. Norepinephrine acts to selectively accentuate specific incoming stimuli in a manner that increases the signal-to-noise ratio. AMYG—amygaloid body; HYPO—hypothalamus; THAL—thalamus. (*From* Manter and Gatz [4].)

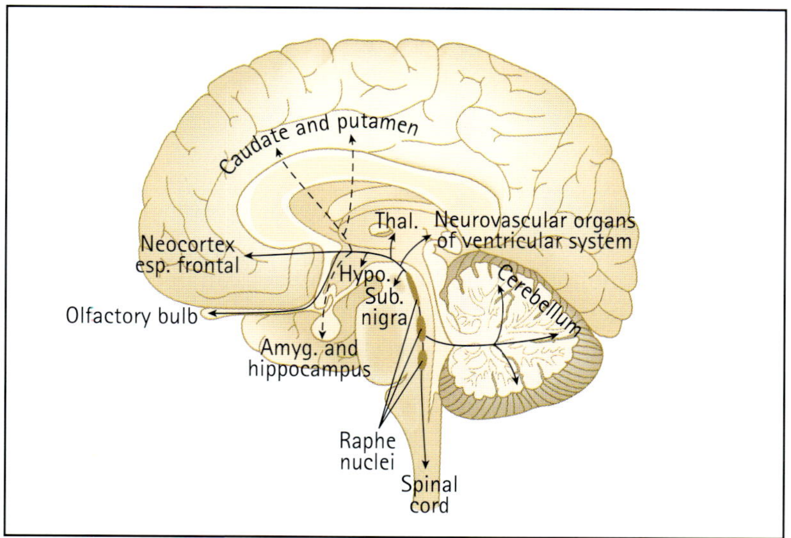

FIGURE 2-25.

The raphe nuclei. The vast majority of cell bodies of origin for serotonin are in the raphe nuclei. Serotonin is also present in mast cells, platelets, and certain gut cells. It is produced from precursor tryptophan. Stimulation in raphe sites inhibits reflex bladder and pelvic nerve activity. Noxious levels of bladder distention increase the firing rate of raphe neurons. Serotonin receptor blockers (5-hydroxytriptamine sub three blockers) decrease volume threshold of fullness sensation, indicating that descending serotonin pathways suppress afferent bladder information. thus inhibiting the micturition reflex. AMYG—amygaloid body; HYPO—hypothalamus; SUB NIGRA—substantia nigra. (*From* Manter and Gatz [4].)

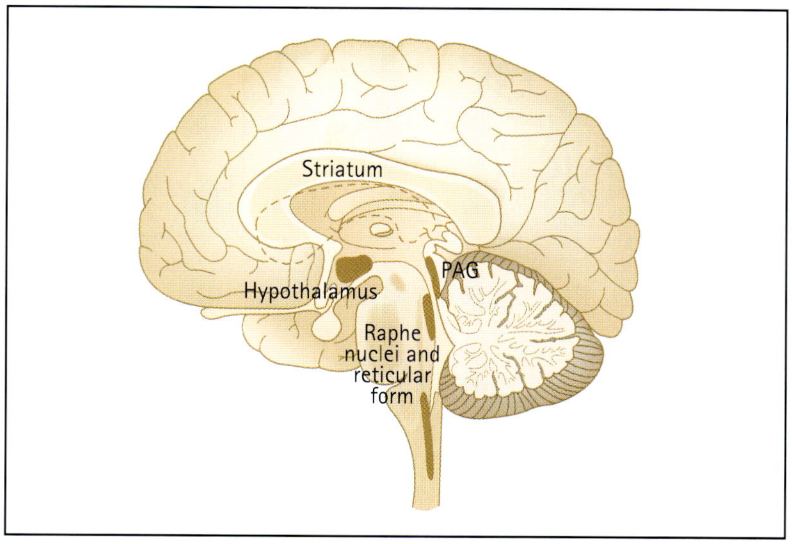

FIGURE 2-26.

Hypothalamus and periaqueductal gray (*PAG*). Anterograde tracers injected into the paraventricular nucleus of the hypothalamus labeled terminals in the sacral parasympathetic nucleus as well as the sphincter motor neurons. Neurons in the anterior hypothalamus project to the pons micturition center. In animals, electrical stimulation of the anterior hypothalamic region induces bladder contraction via medial pontine center parasympathetic pathway and stimulation of the posterior region of hypothalamus inhibits bladder activity by sympathetic inhibitory pathways. Interneurons in the lumbosacral cord project strongly to the PAG, which in turn projects to the pons micturition center, or "M" region. The PAG and the hypothalamus are activated on positron emission tomographic scanning during micturition.

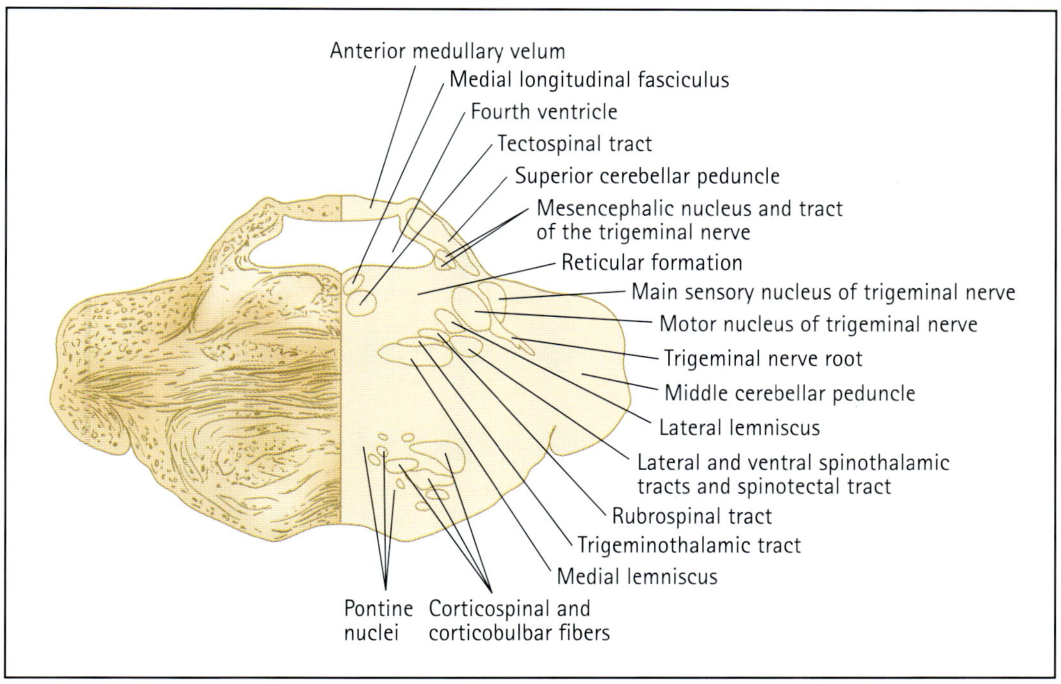

FIGURE 2-27.

Pons. The coordination between sacral cord parasympathetic motor neurons and the nucleus of Onuf motor neurons to the sphincters does not occur in the spinal cord, but in an area of the pons, the "M" region, known as the pontine micturition center (PMC) or Barrington's nucleus. The contraction of the pelvic floor musculature is controlled by another group of neurons in the pons, the "L" region. In the cat, lumbosacral interneurons project to the midbrain periaqueductal gray, which in turn projects to the PMC. The PMC neurons are glutaminergic, excitatory to sacral parasympathetic neurons to produce bladder contraction. PMC terminals on the sacral dorsal commissural gray are excitatory and contact inhibitory gamma-aminobutyric acid neurons, which inhibit motor neurons to external urethral sphincter. The PMC and the "L" region are not interconnected at the pontine level. The PMC is activated on positron emission tomographic studies during micturition. In normal subjects who could not urinate on command, the "L" region was activated. (*From* Manter and Gatz [4].)

REFLEX PATHWAYS

GANGLIONIC REFLEXES

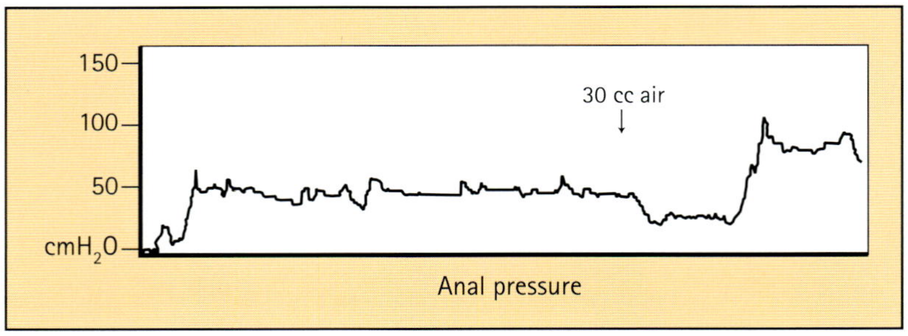

FIGURE 2-28.

Rectal-anal inhibitory reflex. Reflex pathways can occur even in decentralized pelvic organs; hence, the pathway acts through ganglia but in a reflex manner, not incorporating the central nervous system. An example of a clinically testable one is the rectal-anal inhibitory reflex. This relaxation of the internal anal sphincter in response to rectal distention is not abolished by spinal anesthesia. The smooth muscle of the internal anal sphincter, unlike the rest of the intestinal smooth muscle, is contracted by sympathetically mediated alpha-adrenergic activity [16]; hence, this intramural type of reflex is indicative of the ability of prevertebral ganglion neurons to act as an *integrative* station for preganglionic and afferent inputs, important for local and ganglionic reflexes controlling the gut.

CENTRAL NERVOUS SYSTEM REFLEXES

Storage Reflexes

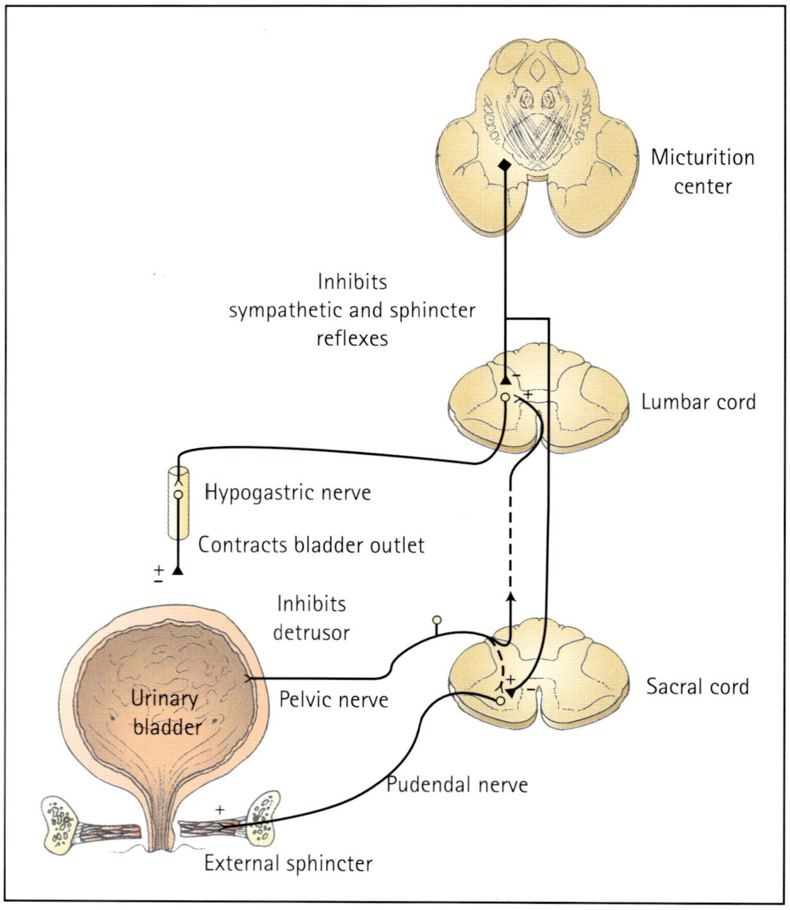

FIGURE 2-29.

Urethral sphincter storage reflexes. The urethral skeletal sphincter muscles have a tonic discharge that increases with bladder filling. This reflex pathway is probably direct spinal, responding to low level bladder afferent input from sensory neurons (see Figure 2-5) that activate Onuf's nucleus (see Figure 2-19).

Sympathetic reflex pathway. During storage, bladder distention produces low level afferent firing with sacrolumbar intersegmental reflex activation of lumbar sympathetic preganglionic neurons (see Figure 2-18). The efferent pathway is via prevertebral hypogastric ganglionic sympathetic nerves that cause bladder outlet contraction and parasympathetic ganglionic inhibition by alpha-receptor activity and detrusor relaxation by beta-receptor activity.

Surgical or pharmacologic sympathetic blockade can reduce urethral resistance, bladder capacity, and compliance and increase bladder contractions. (*From* DeGroat [15]; with permission.)

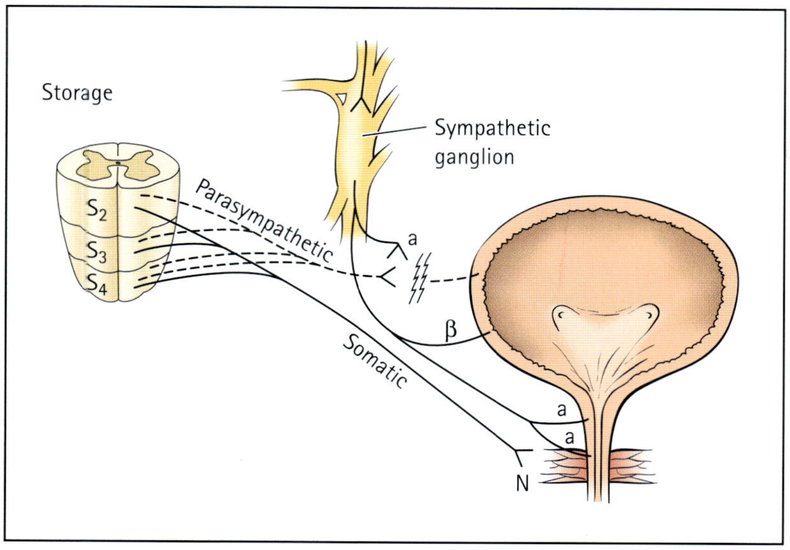

FIGURE 2-30.

Storage.Through spinal reflex pathways, somatic facilitation of the external sphincter, sympathetic contraction of the bladder neck, and sympathetic inhibition of detrusor and parasympathetic ganglia bladder storage is promoted.

Micturition Reflexes

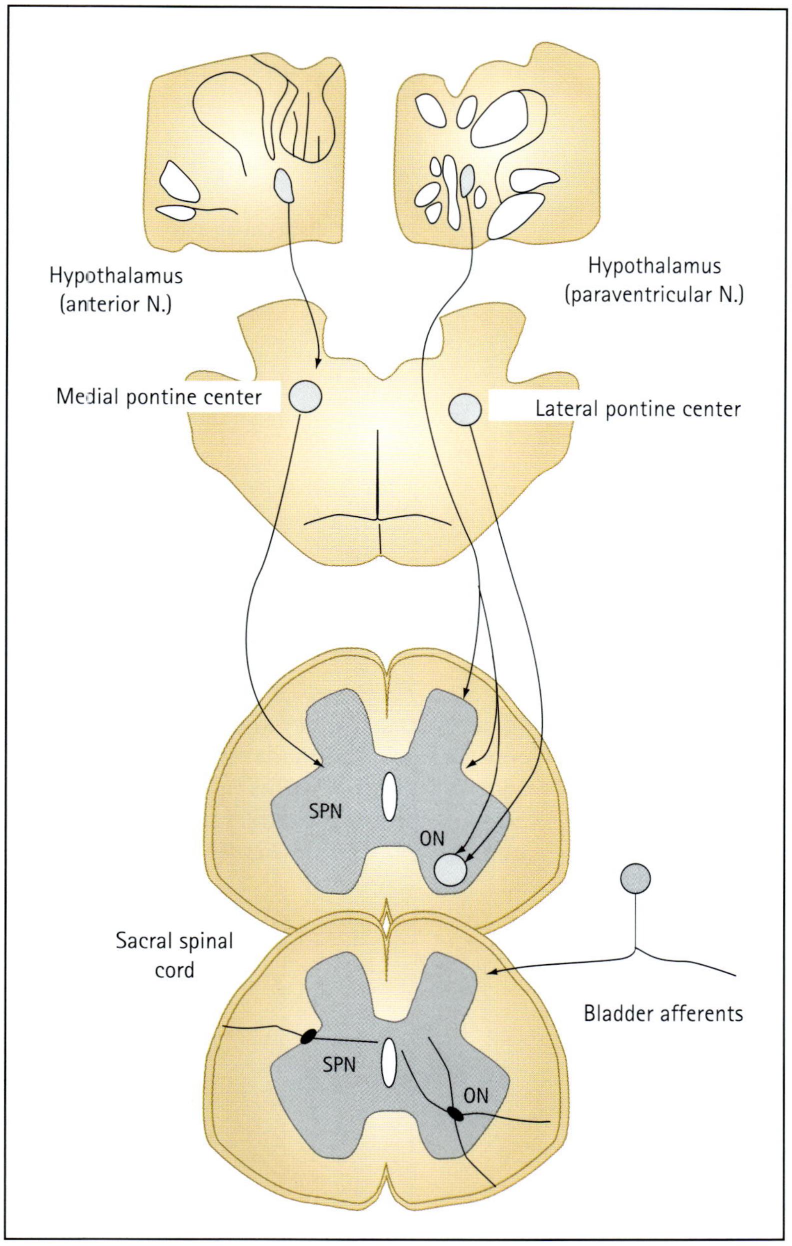

FIGURE 2-31.

Micturition reflexes. The afferent pathways for micturition reflexes are high-level afferent activity via pelvic nerve and, except for the spinal direct reflex activating the sacral parasympathetic preganglionic neurons (see Figure 2-18) involve supraspinal pathways. For inhibition of external sphincter activity, a "set-point" in the pontine micturition center (see Figure 2-27) has tonic inhibitory gamma-aminobutyric acid modulation and when adequately stimulated, urethral sphincter electromyographic activity is inhibited, the first step in micturition, and the sacral preganglionic neurons increase firing with resultant bladder contraction. The parasympathetic efferent outflow to the bladder is activated via the medial pontine center using glutamic acid as neurotransmitter using both N-methyl-D-aspartate (NMDA) and non-NMDA glutaminergic receptors. Inhibition of sympathetic outflow during micturition is probably a function effected through the same pontine center.

Suprapontine controls over the reflexes are largely inhibitory (see Figure 12-18). Frontal cortical areas inhibit the anterior hypothalamus (see Figure 2-23) to prevent activation of medial pontine stimulation of parasympathetic sacral neurons. Paracentral cortical connections with the brainstem and cord activate tonic activity in Onuf's nucleus and reflexly and voluntarily can stop the tonic sphincter activity. This activity may be interrelated with the posterior hypothalamic region, including the paraventricular nucleus, which sends direct sacral projections to parasympathetic (SPN) and Onuf's nucleus (ON). (From DeGroat [15].)

The Bradley Loop Concept

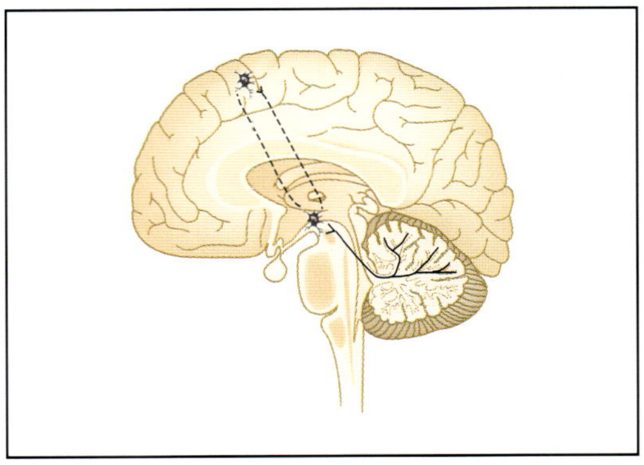

FIGURE 2-32.
The Bradley loop concept of bladder reflexes [17–19]. This theorized concept of micturition has evolved and been widely used clinically. The concepts have been largely complementary to the simultaneously developed concepts of DeGroat, referred to extensively in the previous figure legends. Differences in the concepts are (1) DeGroat stresses more the importance of sympathetic modulation of bladder storage and (2) Bradley has provided data supporting separate neural pathways governing voluntary control of sphincter activity beyond sacral cord phenomena. Bradley loop one: Neuronal connections between frontal lobes and pontine mesencephalic micturition center. (*From* Erlanger [13].)

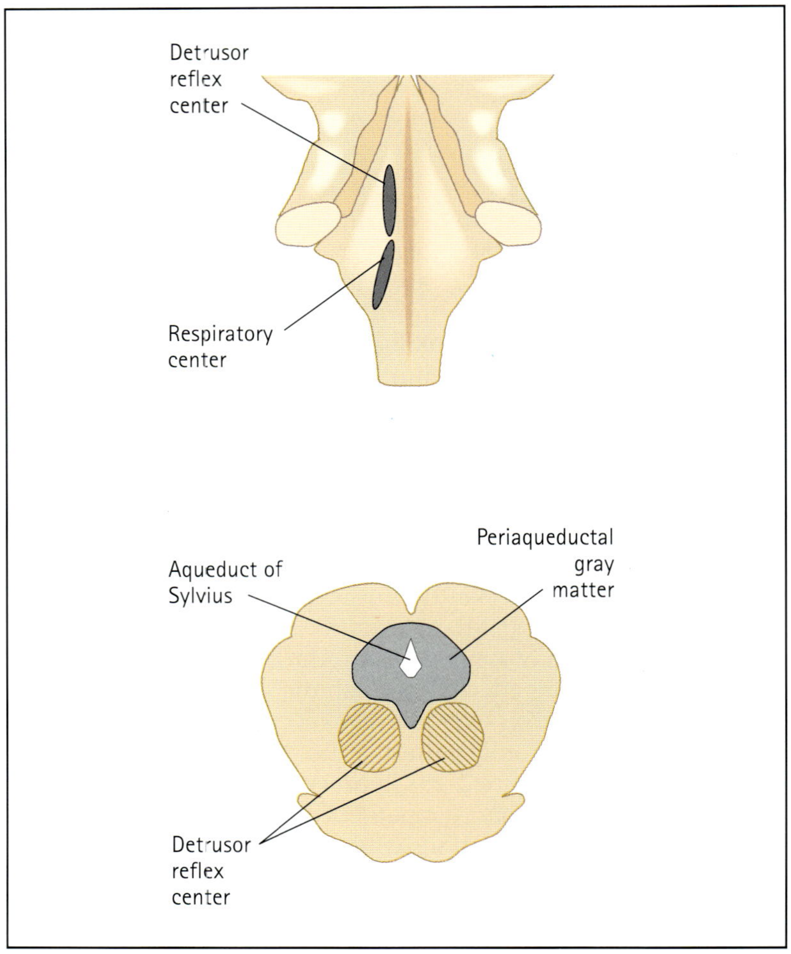

FIGURE 2-33.
Loop one. This provides voluntary control of micturition reflex; interruption causes involuntary bladder contractions which are coordinated with urethral relaxation. (*From* Bradley [17]).

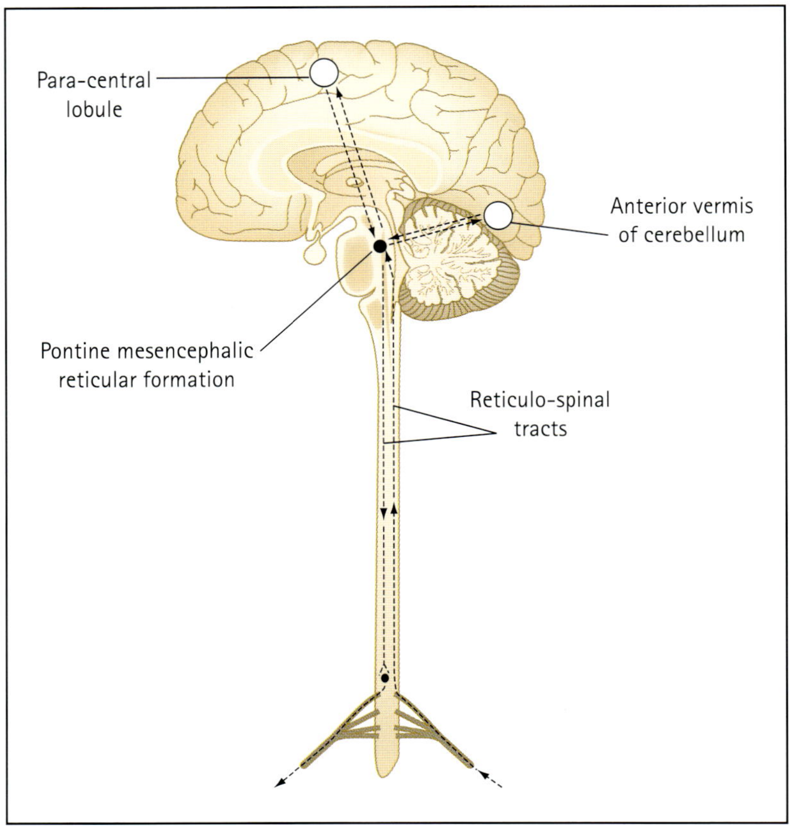

FIGURE 2-34.
Loop two. Long routing of sensory bladder afferents in the spinal cord and brainstem and descending pathways from the micturition center to detrusor motor neurons in sacral gray matter. Interruption causes involuntary bladder contractions not coordinated with urethral relaxation. (*From* Erlanger [13].)

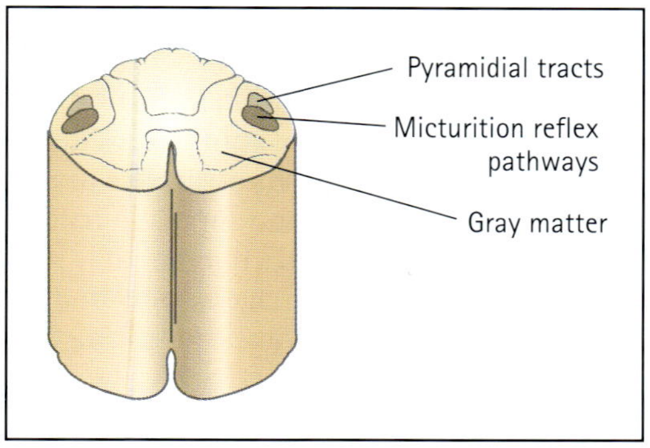

FIGURE 2-35.

Sacral gray matter. Its function is to coordinate and provide for detrusor reflex of adequate temporal duration to allow complete evacuation. Interruption of the pathway produces detrusor areflexia and urinary retention (the correlates of "spinal shock" with acute spinal cord transection. The later development of reflex bladder activity in suprasacral bladder transection is suggested to be due to ephaptic interaction between newly sprouting neurites and axons at the transection level. This "collateral sprouting" theory differs from deGroat's concept of the emergence of a vestigial reflex pathway with spinal transection [20] (see Figure 2-38), the latter concept having compelling evidence. (*From* Bradley [17].)

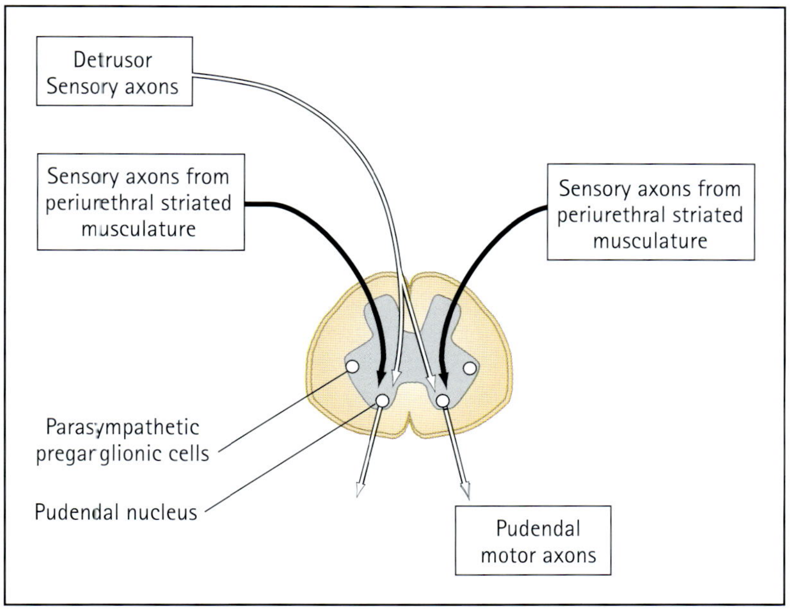

FIGURE 2-36.

Loop three. The peripheral detrusor afferent axons synapsing on pudendal motor neurons provide reflexive urethral relaxation with detrusor contraction. (*From* Bradley [17].)

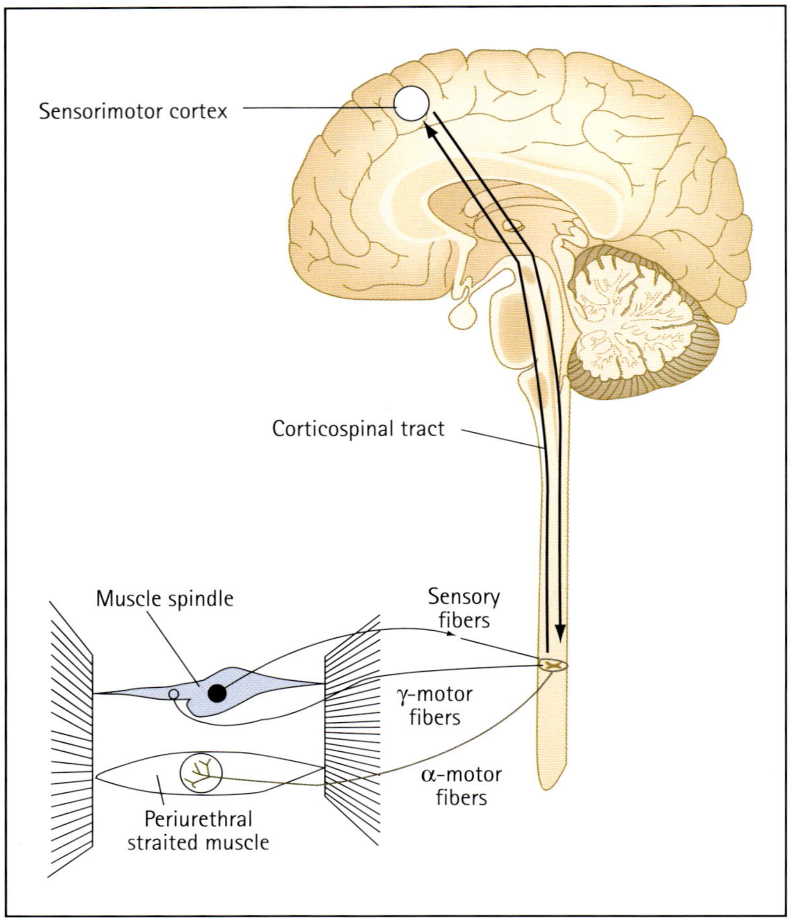

FIGURE 2-37.

Loop four. Suprasacral component. Loop four has two components; one is the suprasacral afferent and efferent innervation of the pudendal motor neurons to the periurethral sphincter. This presumes upper motor neurons control in a fashion similar to limb muscles with neurons from the superior and medial portions of the motor cortex giving rise to pyramidal tract fibers that traverse the lateral cord to Onuf's nucleus. Damage results in an "upper motor neuron" type lesion with preservation of sphincter tone, but loss of volitional activation (as contrasted with lower motor neuron lesion of pudendal nerve with loss of tone). The pathway is also inhibitory, allowing voluntary cessation of the tonic sphincter activity in initiation of micturition. Loss of this ability clinically presents with hesitancy. The Onuf's nucleus differs from other anterior horn cells in having both upper motor neurons of types going to somatic motor cells and autonomic motor cells.

Sacral component: The second portion of loop four consists of afferent fibers from striated muscle fibers that synapse on pudendal motor neurons. In contrast to loop three sphincter relaxation with detrusor contraction, this provides sphincter contraction during filling and is stimulated by sensory impulses from pelvic floor muscle spindle activity. It must differ from simple somatic motor reflexes because the urethral intrinsic skeletal muscle sphincter does not have spindles. (*From* Ostergard [13].)

Pathologic Reflexes in Spinal Cord Transection

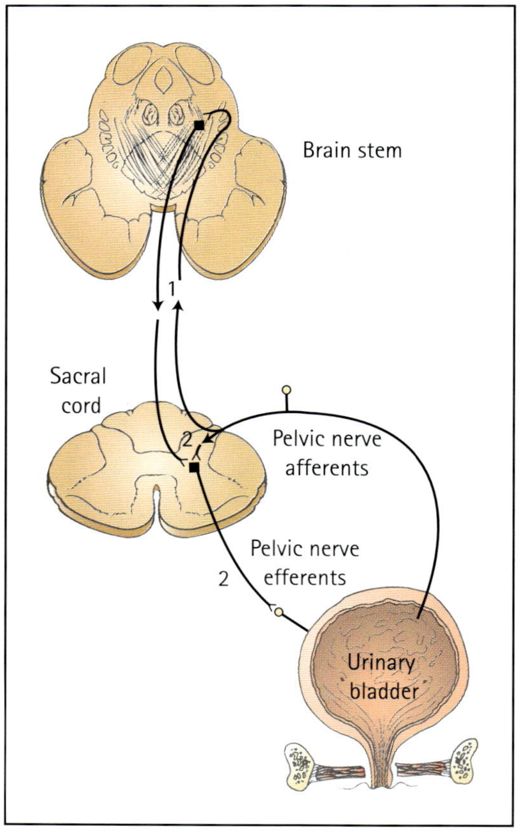

FIGURE 2-38.

Micturition reflex. DeGroat's theories have evolved. The micturition reflex in normal animals (*pathway 1*) with stimulation of myelinated (alpha-delta) afferents from the bladder and recording from postganglionic nerves on the bladder surface had latencies of 100 ms with a demonstrated central delay of 60 to 75 ms, suggesting supraspinal reflex mechanism. This reflex remained present in decerebrate animals but was lost in acute and chronic spinal animals. Sixty percent of animals with an intact spinal cord had a second reflex (*pathway 2*) with latency of 180 to 200 ms with demonstrated central delay of 15 to 40 ms, occurring only at stimulus intensities sufficient to activate unmyelinated afferent fibers (C fibers). This reflex was abolished with spinal cord transection but 3 to 7 days later returned and increased in magnitude in conjunction with development of reflex micturition. Capsaicin, a neurotoxin that disrupts C-fiber function, blocks the bladder contractions induced by bladder distention in chronic spinal cats, but not in normal cats. Thus, chronic spinal animals have facilitation of C–fiber-evoked reflex and lose alpha–delta-evoked reflexes, indicating two distinct central pathways, supraspinal and spinal, using different afferent limbs (alpha-delta and C-fiber, respectively). Clinically this C–fiber-mediated reflex may be tested by instillation of cold water into the bladder, activating C fibers. There is no resulting voiding reflex in normal patients, but reflex voiding in response to the cold water appears in patients with upper motor neuron lesions (multiple sclerosis, cerebrovascular disease, Parkinson's disease, elderly with loss of sensation, normal infants) suggesting that C-fiber afferents are involved in several pathologic conditions associated with bladder overactivity. There are many possible mechanisms for the emergence of C-fiber reflexes in paraplegic cats, for example, cord changes, loss of supraspinal inhibition, changes in neurotransmitters, but there is considerable evidence that one factor of importance is changes in the *afferent* neurons. (*From* Krane and Siroky [8].)

Pathologic Reflexes with Bladder Outlet Obstruction

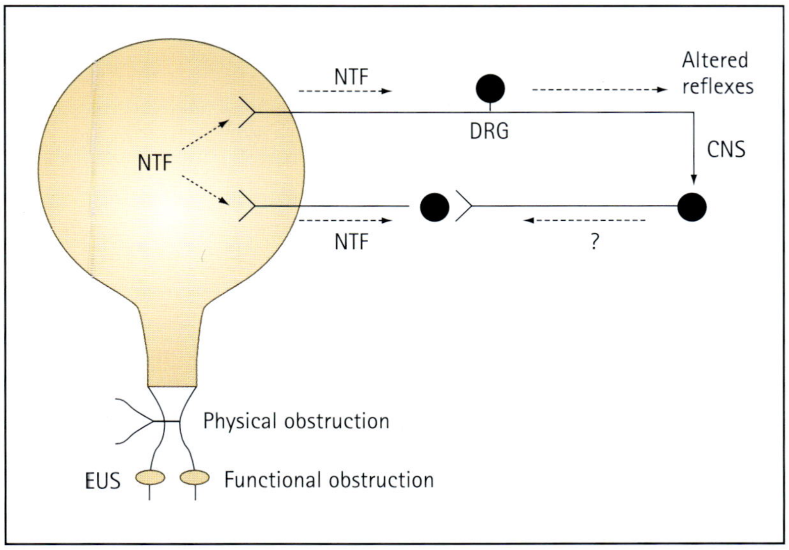

FIGURE 2–39.

Neuroplasticity in bladder neural pathways following partial urethral obstruction. In paraplegic cats that develop reflex voiding, the voiding is inefficient secondary to detrusor-sphincter dyssynergia. The bladder becomes enlarged and the afferent neurons markedly (50%) increase in size. In animals with urinary diversion after spinal transection, the bladder distention and hypertrophy was avoided and the afferent neuron hypertrophy was prevented, suggesting that factors released in the hypertrophied bladder are responsible for the neural changes. Outlet obstruction produced by urethral ligation in cats with intact spinal cords induces hypertrophy of bladder afferent and efferent neurons, and this is accompanied by increased levels of nerve growth factor (NGF). Changes in afferent neuron pathways can also be elicited by other agents (*e.g.*, bradykinin, histamine, nitric oxide) that can be released in the urinary bladder by afferent neurons. Hence, disorders in the central nervous system can increase bladder activity by altering central neural mechanisms; however, central neural mechanisms may also be altered by local bladder conditions, such as obstruction, inflammation, or injury, and lead to overactive bladder. With these conditions, a C–fiber-mediated spinal reflex develops, which can be tested with the ice-water test. An increase in NGF occurs with each of these conditions and if blocked, the urinary frequency following obstruction or inflammation does not occur [21] Manipulating NGF production or blocking its receptors may influence an overactive bladder. DRG—dorsal root ganglia; EUS—external urethral sphincter; MPG—major pelvic ganglia; NTF—neurotropic factors. (*From* DeGroat [15].)

Sacral Neuromodualtion

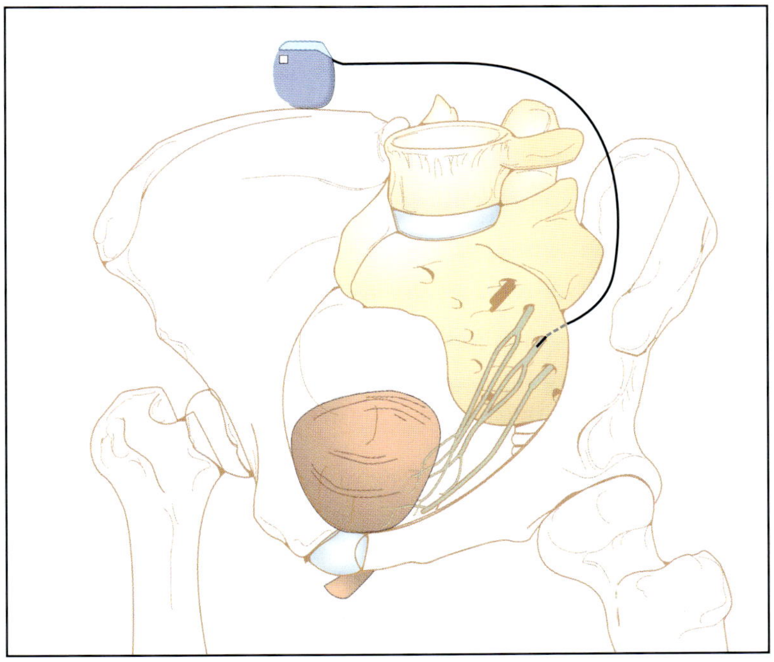

FIGURE 2–40.

Implant therapy. Sacral neuromodulation has been shown to have clinical effectiveness in bladder overactivity and voiding dysfunctions. The mechanisms of action are complex and may involve counteracting the development of new pathologic micturition reflexes. Rat studies [22] using cystometric and electrophysiologic recording and measurements of C–fiber-stored neuropeptides (calcitonin gene-related peptide, substance P, neurokinin A) revealed that the elevation of C-fiber neuropeptides found in the dorsal root ganglia after spinal cord transection was returned to control values with sacral neuromodulation.

CLINICAL STIGMATA OF URINARY TRACT DYSFUNCTION WITH LESIONS OF THE CENTRAL NERVOUS SYSTEM

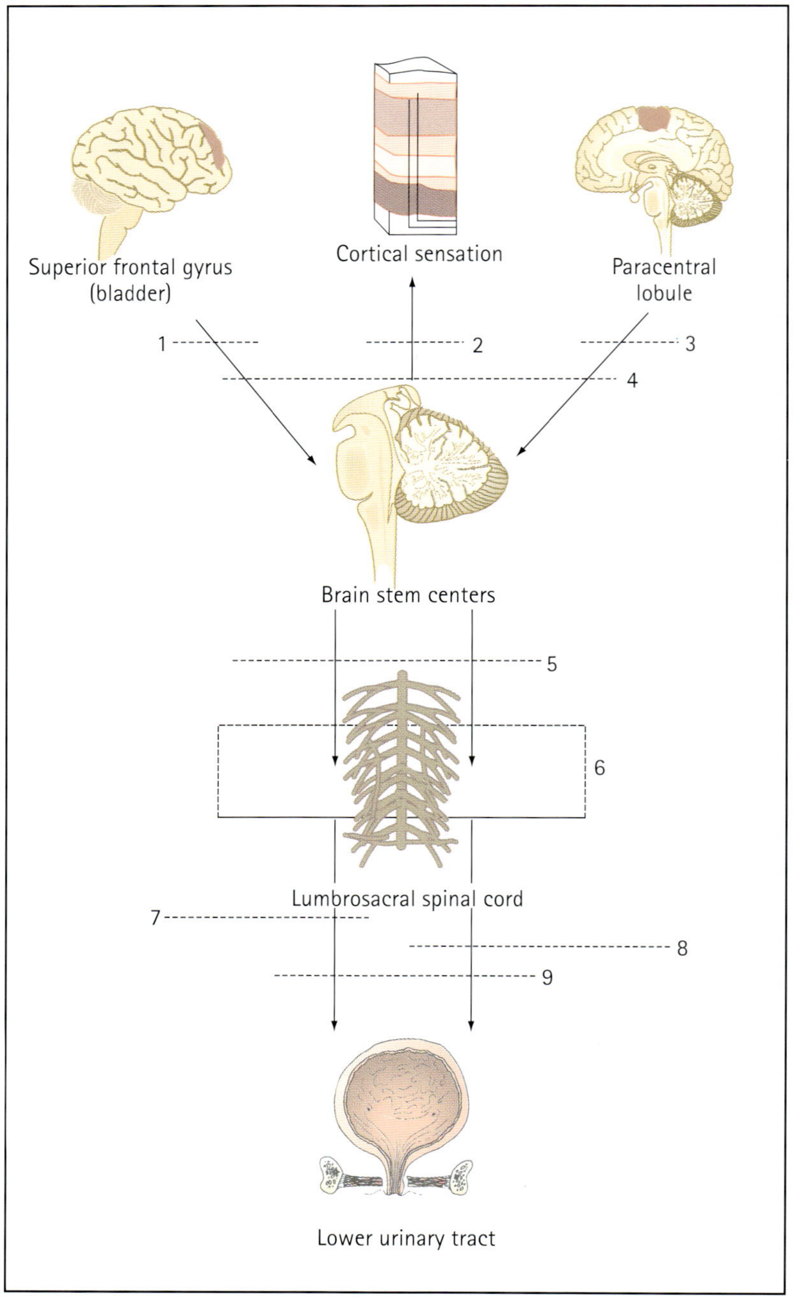

FIGURE 2-41.

Clinical stigmata of lesions relating to the lower urinary tract function:

Simplified scheme of interaction of various levels of the nervous system in micturition. The locations of certain possible nervous lesions are denoted by numbers and explained as follows.

1, Lesions isolating the superior frontal gyrus prevent voluntary postponement of voiding. If sensation is intact, this produces urge incontinence. If the lesion is larger, there is additional loss of social concern about incontinence.

2, Lesions isolating the paracentral lobule, sometimes associated with a hemiparesis, cause spasticity of the urethral sphincter and retention. This will be painless if sensation is abolished. Minor degrees of this syndrome may cause difficulty in the initiation of micturition.

3, Pathways of sensation are not known accurately. In theory, an isolated lesion of sensation above the brainstem would lead to unconscious incontinence. Defective central conduction of sensory information would explain nocturnal enuresis.

4, Lesions above the brainstem centers lead to involuntary voiding that is coordinated with sphincter relaxation.

5, Lesions below brainstem centers but above the lumbosacral spinal cord, after a period of bladder paralysis associated with spinal shock, lead to involuntary reflex voiding that is not coordinated with sphnicter relaxation (detrusor-sphincter dyssynergia).

6, Lesions destroying the lumbosacral cord of the complete nervous connections between the central and peripheral nervous system result in a paralyzed bladder that contracts only weakly in an autonomous fashion because of its remaining ganglionic innervation. However, if the lumbar sympathetic outflow is preserved in the presence of conus or cauda equina destruction, there may be some residual sympathetic tone in the bladder neck and urethra that may be sufficient to be obstructive.

7, A lesion of the efferent fibers alone leads to a bladder of decreased capacity and decreased compliance associated experimentally with an increased number of adrenergic nerves.

8, A lesion confined to the afferent fibers produces a bladder that is areflexic with increased compliance and capacity.

9, Because there are ganglion cells in the bladder wall, it is technically impossible to decentralize the bladder completely, but congenital absence of bladder ganglia may exist, producing megacystitis. (*From* Torrens [23].)

Work by deGroat and others has led to a new era of understanding of neural activity relating to urogynecologic disorders. Together, the clinicians and the scientists, working in conjunction with manufacturers and the interested public, can use the knowledge to dramatically improve patient care .

REFERENCES

1. Elbadawi A: Comparative neuromorphology in animals. In *The Physiology of the Lower Urinary Tract*. Edited by Torrens M. Berlin: Springer-Verlag; 1987:
2. Hale D, Benson JT, *et al.*: Histologic analysis of needle biopsy of urethral sphincter from normal and stress incontinent women with comparison of electromyographic findings. *Am J Obstet Gynecol* (in press)
3. Merrill Life Science, Glencoe Division, Macmillan/McGraw-Hill School Publishing Co., Westerville, OH. 1993.
4. Manter JT, Gatz AJ: In *Essentials of Clinical Neuroanatomy and Neurophysiology*, edn 8. Edited by Gilman S, Newman SW. Philadelphia: FA Davis; 1992.
5. Kimura J: In *Textbook of Histology* edn 10. Philadelphia: WB Saunders; 1975: .
6. Wiesenfield-Hallin Z, Hao JX, Xu, XJ, Hokfelt T: Nitric oxide mediates ongoing discharges in dorsal root ganglion cells after peripheral nerve injury. *J Neurophysiol* 1993, 70:2350–2353.
7. Clemente CD: *Gray's Anatomy*, edn 30. Philadelphia: Lea & Febiger, 1985:940, 1192, 1248.
8. Krane RJ, Siroky MB: *Clinical Neuro-Urology*, edn 2. Boston: Little, Brown, 1991.
9. Elbadawi A, Schenk EA: A new theory of the innervation of bladder musculature. Part 3. Postganglionic synapse in uretero-vesical-urethral autonomic pathways *J Urol* 1971, 105:373.
10. Lundborg G: *Nerve Injury and Repair*. Edinburgh: Churchill Livingstone; 1988:3, 5, 33.
11. Campenot RB: Local control of neurite development by nerve growth factor. *Proc Natl Acad Sci U S A* 1977, 74:4516–4519.
12. Low PA: *Clinical Autonomic Disorders*. Boston: Little, Brown; 1993:21.
13. Erlanger J, Gasser HS: *Electrical Signs of Nervous Activity.* Philadelphia: University of Pennsylavania Press, 1937.
14. Colleselli K, et al.: The female urethral sphincter: a morphological and topographical study. *J Urol* 1998, 160:49–54.
15. DeGroat WC: Neurologic basis for the overactive bladder. *Urology* 1997, 50 (suppl 6A):36–52.
16. Rayner W: Characteristic of the internal anal sphincter and the rectum of the vervet monkey. *J Physiol* 286:383–399.
17. Bradley WE, Teague CT: Spinal cord organization of micturition reflex afferents. *Exp Neurol* 1968, 22:504.
18. Bradley WE, Sundin T: The physiology and pharmacology of urinary tract dysfunction. *Clin Neuropharmacol* 1982, 5:131.
19. Bradley WE, Timm GW, Scott FB: Innervation of the detrusor muscle and urethra. *Urol Clin North Am> 1974, 11:*
20. DeGroat WC, Booth AM: Autonomic systems to the urinary bladder and sexual organs. In *Peripheral Neuropathy*. Edited by Dyck PJ, et al. Philadelphia: WB Saunders; 1984:285–299.
21. Steers WD, Creedon D, Tuttle JB: Immunity to NGF prevents afferent plasticity following hypertrophy of the urinary bladder. *J Urol* 1996, 155:378–385.
22. Hassouna MM: Interstim Continence Control Therapy, Education Program, Minneapolis. March 27, 28, 1998.
23. Torrens M: *The Physiology of the Lower Urinary Tract*, New York: Springer-Verlag; 1987.

CHAPTER 3

Diagnosis of Urinary Incontinence

Mary T. McLennan and Alfred E. Bent

Incontinence affects about 13 million Americans with the prevalence increasing with age. The community-dwelling elderly have a 15% to 30% prevalence rate, which may increase to 50% in residents of nursing homes. The direct economic cost to society is estimated at $16.4 million (1994 dollars). Thus, the health care professional must provide expedient assessment, diagnosis, and management of this disorder. This chapter reviews current assessment modalities for urinary incontinence in women.

Urinary incontinence in itself is a symptom not a diagnosis. Determining the specific type is fundamental in determining the most specific and cost-efficient therapy. All patients should undergo a basic evaluation. It is imperative in the elderly to look for reversible conditions that may cause transient incontinence (*i.e.*, DIAPPERS: delirium, infection, atrophic vaginitis, pharmacologic, psychological, endocrine, restricted mobility, stool impaction).

Basic evaluation should include history, physical examination, assessment of mobility and toilet access (elderly), review of medication, urolog record, cough stress test, and physical examination. History should include general medical, neurologic, and specific genitourinary problems. The chief complaint and history of presenting problem should be first ascertained. Review of the urolog may provide additional information not readily obtained by specific questioning. Examination includes assessment of mental status; mobility; dexterity; neurologic, abdominal, pelvic, and rectal areas; direct observation of urine loss; postvoid residual urine; cotton swab angle, and urinalysis.A simple office cystogram may provide additional information. Based on the above assessment, conservative therapy may be instituted.

Urodynamic testing is not necessarily part of the initial evaluation and should be reserved for patients who meet the criteria outlined in Figure 3-24. Cystoscopy is not indicated in all patients but should be considered in those with a history of previous failed surgery, history suggestive of intrinsic sphincter deficiency, interstitial cystitis, recurrent urinary tract infections, recent onset of frequency, urgency with or without urge incontinence especially in a smoker over 50 years of age, and the presence of hematuria. Radiologic techniques are used when specific diagnoses are suspected, for example, hematuria, impaired compliance, urethral diverticulum, and vesicoureteral reflux.

Electrodiagnostic testing will not be discussed here. The role of these techniques in the diagnosis of incontinence is still under investigation. Similarly, magnetic resonance imaging has certainly clarified our understanding of the anatomy of the pelvis and its supports, but its role in incontinence is unknown.

PATIENT HISTORY

Patient Questionnaire

Please bring this completed form with you at the time of your first visit.

Name ______________________ Date ______________________
Birthdate ______________________ Age ______________________
Please describe your current medical problem: ______________________

____

OBSTRETIC AND GYNECOLOGIC HISTORY

Number of pregnancies	____	Number of children born alive	____
Number of miscarriages	____	Current birth control method	____
Onset of first menstrual period	____	Last menstrual period	____
Length of menstrual cycle	____	Duration between menstrual cycles	____
Are your periods regular? Yes ____	No ____	Have you been through menopause?	____

Have you had any treatment to your cervix? Yes ____ No ____
Cautery ______________________ Other ______________________
Cryosurgery ______________________ If yes, when? ______________________

Do you have any of the following?
- Bleeding between periods; if yes, duration ______________________
- Bleeding after intercourse; if yes, duration ______________________
- Heavy menstrual periods; if yes, duration ______________________
- Pain with periods; if yes, duration ______________________
- Uncontrolled loss of urine; if yes, duration ______________________

Have you ever had any of the following:
- Herpes ____
- Venereal warts ____
- Sexually transmitted diseases ____

Are you sexually active at this time? Yes ____ No ____
Is your sex life satisfactory for you? Yes ____ No ____

PAST MEDICAL HISTORY – PLEASE ANSWER YES OR NO

As a child did you have:

____ Rheumatic fever	____ Rubella (measles)
____ Scarlet fever	____ Other

As an adult have you had:

____ Bladder infections	____ Asthma
____ Chronic fatigue syndrome	____ Heart disease
____ Diabetes	____ Epstein-Barr virus
____ Kidney disease	____ High blood pressure
____ Kidney infection	____ Jaundice
____ Liver disease	____ Mononucleosis
____ Pneumonia	____ Serious injuries or accident
____ Stroke	____ Tuberculosis

Please list all medicines which you are currently taking including contraceptives and vitamins; include dose and frequency. ______________________

____

Do you have any allergies? If so, please list: ______________________

SURGICAL HISTORY

Have you had any operations? Yes ____ No ____
If yes, please list type, and date or age when performed ______________________

____

Have you had any blood transfusions? Yes ____ No ____

HEALTH HABITS

Do you consider yourself healthy?
Do you smoke? Yes ____ No ____ How many packs a day? ______________________
Do you use alcohol? Yes ____ No ____ Do you use any street drugs? ______________________

FIGURE 3-1.

Patient questionnaire. A general medical questionnaire can be sent to the patient for her completion before her visit. This not only expedites the visit but also allows the patient to obtain information regarding previous surgeries or medical conditions. The responses to the forms are then reviewed at the time of the visit.

1. Please describe your current urinary problem
2. Do you lose urine with coughing, lifting, sneezing, straining, aerobics, or exercise? Yes_____ No_____
3. Do you lose urine involuntarily with urgency or without sensation before you reach the toilet? Yes_____ No_____
4. How often on average do you void during the day: every 1/2 h, 1 h, 1 1/2 h, 2 h, 3 h or more than 3 hours, (Circle one)
5. How many times do you get up at night to void? (0, 1, 2, 3, 4, 5 or more)
6. Have you ever wet the bed? Yes_____ No_____
7. Do you leak during sexual intercourse? Yes_____ No_____
   Or with orgasm? Yes_____ No_____
8. Do you wear protection because of urinary leakage? Yes_____ No_____
   If yes, circle one: intermittent, waking hours, continuously
9. Have you had prior treatment for urinary incontinence? Yes_____ No_____
   If yes circle each one that apply:
   Behavioral – Kegels, pelvic floor muscle exercise, biofeedback, and electrical stimulation, bladder retraining drills
   Drugs – which ones?
   Surgery – what surgery?
10. Do you currently have or have you ever had any of the following medical conditions?
    Diabetes Yes_____ No_____
    Stroke Yes_____ No_____
    Parkinson's disease Yes_____ No_____
    Paralysis or weakness Yes_____ No_____
    Multiple sclerosis Yes_____ No_____
    Spina bifida Yes_____ No_____
11. Do you have recurrent urinary tract infections (cystitis)? Yes_____ No_____
    If yes, circle how often: 2/y, 3/y, 4/y, 5/y, more than 5/y
12. Have you ever had blood in your urine? Yes_____ No_____
13. Do you have pain, discomfort, burning, severe urgency, abdominal pain, straining, slow stream when you void? (Circle each that applies)

FIGURE 3-2.

Urinary questionnaire. This urinary questionnaire is also completed before the patient's first visit. Question 1 is open-ended so the patient can describe the problem as she sees it. Question 2 is designed to elicit the symptom of stress incontinence. Questions 3 through 7 usually indicate urge incontinence. Severity is addressed in question 8. Questions 11 and 12 screen for recurrent urinary tract infection or neoplasm. Question 13 screens for infective and inflammatory conditions and voiding dysfunction. Although not listed, patients need to be specifically questioned regarding associated bowel dysfunction: constipation, sense of incomplete emptying, incontinence of gas, and liquid or solid stool, because significant bowel symptoms may be present in up to 30% of patients presenting with urinary incontinence [1].

SUBJECTIVE QUESTIONNAIRES

Urogenital Distress Inventory—Short Form UDI-6

Do you experience, and, if so, how much are you bothered by:

- Frequent urination
- Urine leakage related to the feeling of urgency?
- Urine leakage related to physical activity, coughing, or sneezing?
- Small amounts of urine leakage (drops)?
- Difficulty emptying your bladder?
- Pain or discomfort in the lower abdominal or genital area?

Incontinence Impact Questionnaire—Short Form IIQ-7

Has urine leakage and/or prolapse affected your:

- Ability to do household chores (cooking, housecleaning, laundry)?
- Physical recreation such as walking, swimming, or other exercise?
- Entertainment activities (movies, concerts, etc.)?
- Ability to travel by car or bus more than 30 minutes from home?
- Participation in social activities outside your home?
- Emotional health (nervousness, depression, etc.)?
- Feeling frustrated?

FIGURE 3-3.

Subjective questionnaires. Increasing emphasis is being placed on quality of life issues with respect to patient satisfaction and treatment success. These two forms represent reliable and valid means of assessing subjective aspects of incontinence and its severity [2]. They may be useful in making treatment decisions and evaluating results of both conservative and surgical interventions. These short versions minimize the burden on the patient [3].

Time	Amount Voided	Leak Volume	Urge Present	Activity	Amount/Type of Intake

FIGURE 3-4.

Voiding diary/urolog. A 24-hour voiding diary is a useful supplement to the history. Diaries may vary slightly but basically involve the patient recording the voiding times, volumes, leakage, presence or absence of urge, activity, and type and volume of intake. It helps pinpoint frequency and pattern of voiding and leakage and is more reliable than the patient's memory of such events. It may help to modify the initial diagnostic impression obtained from the history.

Time	Amount Voided	Leak Volume	Urge Present	Activity	Amount/Type of Intake
8:00 a.m.	23 oz		yes	woke up and made coffee	
10:18 a.m.	13 oz		yes	sitting	40 oz coffee
11:18 a.m.	11 oz		yes	working in kitchen	4 oz coffee, 8 oz citrucel, 8 oz orange juice, 4 oz water
11:27 a.m.		1	no	sneezed sitting	
12:40 p.m.	18 oz		yes	sitting	4 oz water
1:38 p.m.	17 oz		yes	walking	4 oz water
4:05 p.m	14 oz		yes	standing	24 oz water, 4 oz watermelon
5:30 p.m.	10 oz		yes	standing	16 oz water
7:38 p.m.	14 oz		yes	standng cooking	42 oz water
9:50 p.m.	17 oz		yes	standing washing dishes	12 oz sparkling wine
11:45 p.m.	11 oz		yes	walked up stairs	4 oz sparking wine, 13 oz water
12:00 a.m.	4 oz		yes	sitting	4 oz water
6:20 a.m.	34 oz		yes	sleeping	

FIGURE 3–5.

Urolog.This 53-year-old woman with a history of chronic allergies complained of leakage with coughing and sneezing and some associated urinary frequency. She denied any urge-associated leakage. Her voiding diary demonstrates that her one leakage episode was with sneezing. She voids frequently but with excellent volumes (average of 490 mL, maximum of 1020 mL), which can be explained by her large fluid intake. The diary supports the clinical diagnosis of stress incontinence.

Date	Time	Amount Voided	Accidents?	Reason for accident	Amount of fluid I drank
10/23	6:30 a.m.	300cc	yes	getting to bathroom	
	9:15 a.m.	300 cc			8 oz
					8 oz
					4-6 oz
	9:45 a.m.	100cc	yes	urge	
	11 a.m.	150 cc			
	12:45 p.m.	200 cc			8 oz
	2:15 p.m.	200 cc	yes	sitting	6 oz
	3:30 p.m.	100 cc	yes	urge	
	5:00 p.m.	150 cc			
	8:00 p.m.	200 cc	yes	eating	8 oz
	10:45 p.m.	100 cc	yes	prepare for bed	8 oz

Number of pads I used today: 4

FIGURE 3-6.
Urolog. The diary of this 51-year-old woman is typical of a patient with urge incontinence. She complained of being unable to make it to the toilet, voiding every 1 to 11/2 hours during the day. Her diary shows that she voids at frequent intervals with small volumes and all leakage episodes were associated with urge.

Time	Amount Voided	Leak Volume	Urge Present	Activity	Amount/Type of Intake
6:00 a.m.	2.5 oz			awakening	
7:01 a.m.	2 oz			awakening	
8:02 a.m.	3 oz			awakening	
8:45 a.m.				resting in chair	6 oz prune juice
9:15 a.m.					8 oz milk, 8 oz water
9:45 a.m.	2 oz				
11:00 p.m.	22 oz			sitting in chair	4 oz water
11:10 a.m.					10 oz water
11:15 a.m.	1 oz			walking	
11:20 a.m.	drops			bowel mvmt	
11:55 a.m.	1.75 oz			reading	
12:45 p.m.	1.5 oz			standing	
1:15 p.m.	1.5 oz			doing laundry	
2:00 p.m.					8 oz water
2:30 p.m.					16 oz iced tea
2:30 p.m.	2 oz			eating lunch	
2:55 p.m.	2 oz			bowel mvmt	42 oz water
3:10 p.m.	3 oz			reading	
3:50 p.m.				ironing	10 oz water
4:00 p.m.	3 oz			ironing	
5:05 p.m.	2 oz			ironing	
6:15 p.m.	2.75 oz			ironing	
6:30 p.m.				eating dinner	12 oz iced tea
7:20 p.m.	3 oz			sitting	
7:37 p.m.	2 oz			walking	
8:15 p.m.	2 oz			resting in chair	
9:00 p.m.	2 oz			folding laundry	
10:00 p.m.				crocheting	1 oz water (with medication)
10:30 p.m.	3 oz			crocheting	
12:15 a.m.	3 oz			resting in chair	
12:35 a.m.	2 oz			folding laundry	
1:50 a.m.	2.5 oz				
2:35 a.m.	2 oz			sleeping	
3:00 a.m.	2 oz			sitting in chair	8 oz milk
4:25 a.m.	3 oz			sleeping	
6:00 a.m.	3 oz			awakening	

FIGURE 3-7.

Urolog. This 60-year-old woman complained of severe frequency every half hour with associated suprapubic pain. She denied incontinence. Her voiding diary showed that she voided extremely frequently both day and night with consistently tiny volumes (drops to a maximum of 90 mL). This is typical of interstitial cystitis, which was confirmed at cystoscopy.

PHYSICIAL EXAMINATION

GENERAL PHYSICAL EXAMINATION

- Demeanor
- Cognition
- Facial Symmetry
- Speech
- Gait
- Manual dexterity
- Edema

FIGURE 3-8.

Physical examination. The general physical examination should attempt to identify any neurologic abnormalities and factors that effect toileting such as cognition, dexterity, and mobility. The examiner should observe the patient's demeanor, facial symmetry, speech, and gait. The presence of edema should be ascertained. Seeing the patient walk into the examining room provides valuable information on her general status.

ABDOMINAL EXAMINATION

- Old incisions
- Distension
- Masses
- Distended bladder
- Flank tenderness

FIGURE 3-9.

Abdominal examination. Abdominal examination may provide information on previous incontinence surgeries and possible contributors to increased intra-abdominal pressure or irritative bladder symptoms such as masses or a distended bladder. The examiner should also assess flank tenderness.

NEUROLOGIC EXAMINATION

- Mental status
- Sensory function
- Motor function
- Deep tendon reflexes
- Sacral reflexes

FIGURE 3-10.

Neurologic examination. Screening for mental status changes can be rapidly done in an informal manner by noting the patient's orientation, recent and past memory, speech and comprehension, sensory and motor function, and deep tendon and sacral reflexes. Patients with altered mental status often present with detrusor instability or overflow incontinence.

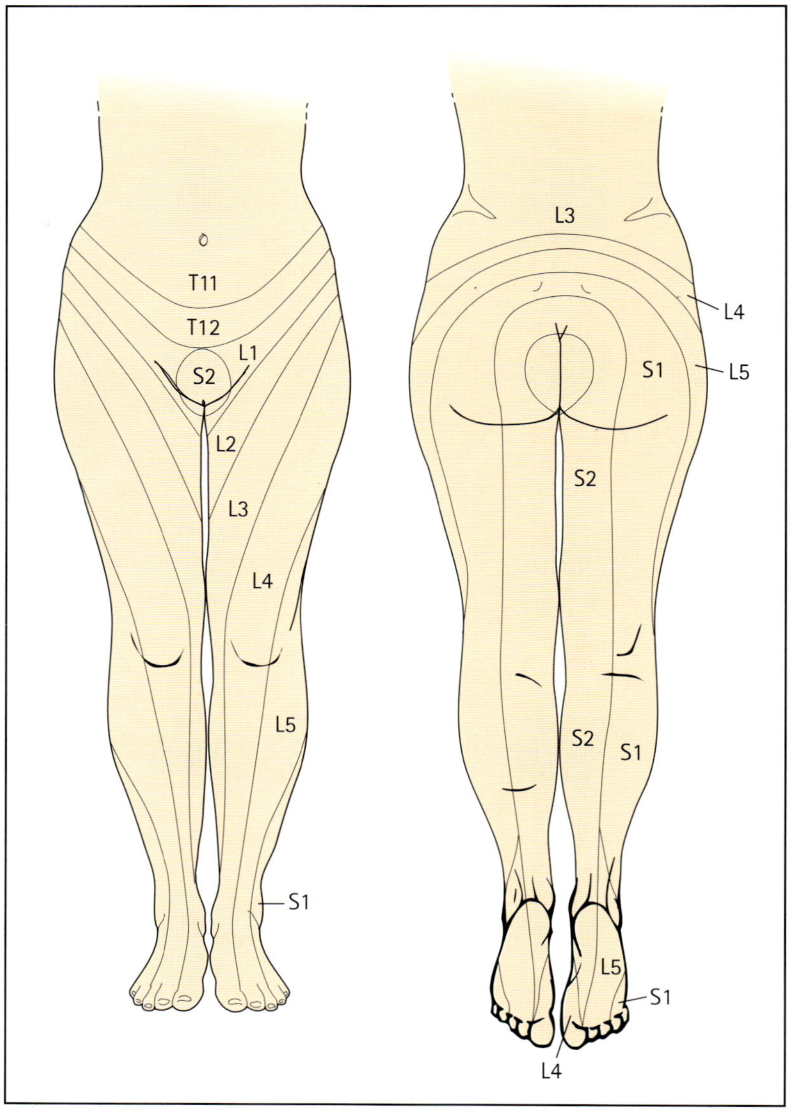

FIGURE 3-11.

Extremity assessment. The proximal and distal extremities and perineum should be tested for light touch and pinprick. The presence or absence and symmetrical nature of responses are noted. (*From* Lind LL, Rosenzweig BA, Bhatia NN: Urologically oriented neurological examination. In: *Urogynecology and Urodynamics*. Edited by Ostergard DR, Bent AE. Baltimore: Williams & Wilkins; 1996:102.)

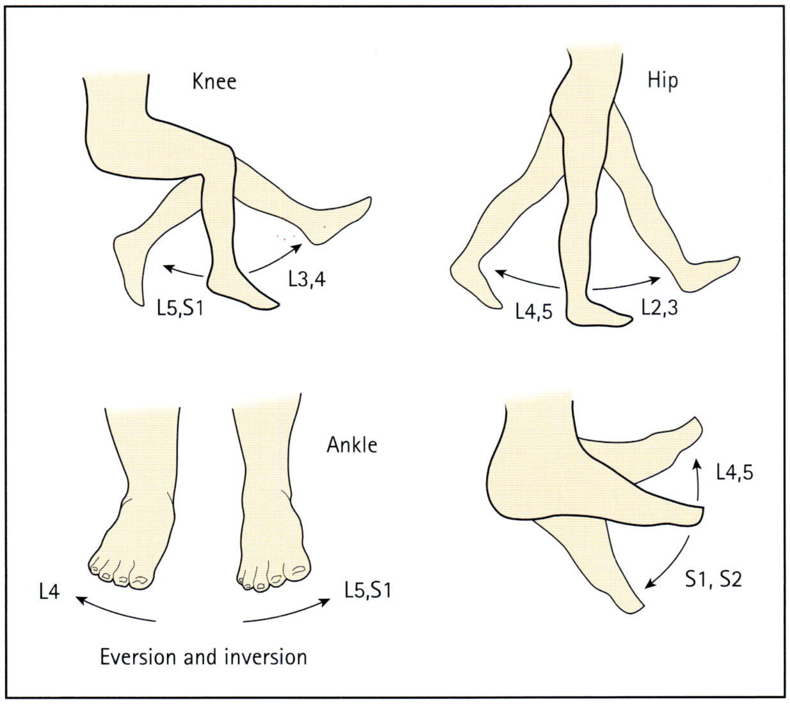

FIGURE 3-12.

For motor function, the lower extremities should be inspected for asymmetry, atrophy, and fasciculation. Asking the patient to move against resistance should test strength of the upper and lower limb and foot. Strength is graded on a scale of 0 to 5; 0, indicates no movement; 1, trace contraction; 2, movement with gravity eliminated; 3, movement against gravity; 4, movement against resistance but less than normal; 5, normal strength. The patella, ankle, and plantar reflexes are tested. Symmetry is noted. It is important for the patient to have the limb relaxed. Ankle reflexes diminish with increasing age. A normal plantar reflex involves plantar flexion of the toes. (*From* Lind LL, Rosenzweig BA, Bhatia NN: Urologically oriented neurological examination. In: *Urogynecology and Urodynamics.* Edited by Ostergard DR, Bent AE. Baltimore: Williams & Wilkins; 1996:101.)

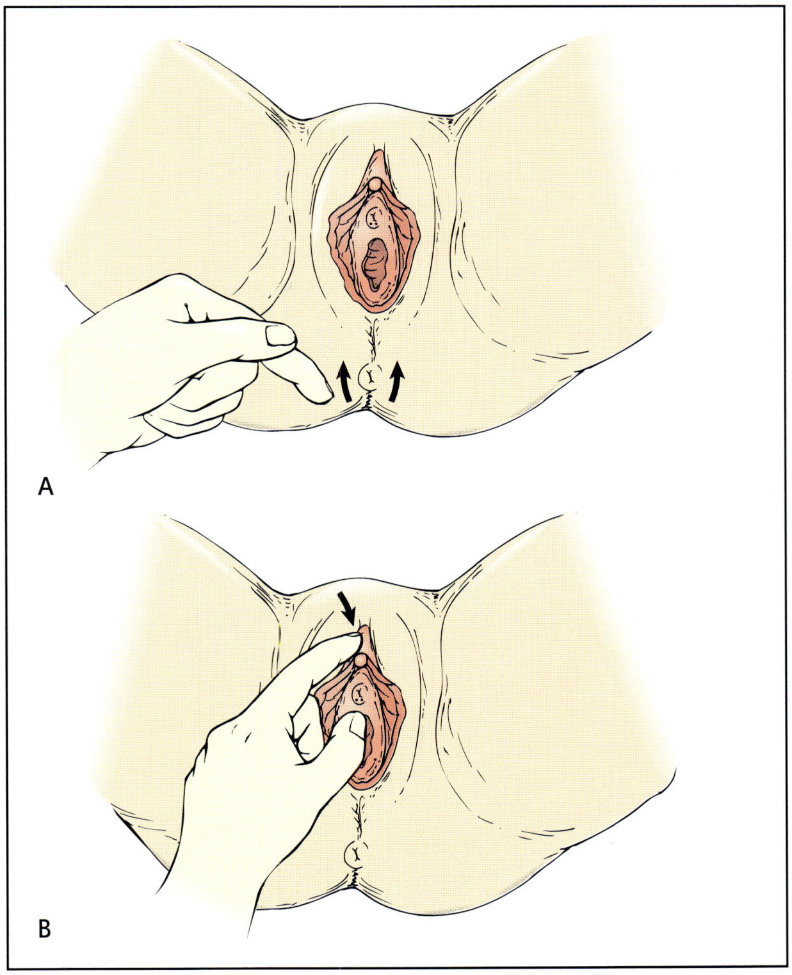

FIGURE 3-13.

Sacral reflexes. Parasympathetic innervation of the detrusor arises from S2-3 with minor contribution from S1-2 traveling as the pelvic nerve. Stimulation results in detrusor contraction. Sympathetic fibers travel in the hypogastric nerve and regulate storage. The periurethral striated muscles are innervated by S1-4 via the pudendal nerve. Rectal examination enables assessment of the tone and voluntary contraction. In the absence of a sphincter tear, preservation of tone but absent volume contraction indicates a suprasacral lesion; decreased tone implies a sacral nerve abnormality. Stroking the skin lateral to the anus results in a contraction (**A**). Similarly, tapping the clitoris and seeing the anal sphincter and perineal muscles contract tests the bulbocavernosus reflex. Pulling on a Foley catheter will result in a similar reflex. Note that these reflexes are absent in up to 30% of neurologically normal women [4]. (*From* Lind LL, Rosenzweig BA, Bhatia NN: Urologically oriented neurological examination. In: *Urogynecology and Urodynamics.* Edited by Ostergard DR, Bent AE. Baltimore: Williams & Wilkins; 1996:103.)

PELVIC EXAMINATION

Signs of hypoestrogenism (urethral caruncle, petechial hemorrhages, thin mucosa, loss of rugal folds)

Pelvic organ prolapse (patient to strain with labia parted both sitting and standing)

Cough stress test—a positive supine stress test with an empty bladder suggests intrinsic sphincter deficiency [5]

Speculum examination

- Obvious pooling in the vagina is indicative of a fistula or ectopic ureter.
- Ask patient to strain for evidence of uterine or vault prolapse.
- Anterior wall—posterior blade of speculum is placed posteriorly and patient asked to strain.
  - If cystocele present, determine if central or lateral by using a lateral wall elevator.
  - If placement reduces cystocele then location of fascial tear is lateral.
  - If cystocele still present then defect is central.
- Posterior wall—posterior blade is placed anteriorly and patient asked to strain.

Bimanual examination

- General examination of uterus and adnexa.
- Specific palpations for tenderness of bladder base as in urethral syndrome.
- Palpation of the anterior vaginal wall and urethra to elicit discharge or mass suggestive of local pathology.

Pelvic floor squeeze

- The index finger placed at the 4 then 8 o'clock position and the patient is asked to squeeze "like you are holding in gas or urine." The response can be graded from 1 to 4: 0, no contraction; 1, slight contraction; 2, stronger contraction; 3, contraction with some elevation; 4, contraction and elevation with resultant closure of the vagina.

Rectal examination

- Assess resting tone and integrity of the sphincter especially anteriorly.
- Ask the patient to contract "as if holding in gas" and assess the pelvic floor muscles and neurologic integrity.
- Rule out masses and impaction.
- A bidigital rectal/vaginal examination with the patient straining may detect an enterocele.

FIGURE 3-14.
Pelvic examination. Physical examination must include all the elements listed. It should focus on excluding neurologic disorders, attempting to reproduce incontinence, excluding pelvic pathology, and assessing pelvic support and rectal sphincter function.

POSTVOID RESIDUAL

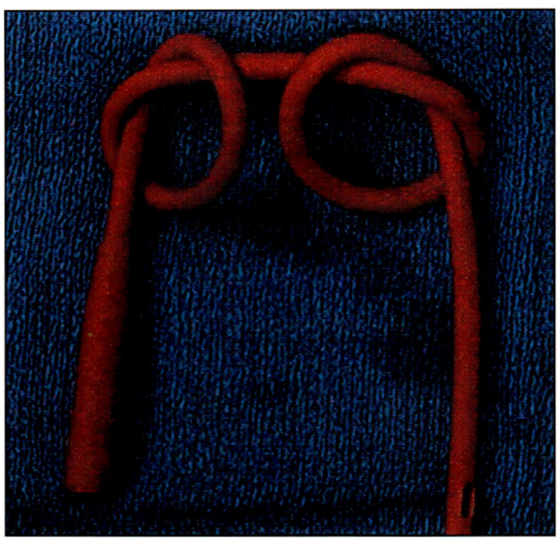

FIGURE 3-15.
Assessment of postvoid residual. Simple catheterization with a 12 or 14F red rubber catheter can be performed shortly after voiding to assess the postvoid residual. Most clinicians consider 50 to100 mL as indicative of normal emptying. An elevated postvoid residual is more difficult to interpret. It should be repeated on several occasions because environment, amount in the bladder prior to voiding, and time lapse to catheterization all affect volume. The incidence of a positive urine culture after a single in-out catheterization ranges from 1% to 20% [6].

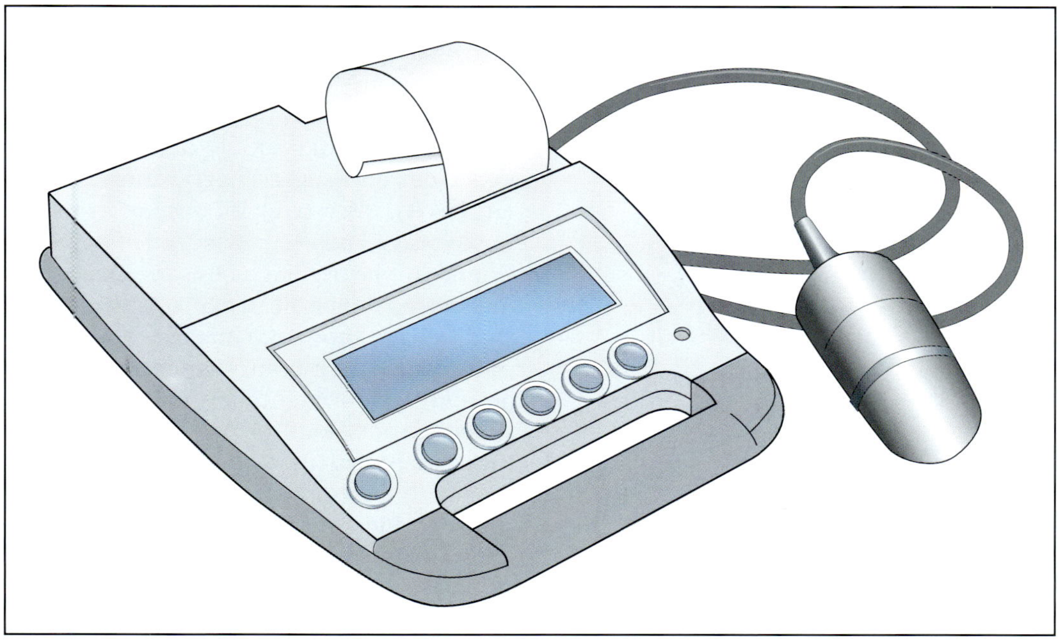

FIGURE 3-16.

Newer sector ultrasound machines provide cross-sectional images of the bladder and automatically calculate bladder volume. With the patient supine, a small amount of gel is placed above the symphysis and the bladder scanner placed firmly and directed toward the bladder. The scanner rotates 360 degrees for 3 seconds and the volume is calculated. Correlation is excellent between catheterized and scanned volumes [7]. This noninvasive instrument avoids the risk of catheterization.

URINE TESTING

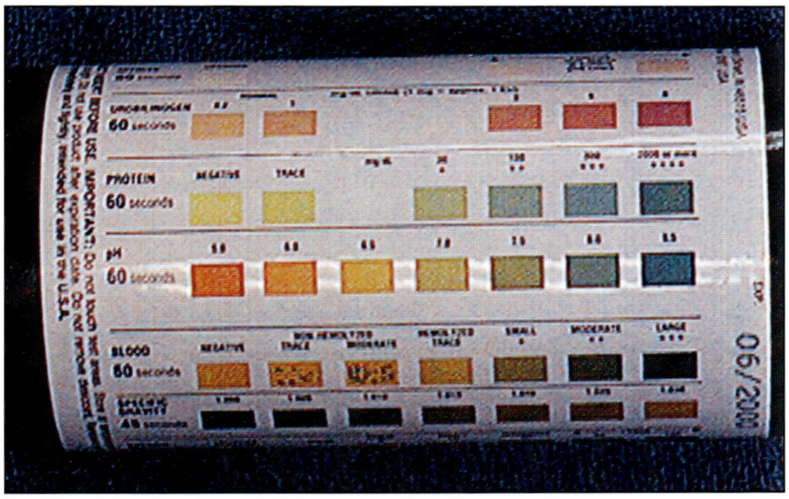

FIGURE 3-17.

Testing methods. Urine "dip" testing is useful for rapid diagnosis but is generally less accurate than microscopy in the detection of infection. The esterase test relies on a color change caused by leukocyte esterase. The nitrate test detects the conversion of nitrate to nitrite by bacteria. Certain bacteria do not convert nitrates. They also depend on bacterial concentrations and are less accurate with decreasing numbers of colonies per milliliter. These tests should be reserved for situations in which an experienced staff member is unavailable to do microscopy. False-positive tests for blood can result from dyes. About 3% of normal individuals will excrete more than three erythrocytes per high-power field [8].

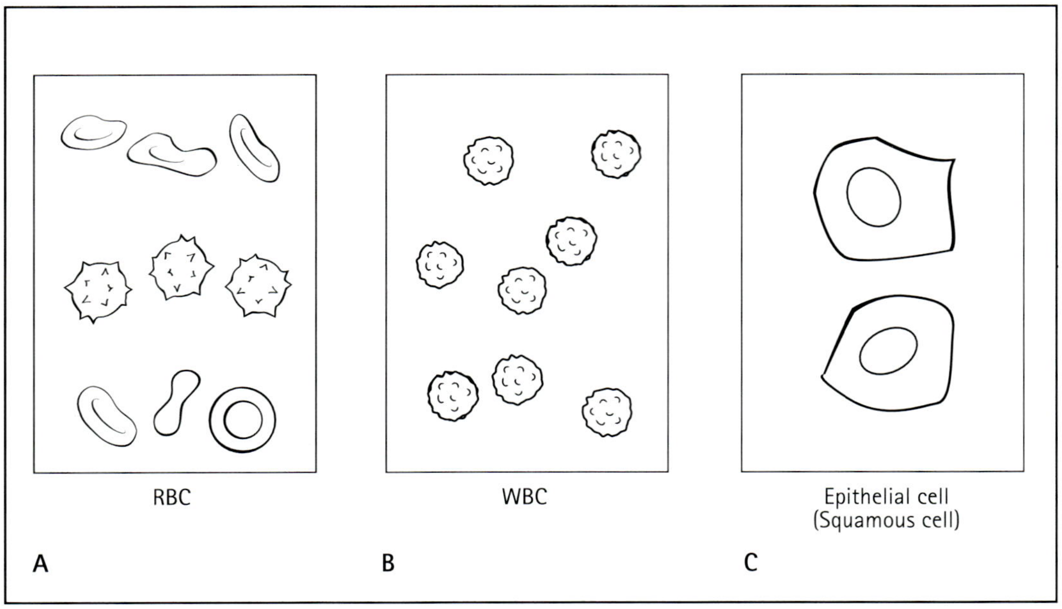

FIGURE 3-18.
Microscopic investigation. Urine microscopy is useful in the detection of hematuria, pyuria, and bacteriuria. These conditions do not typically cause incontinence but may suggest aggravating factors (**A** and **B**). Microscopy of unspun urine is inexpensive and easy. Evidence of pyuria should not be used as a basis for treatment in elderly asymptotic patients. Several studies have shown no increased morbidity or mortality from nontreatment in this group [9]. No evidence in the literature supports routine urine cytology in the incontinent patient. Cytology should be limited to high-risk groups (history of cervical cancer treated with radiation, exposure to aromatic amines, long-term catheter usage, and previous cyclophosphamide treatment). **C**, It is a poor screening tool and well-differentiated tumors often shed minimally. Cells may appear normal while the false-negative rate may be as high as 20% even with high-grade lesions [8].

MOBILITY OF URETHROVESICAL JUNCTION

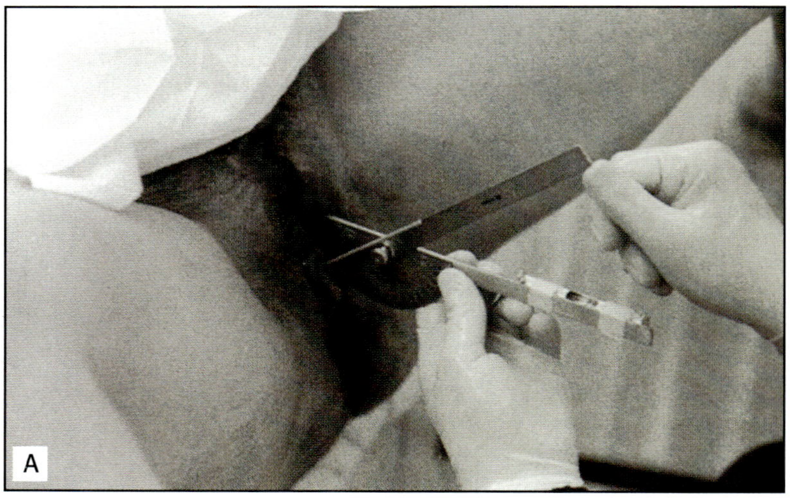

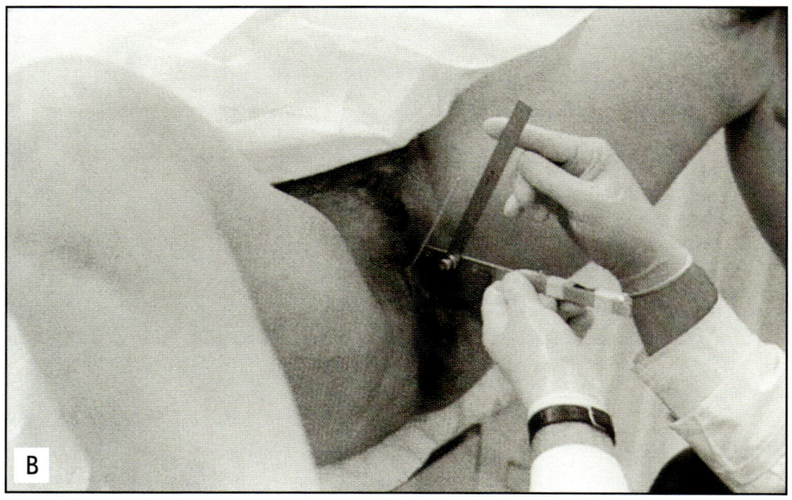

FIGURE 3-19.
Cotton swab test. The cotton swab test is the simplest means of assessing mobility. With the patient supine, the external urethral meatus is cleansed with povidine-iodine. The sterile swab is lubricated with 1% lidocaine jelly, introduced through the urethra into the bladder, then slowly withdrawn until resistance is met. **A**, The swab is now at the urethrovesical junction (UVJ). The patient is asked to strain and the degree of deflection from the horizontal is recorded using a goniometer. **B**, An angle greater than 30 degrees indicates mobility. Mobility of the UVJ appears to be an etiologic factor in the development of stress incontinence [10]. It is also a prognostic factor for success for various surgical procedures [11]. (*From* Agosta AM: Clinical evaluation. In: *Female Pelvic Floor Disorders. Investigation and Management.* Edited by Benson JT. New York: Norton; 1992:64; with permission.)

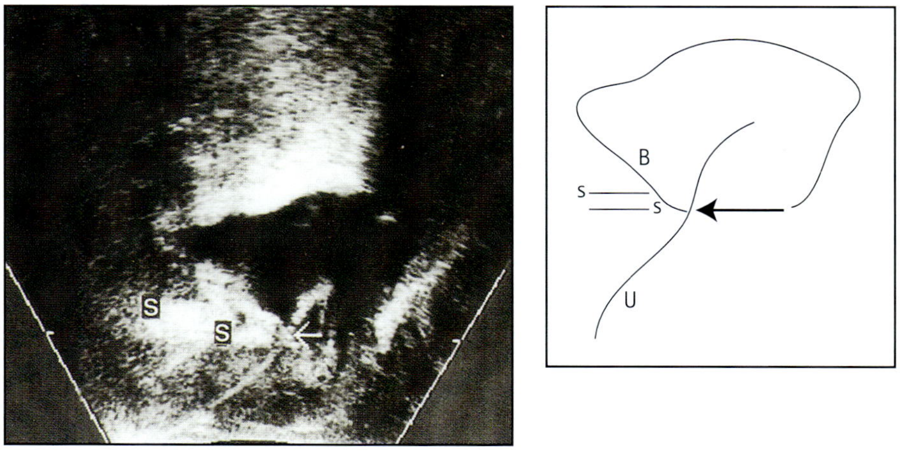

FIGURE 3-20.

Ultrasound examination. Perineal (introital) ultrasound allows good visualization of the bladder base and urethrovesical junction (*arrow*). Vaginal probe ultrasound can cause the bladder neck to rise and impair descent during the Valsalva maneuver. A 3.5- to 5-mHz transducer is placed between the labia inferior to the urethral meatus. A Foley catheter or microtip transducer can be placed in the urethra (*U*) to aid visualization. This does, however, negate one of the arguments for the test being noninvasive. With the patient in the supine and erect position, she is asked to do the Valsalva maneuver. The distance between the urethrovesical junction at rest and strain reflect mobility. Mobility is defined as movement greater than 10 mm [12]. There appears to be good correlation between ultrasound and radiologic imaging [13]. However, a recent study suggests the cotton swab test underestimates mobility compared with visualization with ultrasound [12]. The role of ultrasound is still to be delineated. B—bladder; S—symphysis. (*From* Caputo and Benson [12]; with permission.)

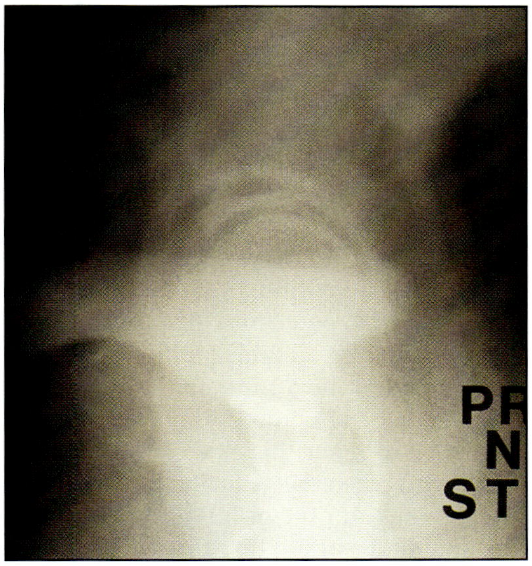

FIGURE 3-21.

Chain cystourethrography. This procedure has largely been superceded because of its invasive nature, exposure to radiation, and often-difficult interpretation of landmarks. A chain is placed in the urethra and lateral x-rays are taken with the patient at rest and straining. The test can be done without a chain.

ADDITIONAL SIMPLE OFFICE TESTS

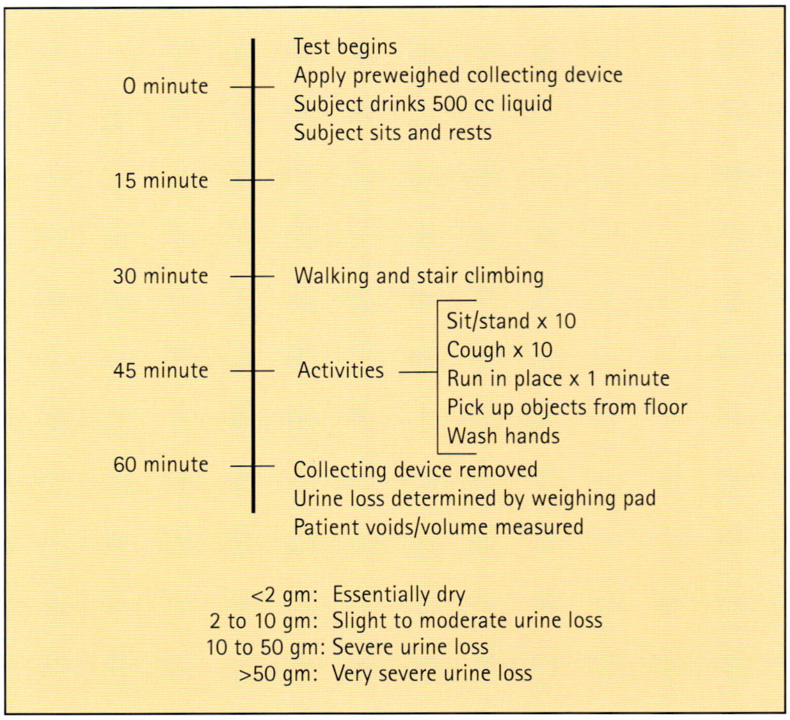

FIGURE 3-22.

Pad test. The pad test is useful to grade the severity of incontinence and demonstrate leakage when other tests have failed to demonstrate incontinence. The 1-hour pad test has been standardized by the International Continence Society. It is diagrammatically represented in this figure. The 12-hour test is performed at home and may provide additional benefits by demonstrating precipitating events, relationship to activity, impact , or other clues as to the cause or possible interventions. A pad weight increase of greater than 1g/h is abnormal. (*From* Pierson CA: Pad testing, nursing interventions and urine loss appliances. In: *Urogynecology and Urodynamics,* edn 4. Edited by Ostergard DR, Bent AE. Baltimore: Williams & Wilkins; 1996:252.)

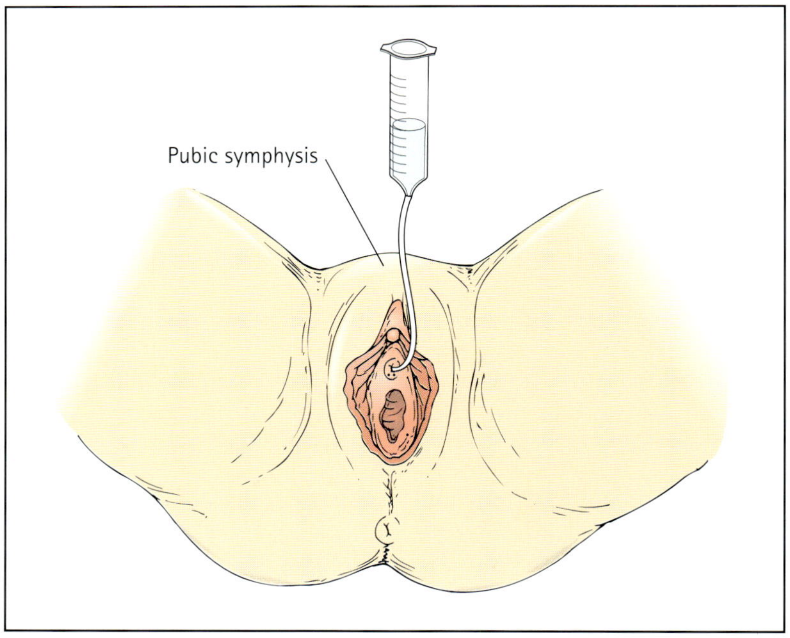

FIGURE 3-23.

Cystometry. Informal simple office cystometry can be performed at the time of the initial consultation to provide additional information. With the patient in the supine position a bulb syringe can be attached to the catheter used to determine the postvoid residual. Room temperature sterile water is added at 50-mL increments. The syringe is elevated so the 50-mL mark is about 15 cm above the symphysis. The meniscus represents the intravesical pressure. The patient is asked to report her first sensation, fullness, and maximum capacity as the syringe is filled. A sudden rise in the meniscus associated with an urge or leakage indicates a detrusor contraction. The abdomen should be palpated to ensure that abdominal strain is absent. Several studies have found reasonable sensitivity (75–88%) and specificity (75%) for the diagnosis of detrusor instability compared to multichannel urodynamics [14]. Beware that small contractions may be missed and that the supine position is less provocative for detrusor instability. On completion of filling, the catheter is removed and the patient asked to cough while supine. Instantaneous leakage represents a positive stress test. Leakage that continues after the cough may indicate the need for more detailed testing. If incontinence is not demonstrated, the patient should be provoked in the standing position. This simple procedure may provide sufficient information to assist in conservative management decisions. Patients requiring operative intervention require more detailed testing. (*From* Bent AE, McLennan MT: Geriatric urogynecology. In: *Urogynecology and Urodynamics.* edn 4. Edited by Ostergard DR, Bent AE. Baltimore: Williams & Wilkins; 1996:446.)

MULTICHANNEL URODYNAMIC TESTING

CRITERIA FOR URODYNAMIC TESTING
Patient complains of incontinence but none is demonstrated
Objective findings do not correlate with symptoms
Frior screening normal or inconclusive
Not responding to conservative therapy
Operative intervention especially if previous failed surgery
Mixed incontinence where clinically difficult to determine which is major contributor to symptoms
Patient with previous radical pelvic surgery
Patient with known or suspected neurologic disorders (multiple sclerosis, herniated disk, spinal cord injury, myelodysplasia)
Pelvic organ prolapse to hymen or beyond
Elevated postvoid residual

FIGURE 3-24.

Urodynamic testing. This type of testing is not necessarily part of the initial evaluation of incontinence. Many patients can be successfully treated conservatively without initial testing. The criteria are guidelines for patients in need of a more specific diagnosis. Urodynamic testing is made up of several parts.

UROFLOWMETRY

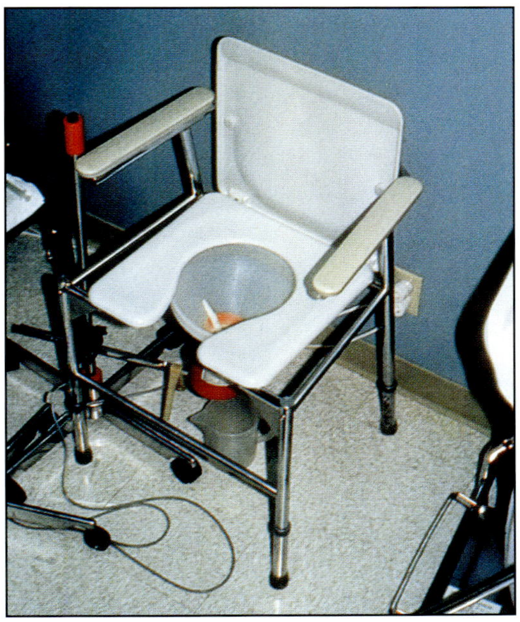

FIGURE 3-25.

Uroflowmetry. The patient is asked to present with a comfortably full bladder. She is asked to void as normally as possible in a chair as seen here. The following measurements are obtained: maximum flow rate (mL/s); average flow rate (mL/s); flow time in seconds; and voided volume (mL). Flow time and maximum and average flow rate increase with increasing voided volume up to 200 mL. There is no consensus of normal voiding parameters; however, most clinicians believe a normal voiding study consists of a voided volume of at least 200 mL, voided over 15 to 20 seconds with a maximum flow rate of 20 mL/s or greater with a smooth continuous curve. Uroflowmetry is used to identify patients with voiding dysfunction and is not useful in the diagnosis of incontinence. (*From* Karram MM: Evaluation of incontinence. In: *Clinical Urogynecology.* Edited by Walters MD, Karram MM. St. Louis: Mosby; 1993:78; with permission.)

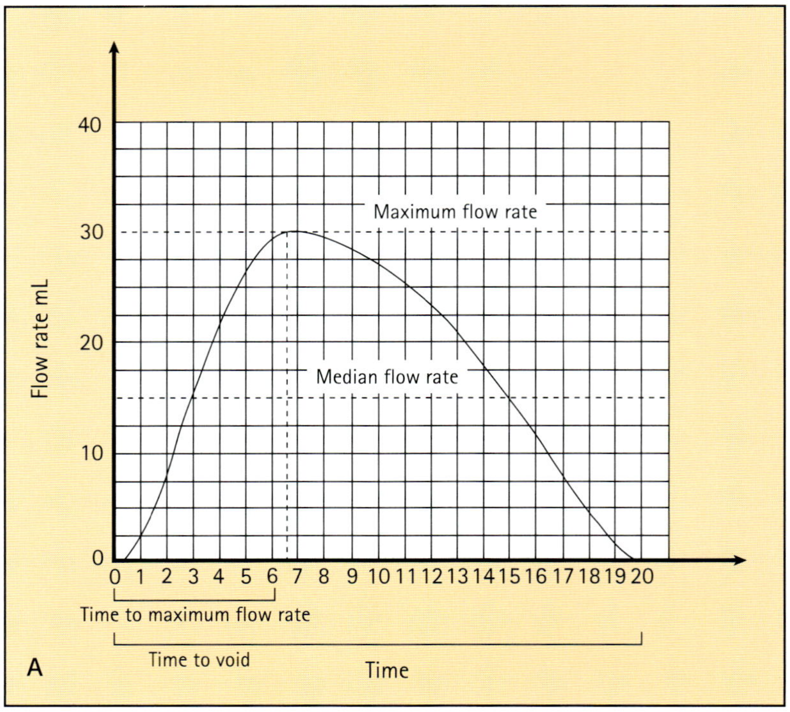

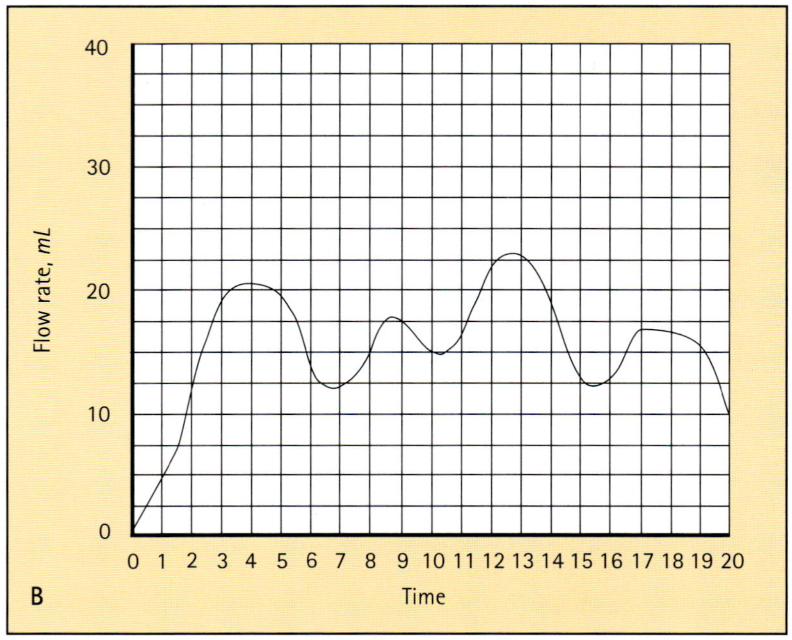

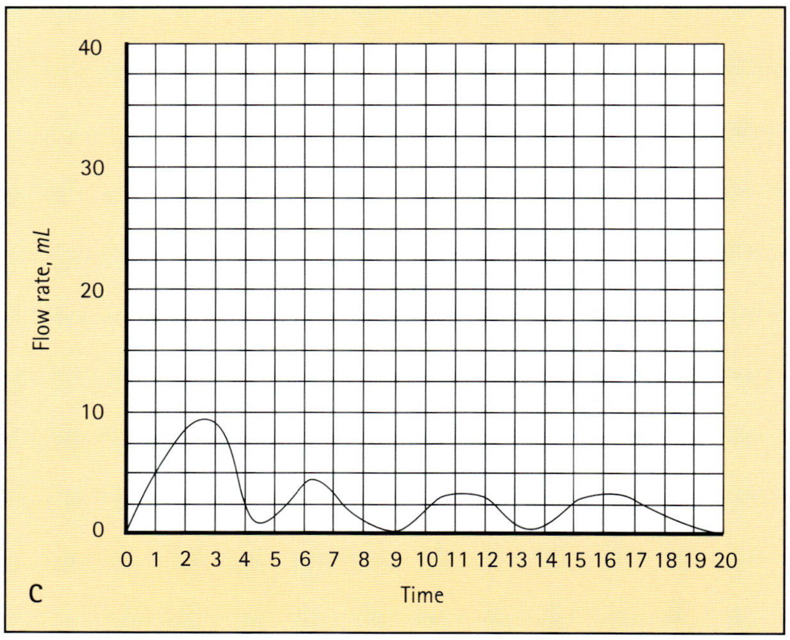

FIGURE 3-26.

Uroflow curve. **A**, normal uroflow curve shows continuous flow with minimal fluctuations with the maximal flow reached within one third of the total voiding time. **B**, Rather than absolute values, the shape of the curve may be a better indicator of voiding dysfunction. Intermittent and interrupted flow patterns characteristically show increasing and decreasing flow rates as manifested by multiple peaks and valleys on the tracing. With the "intermittent" pattern, the downward deflection does not drop below 2 mL/sec. If the deflection falls below this level, it is referred to as "interrupted" (**C**). (*From* Karram MM: Evaluation of incontinence. In: *Clinical Urogynecology.* Edited by Walters MD, Karram MM. St. Louis: Mosby: 1993:78.)

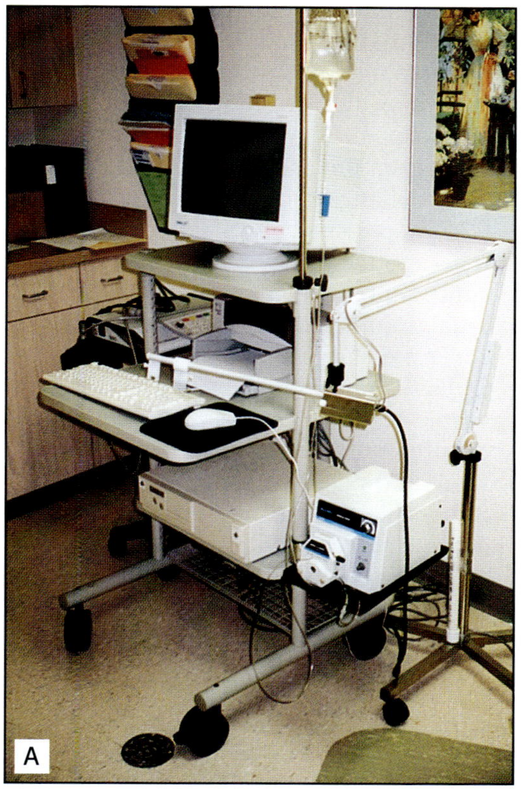

FIGURE 3-27.

Urodynamic unit (**A**). Even a good history may be inadequate for the diagnosis of a particular type of incontinence. A meta-analysis study on the role of patient history in the diagnosis of urinary incontinence found that relying on history alone for the diagnosis of stress incontinence resulted in misdiagnosis in 25% of patients. The incidence of stress-induced detrusor contractions was between 9% and 52% [15]. Symptoms of urge incontinence were even worse predictors with a diagnosis rate of 45%. Other authors have found surgical failure due to persistence of detrusor instability [16]. Identifying these patients allows the physician to counsel the patent regarding her chance of cure and persistence of symptoms postoperatively. Several investigators have compared single (**B**) to multichannel urodymanic studies (**C**). Although the specificity of a single-channel study has been consistently high (82–100%), the sensitivity has been inconsistent [17]. The single-channel study is more difficult to interpret because increases in intra-abdominal pressure may be interpreted as detrusor contractions. Any movement will be shown as an increase in intra-abdominal pressure. It relies more on the operator's technical and interpretive skills.

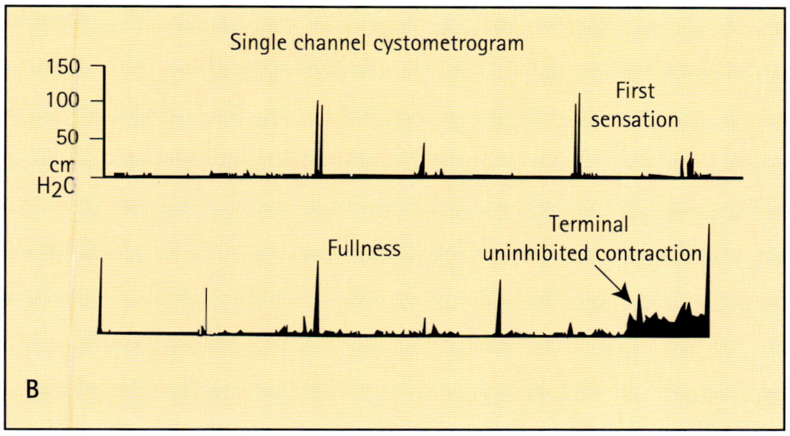

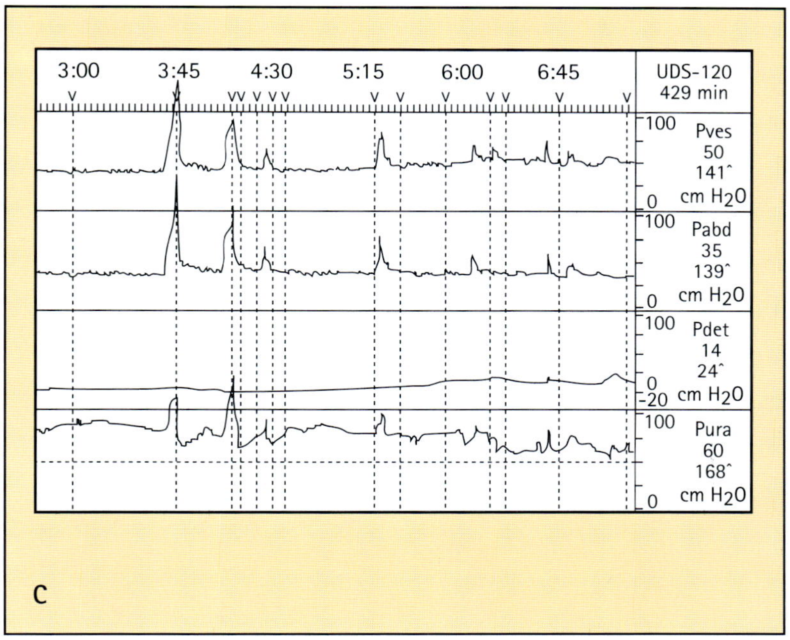

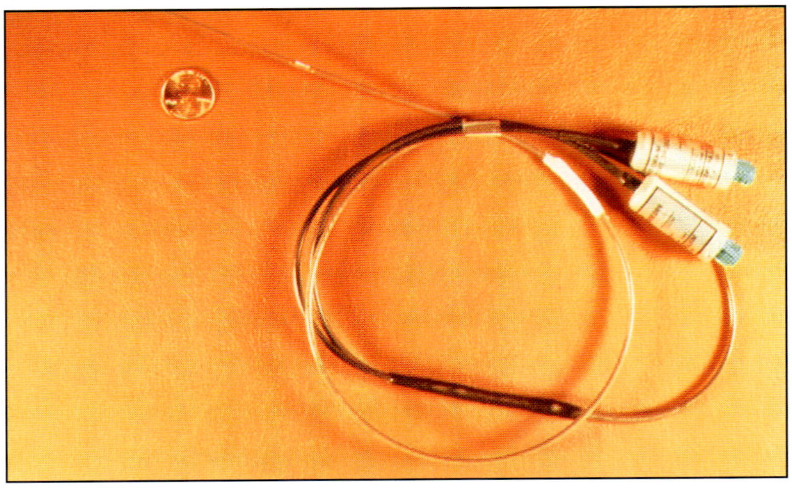

FIGURE 3-28.

Microtransducer. After uroflowmetry, the patient is catheterized and 50 mL sterile water infused. A dual-tip 8F microtransducer (Millar Instruments, Houston, TX) is placed with the distal transducer in the bladder and proximal transducer at point of maximum urethral pressure. The single transducer is placed in the vagina or rectum if a grade 3 or 4 prolapse is present. The patient is placed in the upright position and a 2-minute resting tracing is performed to detect patients with urethral instability. Medium-fill (80 mL/s) cystometry is performed. The patient is asked to report her first sensation to void, fullness, and maximum capacity. Provocative maneuvers at maximum capacity, for example, handwashing, running water, and heel bounce, may be useful in precipitating detrusor instability. Valsalva leak point pressures are performed at 150 mL and 200 mL by asking the patient to slowly perform the Valsalva maneuver and the exact point at which leakage occurs is recorded. If there is no leakage, then the patient can be asked to cough incrementally. The lowest change in vesical pressure needed to cause leakage is the "leak point pressure." At maximum capacity, both transducers are placed back in the bladder and withdrawn on a pulley arm at a rate of 1 mm/s and the maximum urethral pressure is measured. The maximal urethral closure pressure is calculated by subtracting the bladder pressure from the maximum urethral pressure. Cough profiles are performed by asking the patient to cough at each quartile as the catheter is withdrawn in a similar manner as for the closure pressure. The distal transducer is placed at the point of maximal urethral pressure and the patient is asked to void as normally as possible and pressure-flow studies are obtained. Examples of all of these components are detailed in the following clinical cases. (*From* Karram MM: Urodynamics: cystometry. In: *Clinical Urogynecology.* Edited by Walters MD, Karram MM. St. Louis: Mosby; 1993:67.

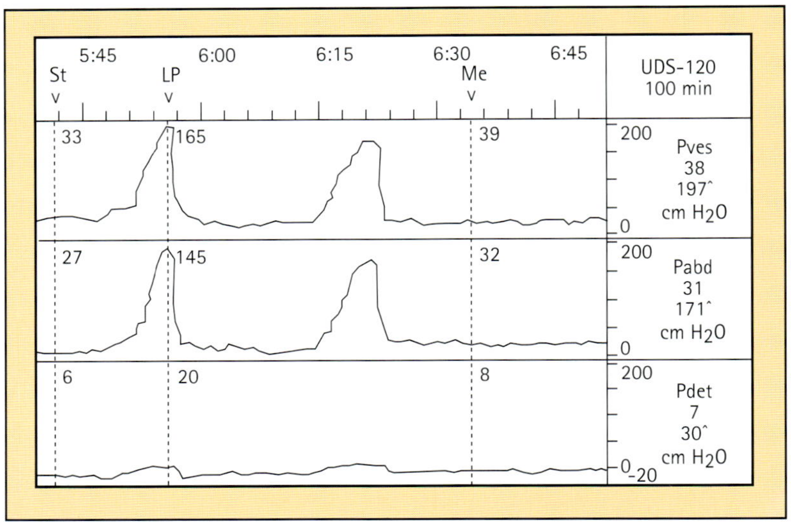

FIGURE 3-29.

Clinical cystometry. This 44-year-old nulliparous woman had a 2-year history of leakage with lifting, coughing, and sneezing that had begun after a hysterectomy. Her postvoid residual was 5 mL and her cotton-tip strain angle was 50 degrees. Cystometry showed a positive leak point pressure (LPP) of 132 cm at 150 mL. Her maximum urethral closing pressure was normal at 42 cm. A diagnosis of genuine stress incontinence with hypermobility was made and she was successfully treated with a laparoscopic Burch retropubic urethropexy procedure.

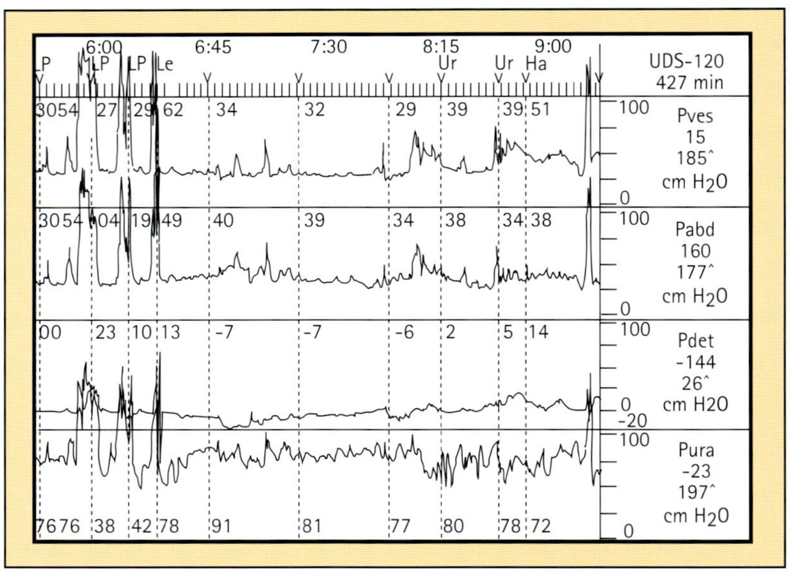

FIGURE 3-30.

Clinical cytometery . This 40-year-old P3013 had a history of mixed incontinence that she desired to have fixed. Clinically, it was difficult to determine which component was most bothersome. Her postvoid residual was 3 mL and her cotton-tip strain angle was 60 degrees. Cystometry showed a positive leak point pressure of 93 cm at 150 mL. She also had multiple detrusor contractions at her maximum capacity. A diagnosis of genuine stress incontinence and detrusor instability was made. Because her urge component appeared to be more severe, initially she was successfully treated medically. She subsequently elected to have surgical correction of her stress component with an open Burch retropubic urethropexy. This cured her stress incontinence and at 3 months postoperatively her urge incontinence has also resolved.

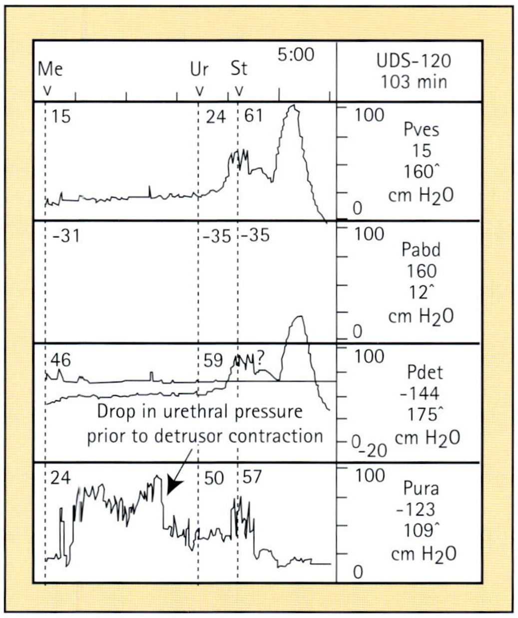

FIGURE 3-31.

Clinical cystometry. This 52-year-old nulliparous patient presented with urgency and frequency. A 6-week course of anticholinergic medication improved her frequency but failed to significantly relieve the urgency. A cystometrogram (CMG) showed an acute drop in her urethral pressure that just preceded an increase in detrusor pressure. These urethral pressure changes would have been missed on a single-channel study. The addition of an α–agonist has markedly improved her symptoms.

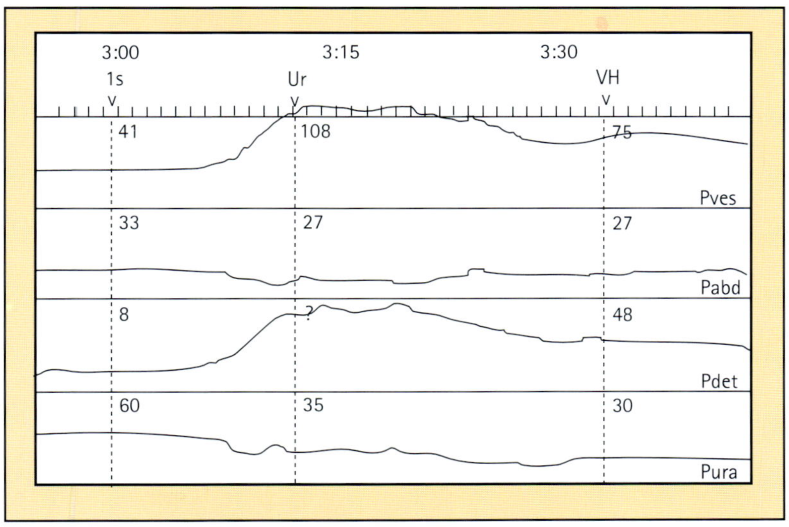

FIGURE 3-32.

Misdiagnosis. This tracing represents a case of a clinical misdiagnosis. This 40-year-old P4014 was scheduled for a retropubic suspension based on a history of stress incontinence. Urodynamic testing demonstrated multiple contractions from 150 mL onward. Further questioning revealed that she suffered from severe urgency. Treatment with an anticholinergic medication resulted in resolution of her symptoms and her surgery was cancelled. CMG—cystometrogram.

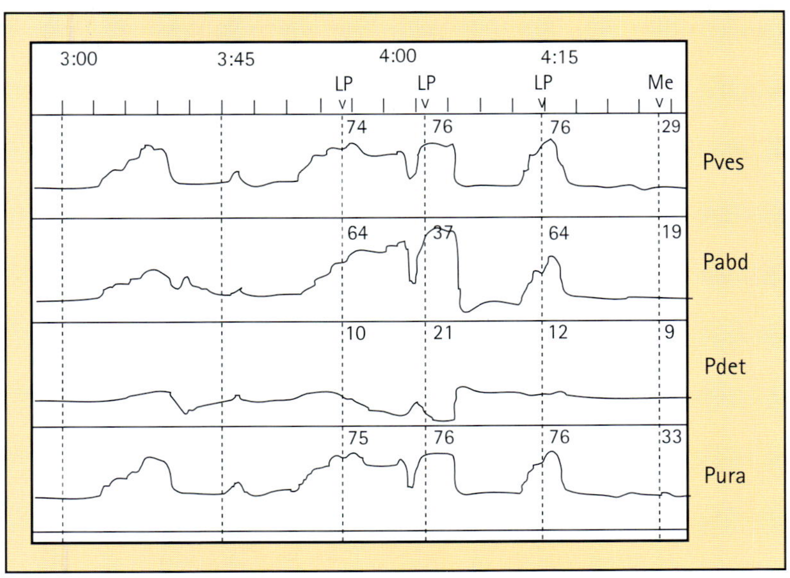

FIGURE 3-33.

Sphincter deficiency. This 72-year-old P2002 was diagnosed as having intrinsic sphincter deficiency based on both a low leak point pressure (LPP) and low maximum urethral closing pressure (MUCP). Clinically she had leakage with cough, sneezing, and lifting even when her bladder was empty. Her postvoid residual was normal and her cotton-tip demonstrated hypermobility at a strain angle of 80 degrees. From the tracing you can see that her LPP at 150 mL was 45 cm. Her MUCP was 20 cm. She was successfully treated with a fascia lata sling.

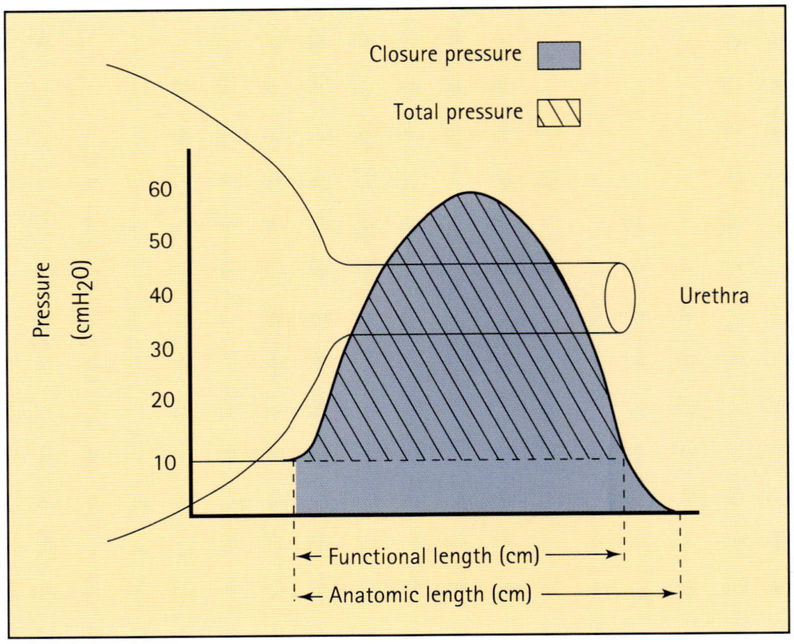

FIGURE 3-34.

Urethral pressure. This is a graphic representation of the urethral pressure along its length. Orientation of the transducer is critical. The urethral pressure is not uniform around its circumference. It is highest anteriorly and lowest posteriorly. It is recommended that the transducer be in the lateral position for this study. A static profile is performed at maximum capacity by placing both transducers in the bladder. The catheter is attached to a pulley arm, which is withdrawn at a constant speed of 1 mm/s, and the pressure recorded. The following measurements are usually obtained: vesical pressure, urethral pressure, functional urethral length, and anatomic length. The maximum urethral closing pressure (MUCP) is calculated by subtracting the vesical pressure form the maximal urethral pressure. A MUCP greater than 20 cm is considered normal in the current literature. The average functional length is 2 to 5 cm. (*From* Karram MM: Manometric investigation—urodynamics. In: *Female Pelvic Floor Disorders—Investigation and Management.* Edited by Benson JT. New York: Norton; 1992:110.)

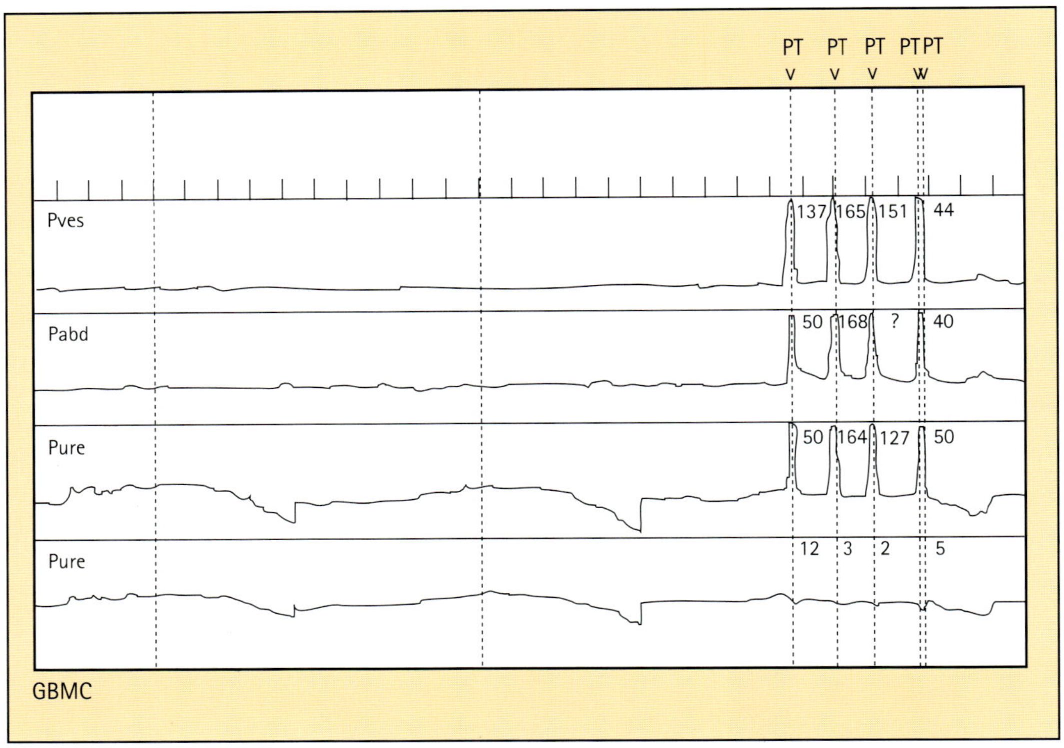

FIGURE 3-35.

Low-pressure urethra. There is no consensus as to the definition of intrinsic sphincter deficiency (ISD). Many clinicians still equate it to a maximum urethral closing pressure (MUCP) of less than 20 cm because patients with a low closure pressure were found in a retrospective study to have a higher failure rate for a standard incontinence procedure [18]. This 70-year-old P2002 has a low MUCP of 14 cm. She has a history of having failed a previous anterior repair and vaginal wall sling. Cotton-tip testing demonstrated persistent hypermobility at a strain angle of 45 degrees. She was successfully treated with a fascia lata sling until 13 months at which time she developed a large enterocele and a recurrence of her stress incontinence (but less than previously) and urge incontinence. UCPP—urethral closure pressure profile.

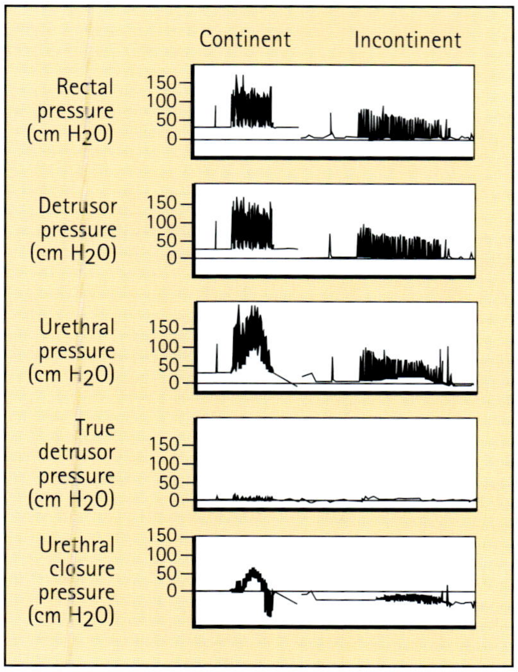

FIGURE 3-36.

Genuine stress incontinence (GSI). The diagnosis of GSI can be further improved by the use of cough profiles. Here the patient is asked to cough at the various quartiles as the transducer is withdrawn. The test provides an objective assessment of the transmission of abdominal pressure along the urethra during stress. For continence, the urethral pressure must remain higher than the bladder pressure. The profile is positive if there is equalization of pressure along the urethra with each cough. The pressure transmission ratio (PTR) is calculated by dividing the amplitude of the urethral pressure increase by the amplitude of the bladder pressure increase and multiplying by 100. Several authors have found that the PTR ratio discriminates well between those patients with GSI and those without using a cut-off of 90% to 95% [19]. Pressure equalization has a high specificity and positive predictive value but low sensitivity for the diagnosis of GSI [20]. However, patients with GSI do not always have equalization. The test is used as an adjunct for the diagnosis. (*From* Jensen JK: Urodynamic evaluation. In: *Urogynecology and Urodynamics,* edn 4. Edited by Ostergard DR, Bent AE. Baltimore: Williams & Wilkins; 1996:133.)

Pressure Flow Study

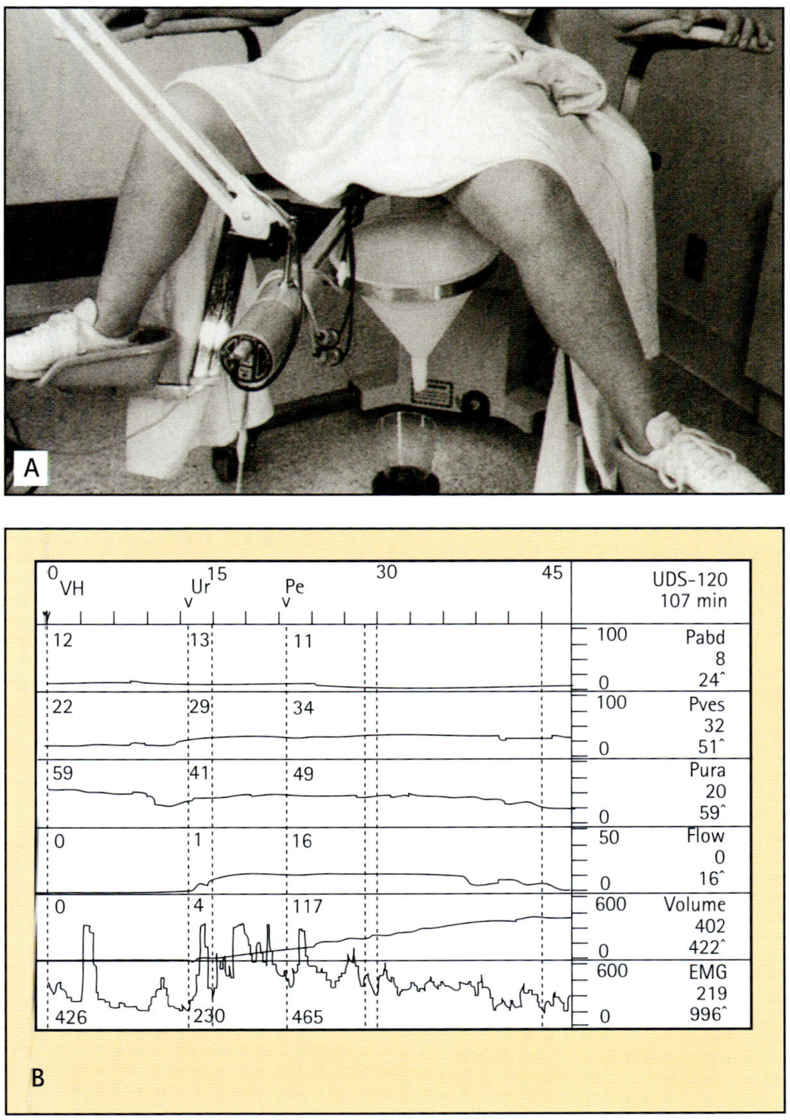

FIGURE 3-37.

Pressure voiding study. The multichannel pressure voiding study simultaneously measures vesical, urethral, and abdominal pressure and electromyographic (EMG) and flow parameters. It objectively demonstrates the patient's voiding mechanism. It is performed at maximum capacity after completion of the urethral pressure profiles. The patient is asked to void with the catheters in place. **A**, A significant percentage of patients (20–30%) are unable to void with the catheter in place. It is also very difficult to know whether voiding in a strange place, in a strange chair with a "tube" in the urethra represents normal voiding for the patient. During normal micturition, urethral relaxation is followed by a detrusor contraction. **B**, Other mechanisms are considered normal, but they should always include a component of urethral relaxation (i.e., urethral relaxation alone, urethral relaxation with detrusor contraction with or without Valsalva maneuver). Bergman defined normal voiding parameters: adequate detrusor contraction, an increase in detrusor pressure of at least 15 cm of water, Valsalva voiding, an increase in abdominal pressure of at least 10 cm, adequate urethral relaxation, and a decrease in urethral pressure of at least 25 cm [21]. The prime role of this test is in the patient with symptoms of voiding dysfunction. Detrusor sphincter dyssynergia occurs when urethral contraction occurs simultaneously with a detrusor contraction. The EMG will show increased activity corresponding to the increase in urethral pressure. Low flow rate associated with minimal or no increase in detrusor pressure is most likely secondary to a weakened detrusor muscle. Distinguishing between the two is important for treatment. (*From* Karram MM. Manometric investigation: urodynamics. In: *Female Pelvic Floor Disorders—Investigation and Management.* Edited by Benson JT. New York: Norton; 1992:107; with permission.)

CYSTOURETHROSCOPY

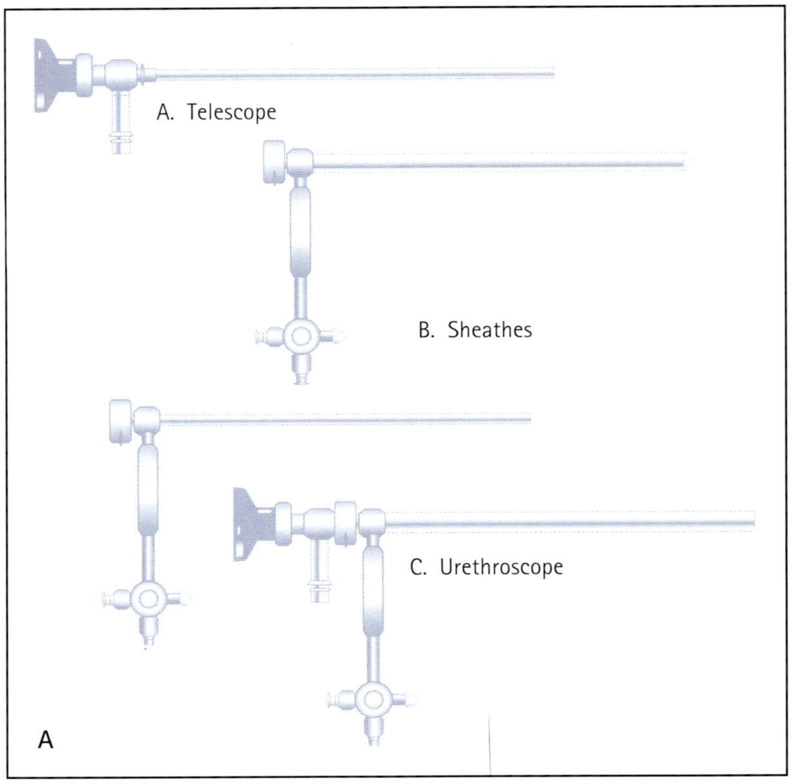

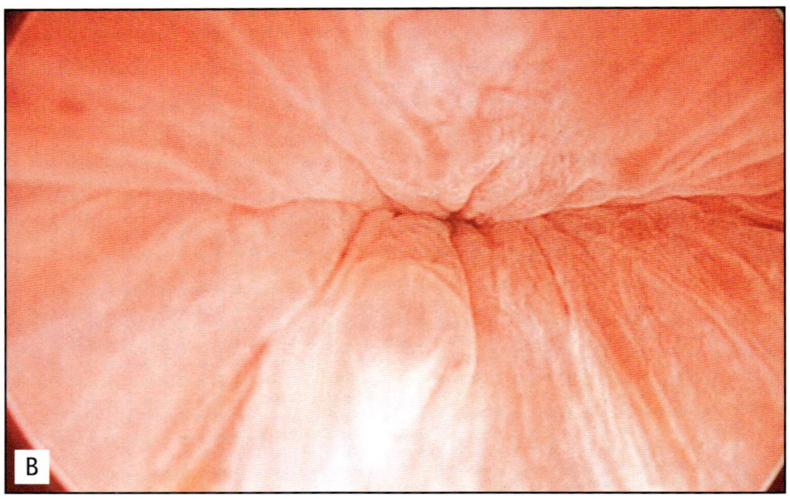

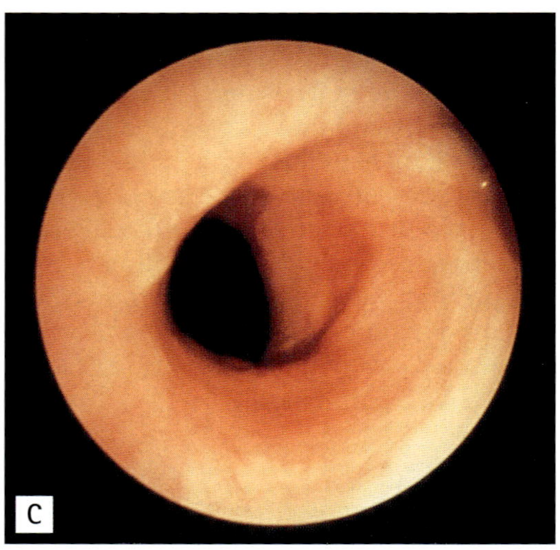

FIGURE 3-38.

Bladder and urethra assessment. Cystourethroscopy allows anatomic assessment of the bladder and urethra and diagnosis of benign and malignant lesions that would remain undiagnosed by history, examination, and urodynamics. Not all incontinent patients always require endoscopic assessment, but patients with prior failed surgery, history suggestive of intrinsic sphincter deficiency, and irritative voiding symptoms especially in a smoker over 50 and a recent onset of symptoms merit evaluation. Urethroscopy is initially performed with a short 0(scope. **A**, The urethral meatus is cleansed with betadine and the instrument introduced under water distention. The lumen is visualized to the urethrovesical junction (UVJ). **B**, The urethroscope is withdrawn to just distal of the UVJ. The dynamics of the UVJ can be seen by asking the patient to cough, strain, and "squeeze like you are holding in urine or gas." With severe dysfunction it may sit widely open. **C**, The instrument is then placed back into the bladder. With one finger occluding the lumen proximally, the tip of the scope is slowly withdrawn.

(*Continued on next page*)

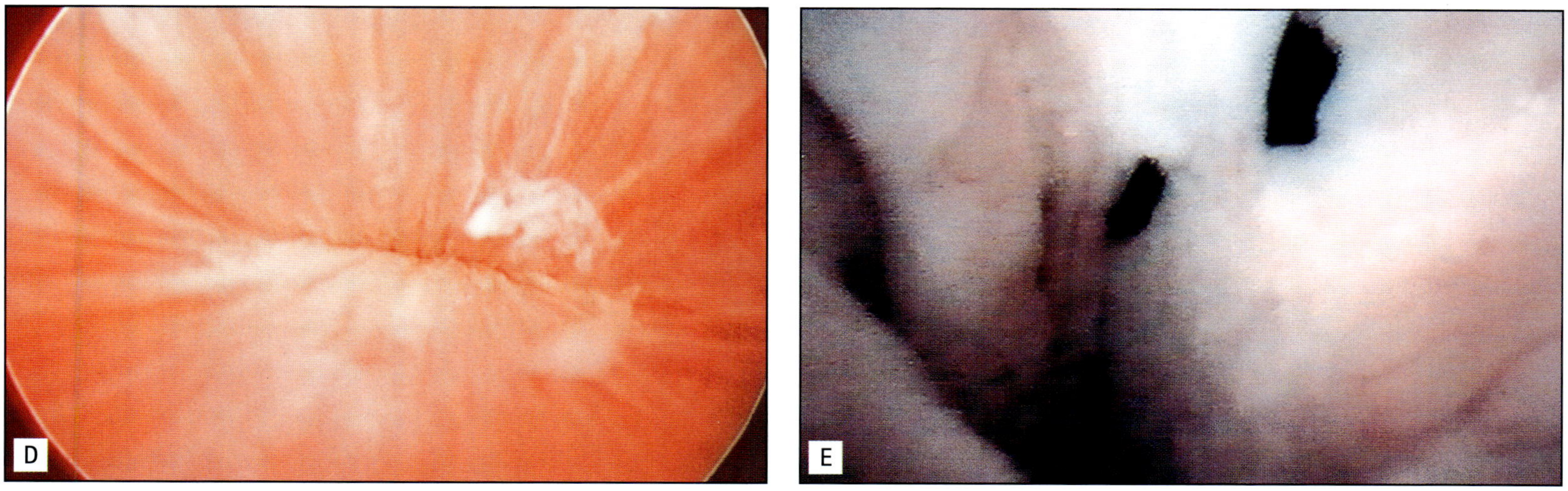

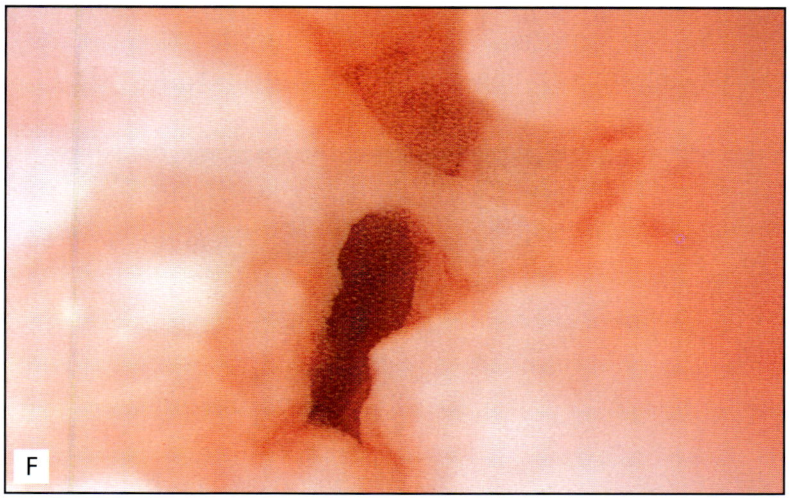

FIGURE 3-38. *(Continued)*
This allows maximum distension for visualization of the mucosa looking for discharge (**D**), diverticuli (**E**), and fistula (**F**).

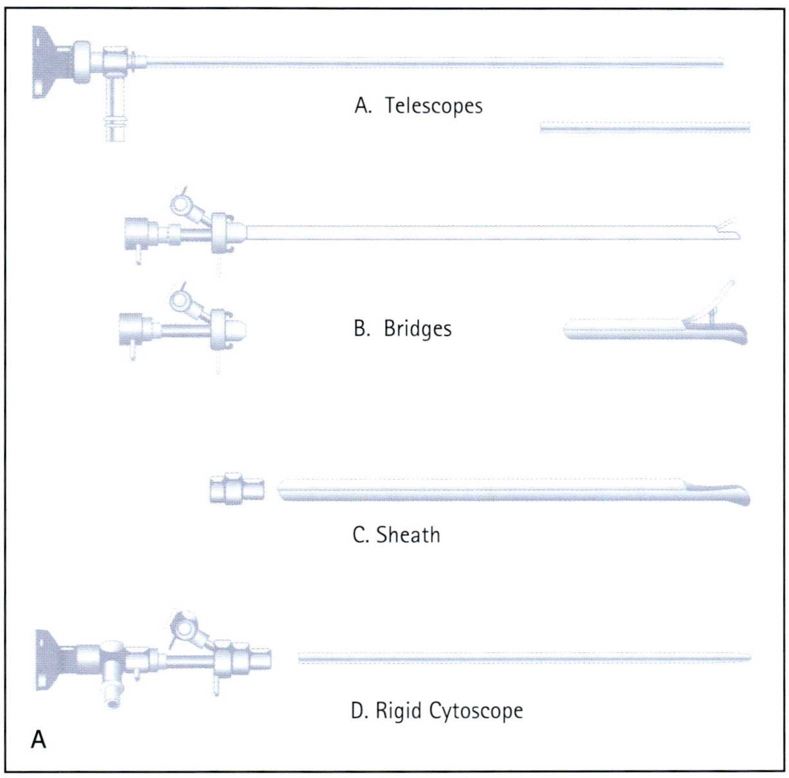

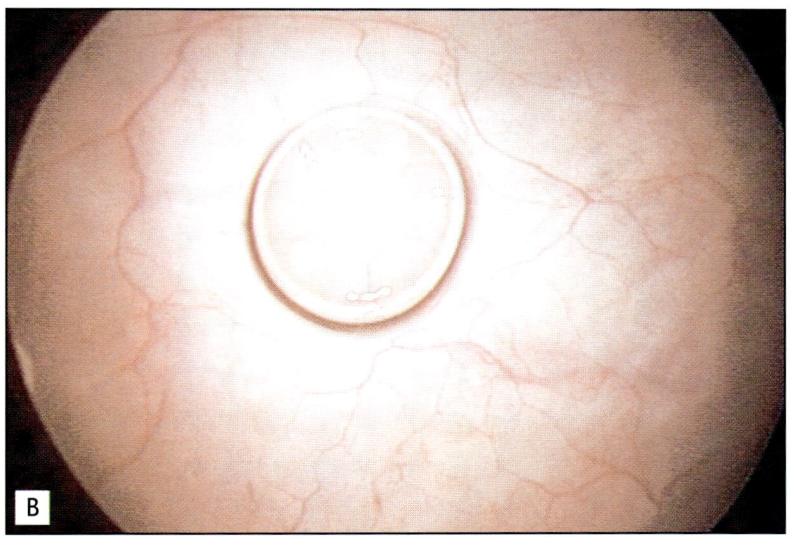

FIGURE 3-39.
Procedure. Cystoscopy is performed with a 30 degree or 70 degree telescope in a 17F sheath (**A**). Xylocaine gel can be used as a lubricant and local anesthetic. Infusion of fluid to 200 to 300 mL will usually provide adequate visualization. **B**, The air bubble is used for orientation and serial sweeps from this central point allow complete assessment of the bladder wall.

(*Continued on next page*)

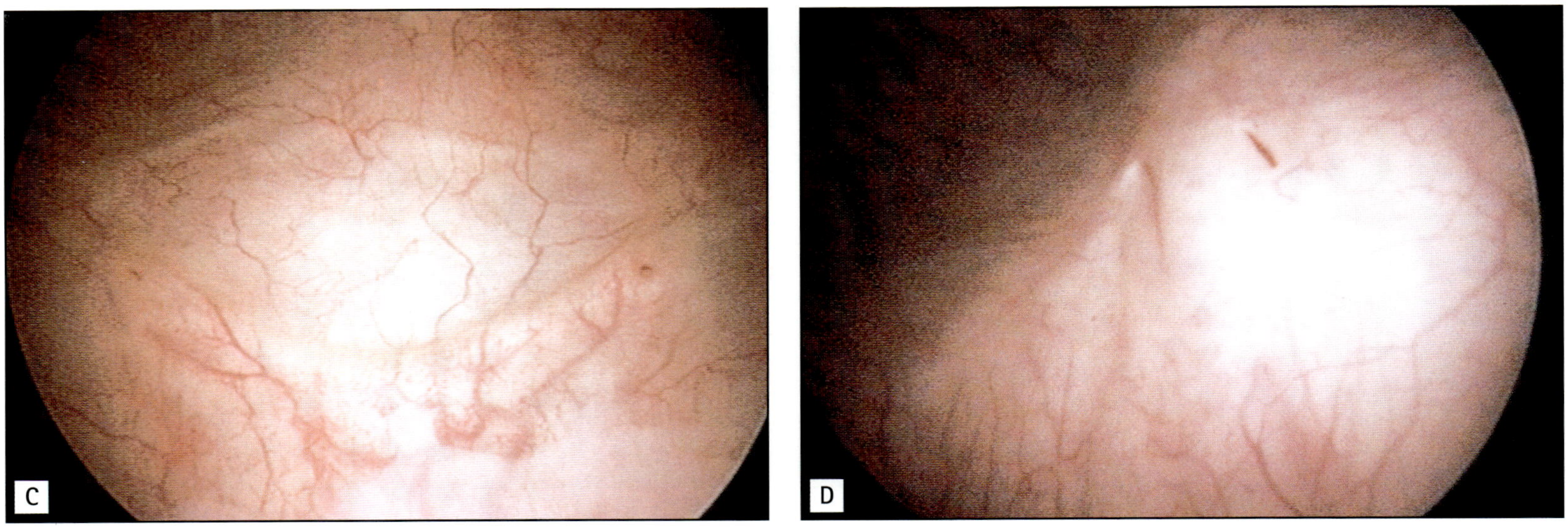

FIGURE 3-39. *(Continued)*
Both ureters should be visualized and patency noted. **C**, The presence of a double ureter is important to detect preoperatively (**D**).

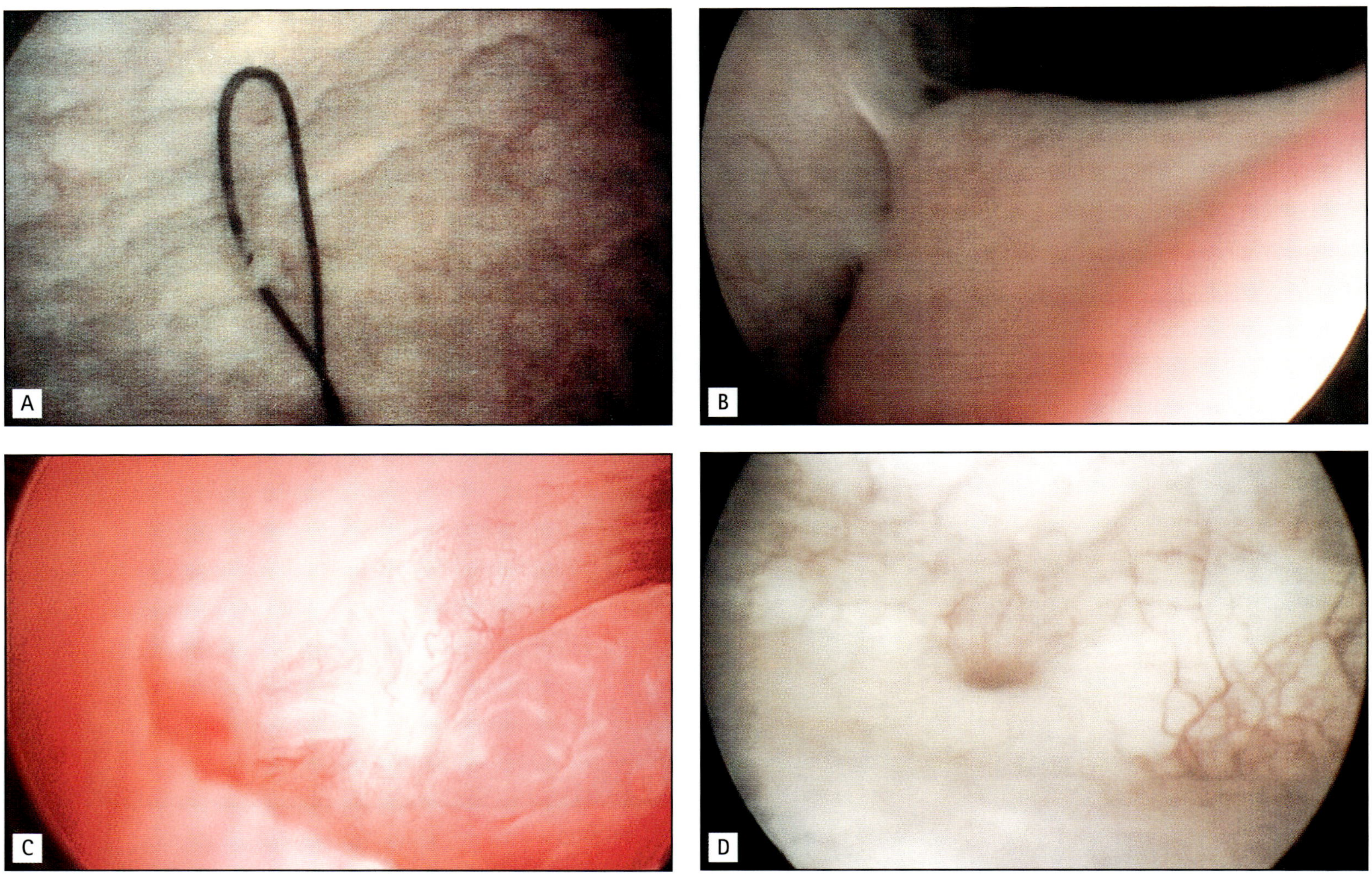

FIGURE 3-40.
Mucosal lesions. In a study of women undergoing combined urodynamic testing and cystoscopy, endoscopy was considered important to the final diagnosis in 19% [22]. Specifically it can provide information on anatomic abnormalities including intravesical suture (**A** and **B**), and intravesical lesions (**C**), and fistula (**D**).

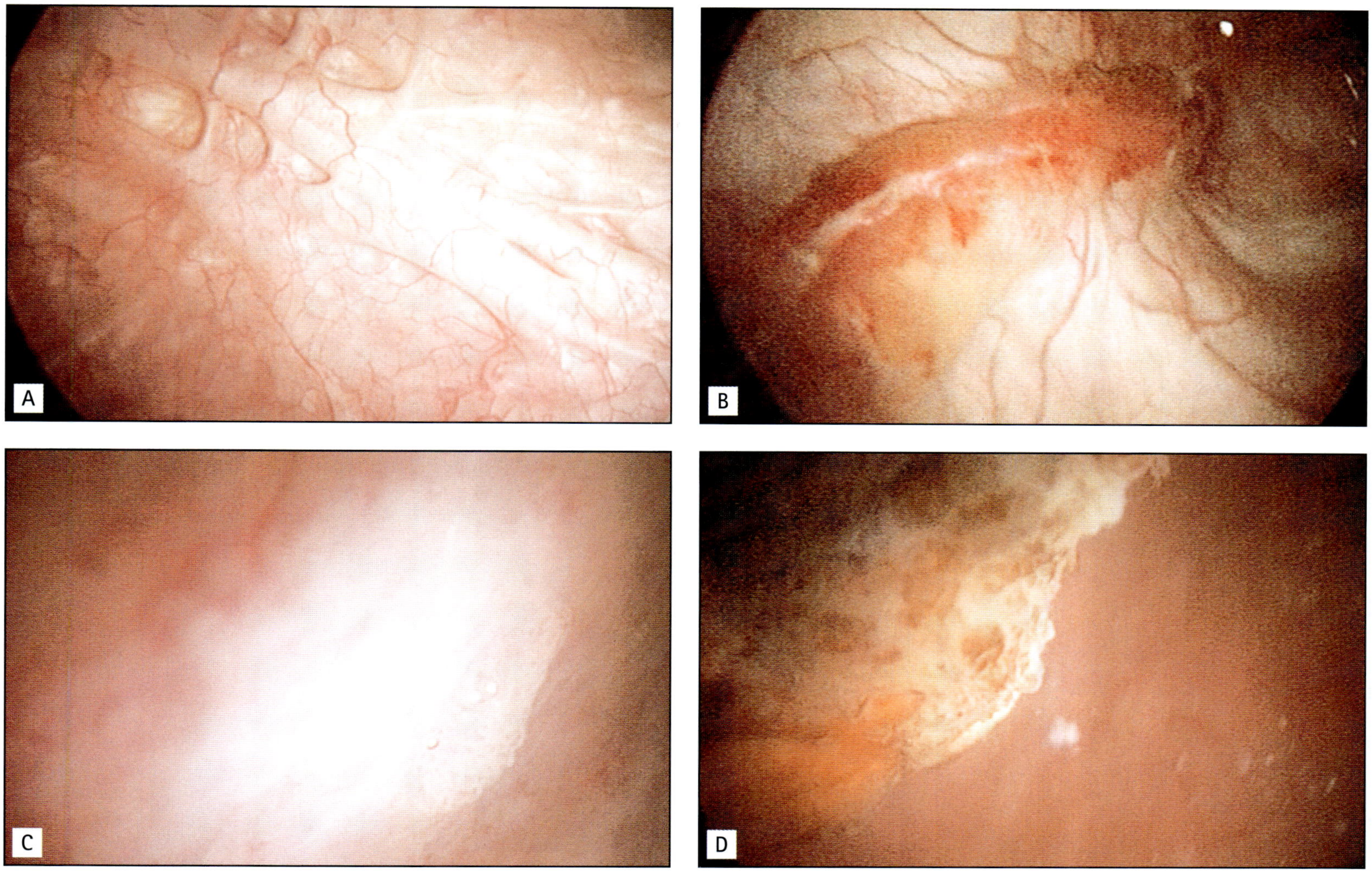

FIGURE 3-41.

Detrusor instability. Trabeculations are common in detrusor instability though not diagnostic. **A**, An injury or suture can present as detrusor instability. **B**, The second most common presenting symptom of bladder cancer is detrusor instability. **C**, The patient shown in **D** was a 62-year-old smoker who presented with a 4-month history of urgency, frequency, and urge incontinence. This was a very aggressive grade III, stage III tumor and the patient died 3 months after the diagnosis.

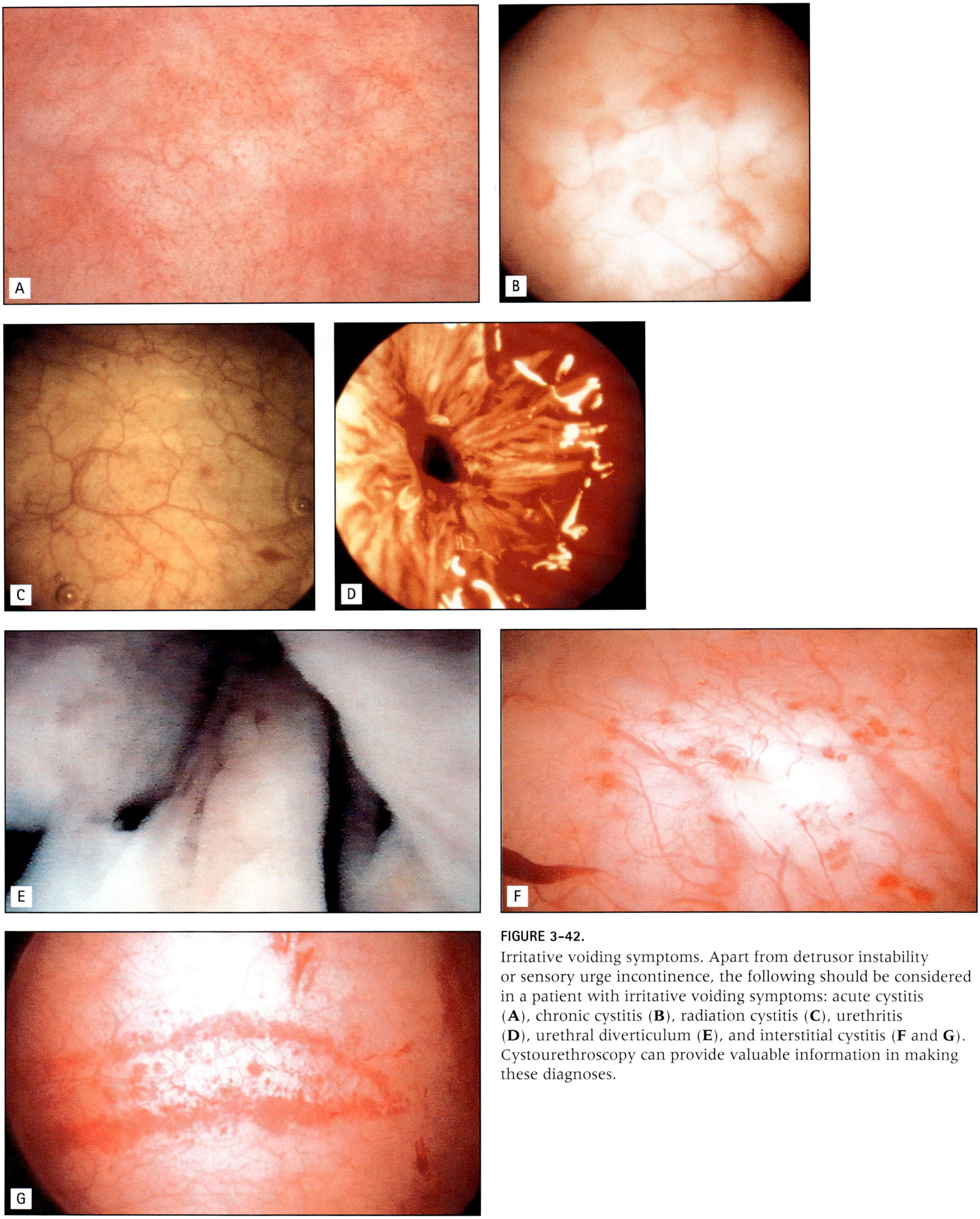

FIGURE 3-42.
Irritative voiding symptoms. Apart from detrusor instability or sensory urge incontinence, the following should be considered in a patient with irritative voiding symptoms: acute cystitis (**A**), chronic cystitis (**B**), radiation cystitis (**C**), urethritis (**D**), urethral diverticulum (**E**), and interstitial cystitis (**F** and **G**). Cystourethroscopy can provide valuable information in making these diagnoses.

IMAGING TECHNIQUES:

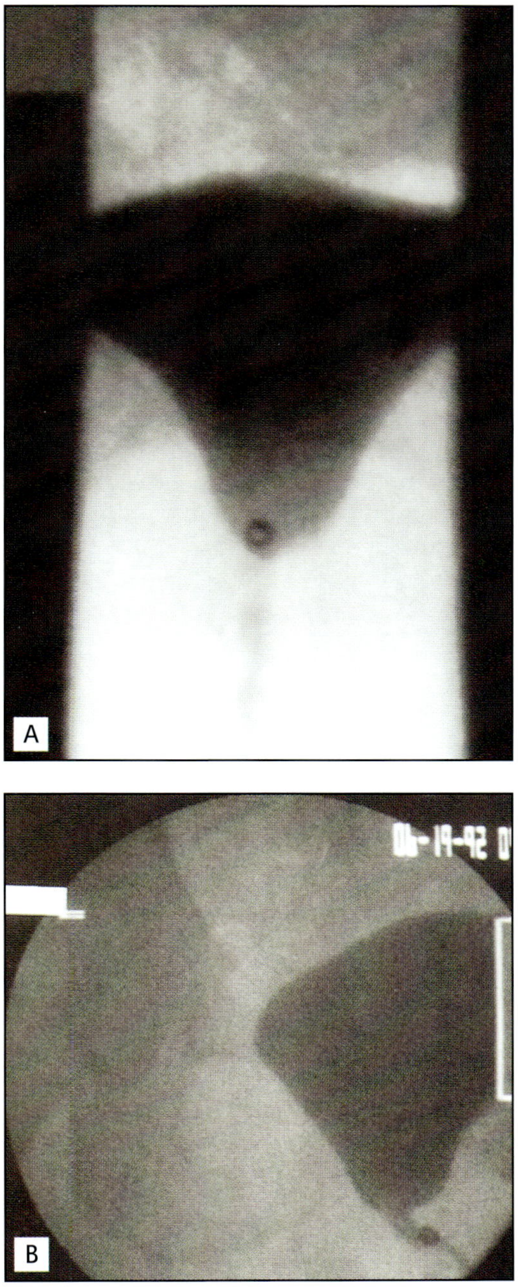

FIGURE 3-43.

Videourodynamics. Videourodynamics combines cystometry with fluoroscopy. Testing can demonstrate leakage and allow assessment of the urethrovesical junction (UVJ) and bladder base. It exposes the patient to 800 mrad of radiation and the equipment is much more expensive. With the patient in the supine position, the bladder is filled at 50 to 100 mL/min with 20% iodinated contrast material. The intravesical and intrarectal (= intra-abdominal) pressures are simultaneously recorded. Studies have shown no significant difference in diagnosis between urodynamics and videourodynamics. The possible exceptions to this are in the patient with postvoid dribbling where diverticuli may be detected (remember urethroscopy will detect about 90%) or the patient complaining of incontinence on standing. In the latter situation it is helpful in distinguishing between intrinsic sphincter deficiency and positionally induced detrusor instability [23]. It also allows more precise measurement of the leak point pressure (LPP) because the exact moment of leakage can be visualized and recorded. **A**, Leakage occurs at a low LPP of 64 cm. There is mobility of the UVJ. A lateral view (**B**) of a different patient demonstrated a LPP of 136 cm. On straining, the urethra and bladder can be seen to first move inferiorly then posteriorly followed by leakage. (*From* Raz S: *Female Urology,* edn 2. Philadelphia: WB Saunders; 1996:109–111; with permission.)

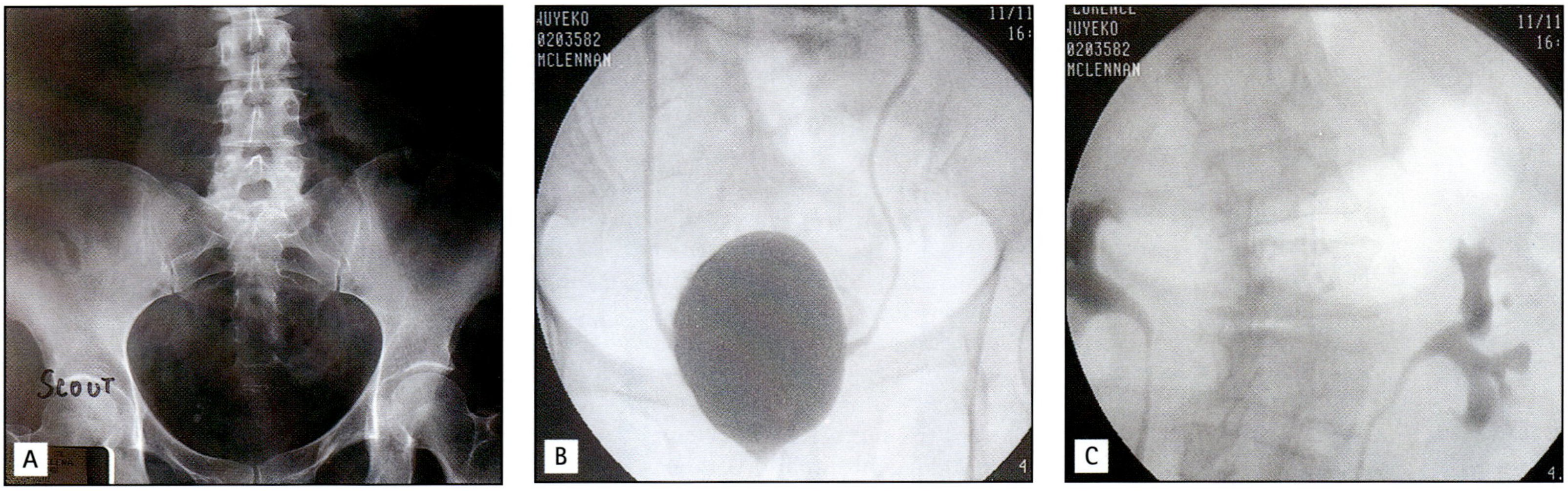

FIGURE 3-44.

Pyelogram. An intravenous pyelogram is not routinely performed in the assessment of incontinence. It should be performed to assess the upper tracts in patients with hematuria, persistent bacteriuria, recurrent urinary tract infections, impaired compliance, and markedly reduced bladder capacity. **A**, A large staghorn calculus is seen in a 52-year-old patient with recurrent urinary tract infections. Renal scan showed only 20% normal function in that kidney. **B** and **C**, Severe reflux is seen in a 79-year-old woman with severe interstitial cystitis who had a maximum capacity on 60 mL under anesthesia.

REFERENCES

1. Jackson SL, Weber AM, Hull TL, *et al.*: Fecal incontinence in women with urinary incontinence and pelvic organ prolapse. *Obstet Gynecol* 1997, 89:423–427.
2. Shumaker SA, Wyman JF, Uebersax JS, et al.: Health-related quality of life measures for women with urinary incontinence: the incontinence impact questionnaire and the urogenital distress inventory. Quality of Life Research 1994, 3:292306.
3. Uebersax JS, Wyman JF, Shumaker SA, *et al* and the Continence Program for Women Research Group: Short forms to assess life quality and symptom distress for urinary incontinence in women: the incontinence impact questionnaire and urogenital distress inventory. *Neurourol Urodyn* 1995, 14:131–139.
4. Blaivas JG: The bulbocavernosus reflex in urology: a prospective study of 299 patients. *J Urol* 1981, 126:197.
5. McLennan MT, Bent AE: Supine empty stress test as a predictor of low Valsalva leak point pressure. *Neurourol Urodyn* 1998. 17:121–127.
6. Fowler JE Jr: Nosocomial catheter-associated urinary tract infection. *Infect Surg* 1993, 2:43–53.
7. Bent AE, Nahhas DE, McLennan MT: Portable ultrasound determination of urinary residual volume. *Int Urogynecol J* 1997, 8:200–2002.
8. Catalona WJ: Urothelial tumors of the urinary tract. In: *Campbell's Urology*, edn 6. Edited by Walsh PC, Retik AB, Stamey TA, Vaughan ED. Philadelphia: WB Saunders; 1992:1094–1115.
9. Eberle CM, Winsemius D, Garibaldi RA: Risk factors and consequences of bacteriuria in non-catheterized nursing home residents. *J Gerontol* 1993, 6:266–271.
10. Enhorning G: Simultaneous recording of intra vesical and intra urethral pressure: a study on urethral closure pressure in normal and stress incontinent women. *Acta Chir Scand Suppl* 1971, 271:1–68.
11. Summitt RL, Bent AE, Ostergard DR, Harris TA: Stress incontinence and low urethral closure pressure. Correlation of preoperative urethral hypermobility with successful suburethral sling procedures. *J Reprod Med* 1990, 35:877–880.
12. Caputo RM, Benson JT: The Q-Tip test and urethrovesical junction mobility. *Obstet Gynecol* 1993, 82:892–896.
13. Gordon D, Pearce M, Norton P, Stanton S. Comparison of ultrasound and lateral chain urethrocystography in the determination of bladder neck descent. *Am J Obstet Gynecol* 1989;160:182–185.
14. Ouslander J, Leach G, Abelson S, *et al.*: Simple vs. multichannel cystometry in the evaluation of bladder function in an incontinent geriatric population. *J Urol* 1998, 140:1482–1486.
15. Jensen JK, Neilsen FR, Ostergard DR: The role of patient history in the diagnosis of urinary incontinence. *Obstet Gynecol* 1994, 83:904–910.
16. Sand PK, Bowen LW, Ostergard DR, *et al.*: The effect of the retropubic urethropexy on detrusor instability. *Obstet Gynecol* 1988, 71:818–822.
17. Sutherst JR, Fischer, M.D., Brown MC: Comparison of single and multichannel cystometry in diagnosing detrusor instability. *Br J Med* 1984, 288:1720–1722.
18. Sand PK, Bowen LW, Panganiban R, Ostergard DR: The low pressure urethra as a factor in failed retropubic urethropexy. *Obstet Gynecol* 1987, 69:399–402.
19. Bump RC, Copeland WE, Hurt WG, et al.: Dynamic urethral pressure profilometry pressure transmission ratio determinations in stress-incontinent and stress continent subjects. *Am J Obstet Gynecol* 1988, 159:749–755.
20. Hilton P, Stanton SL: Urethral pressure measurements by microtransducer: the results in symptom-free women and those with genuine stress incontinence. *Br J Obstet Gynaecol* 1983, 90:919–933.
21. Bhatia NN, Berman A: Urodynamic predictability of voiding following incontinence surgery. *Obstet Gynecol* 1984, 63:85–91.
22. Cundiff GW, Bent AE: The contribution of urethrocystoscopy to evaluation of lower urinary tract dysfunction in women. *Int Urogynecol J* 1996, 7:307–311.
23. Stanton S, Krieger M, Ziv E: Videocystourethrography: its role in assessment of incontinence in the female. *Neurourol Urodyn* 1988, 7:712–713.

CHAPTER 4

Evaluation of Fecal Incontinence

Dee Fenner

Fecal incontinence is the inability to defer the elimination of stool or gas until there is a socially acceptable time and place to do so. Because maintaining fecal continence is a complex physiologic process that requires a person's ability to perceive the type of fecal bolus, store or retain when necessary, and excrete when desirable, the loss of that ability is equally as complex. Fecal continence requires normal stool consistency and volume, normal colonic transit time, a compliant rectum, innervation of the pelvic floor and the anal sphincters, and the interplay between the puborectalis muscle, rectum, and anal sphincters [1]. Loss of one or more of these abilities can lead to fecal incontinence.

Fecal incontinence can be socially debilitating for the patient. The emotional and psychological impact on the quality of life can be devastating for the patient and her family. In the evaluation of fecal incontinence, the physician and patient must communicate sufficiently to have a clear understanding of the patient's symptoms, including loss of flatus or stool, frequency of incontinence, and impact on the quality of the patient's life. Evaluation and treatment should be based on the severity of the patient's symptoms.

The estimated prevalence of fecal incontinence ranges from 1.3% to 11% of women older than 64 years of age. Over 30% of women reporting urinary incontinence also report fecal incontinence or dual incontinence [2–4].

The most common cause of fecal incontinence in women is damage to the anal sphincters at the time of vaginal delivery with or without neuronal injury. Damage can occur by mechanical disruption or separation of the internal anal sphincter or external anal sphincter or by damage to the muscle innervation by stretching or crushing the pudendal and pelvic nerves. Sultan *et al.* [5] showed that 13% of primiparas and 23% of multiparas developed fecal incontinence or fecal urgency postpartum. By anal ultrasound, all but one woman had evidence of anal sphincter disruption. The chance of muscular injury is increased with midline episiotomy, forceps delivery, and vaginal delivery of larger infants. Not all risk factors are known and not all women are susceptible to pelvic floor damage. Further study is needed to accurately predict which women are at risk.

Evaluation of fecal incontinence should include history, physical examination, prior treatment, and proposed therapy. In addition, certain tests, such as nerve conductance studies, may be helpful in counseling patients before surgical therapy in terms of expected outcomes.

CAUSES OF FECAL INCONTINENCE

COMMON CAUSES OF FECAL INCONTINENCE

Obstetric injury
- Disruption of internal anal sphincter
- Disruption of external anal sphincter
- Pelvic floor denervation

Trauma
- Pelvic fracture
- Accidental injury
- Anorectal surgery
- Rectovaginal fistula

Diarrheal states
- Infectious diarrhea
- Inflammatory bowel disease
- Short-gut syndrome
- Laxative abuse
- Radiation enteritis

Rectal neoplasia

Rectal prolapse

Rectocele

Overflow
- Impaction
- Encompresis

Neurologic disease
- Congenital anomalies (*ie*, myelomeningocele)
- Multiple sclerosis
- Diabetic neuropathy
- Neoplasms or injury of brain, spinal cord, cauda equina
- Pudendal neuropathy (childbirth, chronic straining, perineal descent)

Congenital anomalies of anorectum/pelvis

FIGURE 4–1.
Common causes of fecal incontinence.

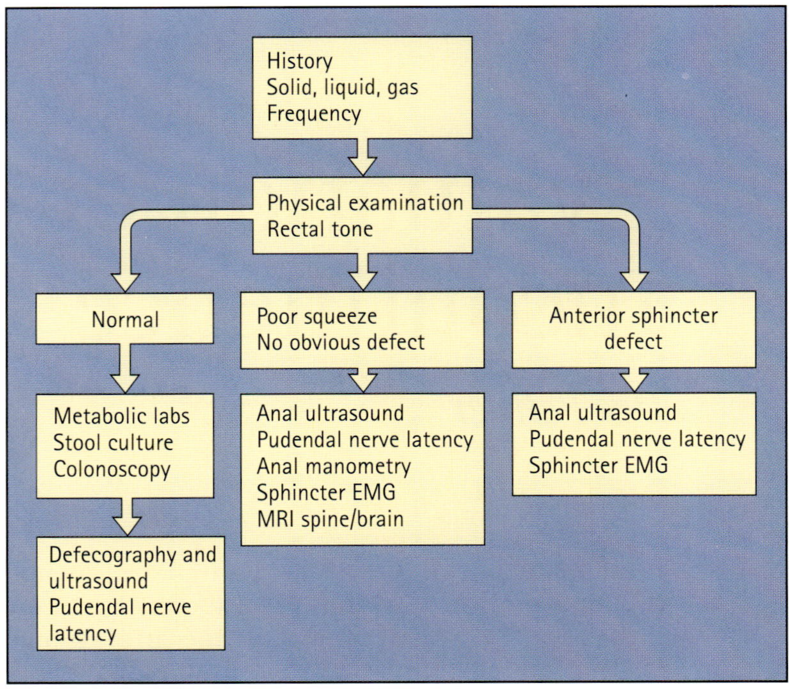

FIGURE 4–2.
Evaluation of fecal incontinence. A detailed history differentiates incontinence of gas, liquid, or solid stool, along with frequency, onset, and effect on the patient's quality of life. The history should assess the possibility of Crohn's disease, ulcerative colitis, irritable bowel syndrome, radiation to the pelvis, neurologic diseases such as multiple sclerosis, and prior anorectal surgeries. A detailed obstetric history should include type of delivery, weight of largest infant, length of second stage, episiotomy or lacerations, and use of forceps or vacuum extraction. Rectal examination should assess resting and squeeze tone, presence of a rectocele or rectal mass, and fecal impaction. Inspection of the rectum and vagina should evaluate for a rectovaginal fistula, prolapsing hemorrhoids, or rectal prolapse. Further evaluation, including radiologic and physiologic tests have been shown in a prospective study at a tertiary colorectal referral clinic to alter the final diagnosis of the cause of fecal incontinence in 19% of the cases [6]. EMG—electromyography, MRI—magnetic resonance imaging.

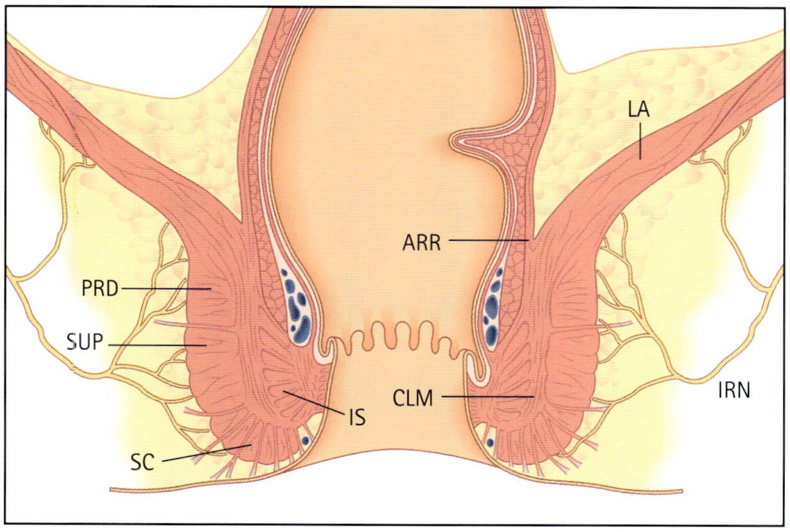

FIGURE 4-3.

A coronal section of the anal canal and lower rectum. It is important to understand the normal anatomy and function of the anal sphincters and nerve supply. ARR—level of anorectal ring, CLM—conjoined longitudinal muscle, IRN—inferior rectal nerve (terminal branch of the pudendal nerve innervation the external anal sphincter), LA—levator ani muscles, PRD—puborectalis/deep external sphincter complex, SC—subcutaneous external sphincter; SUP—superficial external anal sphincter. (*From* Pearl RK: *Practical Guide to Anorectal Testing.* Edited by Smith L. New York: Igaku-Shoin; 1995, with permission.)

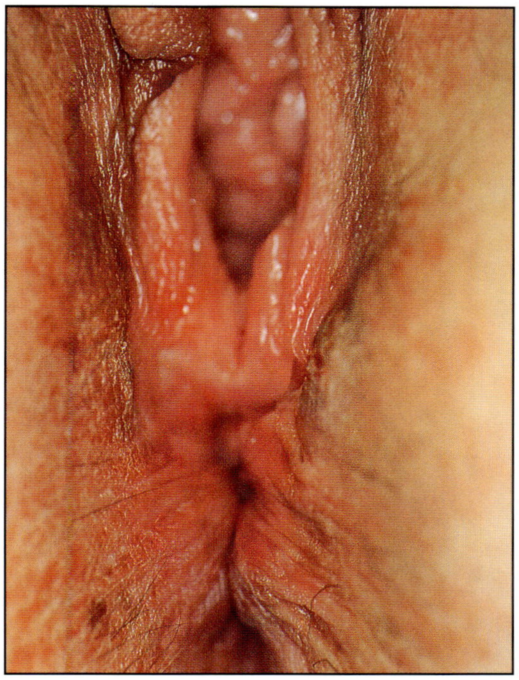

FIGURE 4-4.

Perineum with chronic laceration of external anal sphincter (EAS). Inspection of the perineum shows the classic "dovetail" sign with loss of the anal skin creases anteriorly due to a chronic third-degree laceration of the EAS. Normally, with an intact sphincter, the skin creases are arranged radially around the anus.

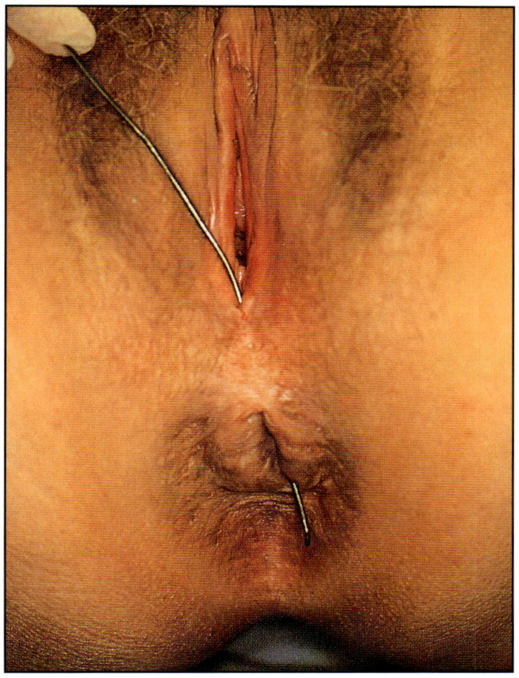

FIGURE 4-5.

Rectovaginal fistula. A rectovaginal fistula should be considered in a patient who has had a recent vaginal delivery with or without known lacerations, a recent pelvic surgery, or a history of inflammatory bowel disease. Patients generally complain of constant stool drainage or vaginal discharge. Anal sphincter injuries are commonly found in conjunction with fistulas, so the entire sphincter mechanism should be fully evaluated before a surgical repair is attempted.

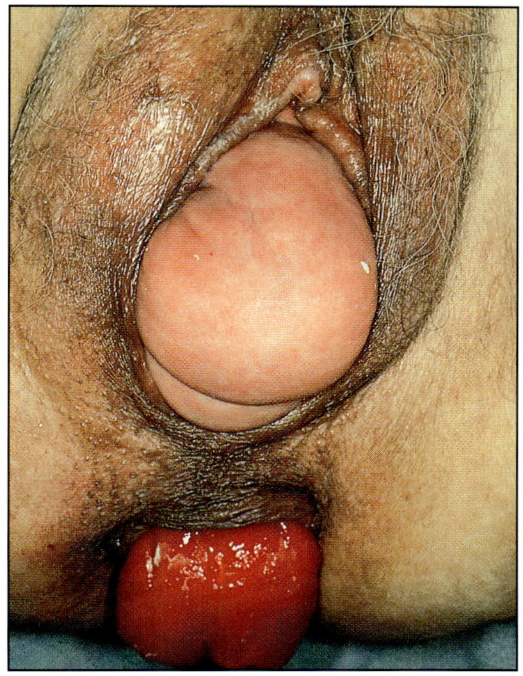

FIGURE 4-6.

Rectal prolapse. Rectal prolapse is accompanied by fecal incontinence in 40% to 60% of patients and may be due to stretching of either the internal anal sphincter by the prolapse or the pudendal nerves as a consequence of chronic straining and perineal descent. Following prolapse repair, continence improves in about 50% of patients [7]. This patient also has vaginal vault prolapse, commonly seen in conjunction with rectal prolapse due to straining and loss of pelvic floor function.

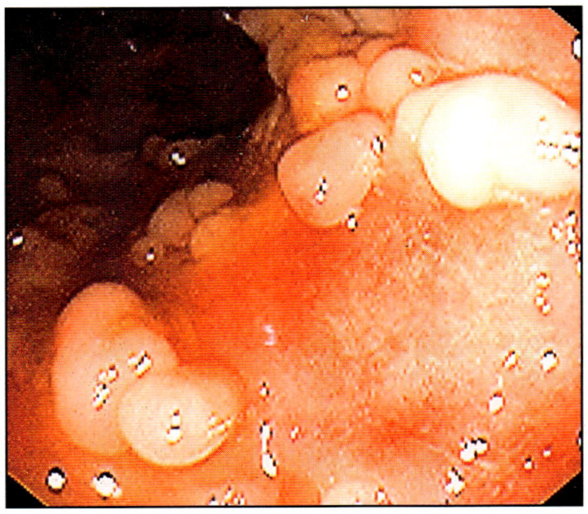

FIGURE 4–7.

Crohn's disease. Crohn's disease on colonoscopy shows areas of normal bowel with pseudopolyps from chronic inflammation. The severity of incontinence from chronic diarrhea resulting from inflammatory bowel disease or irritable bowel syndrome is dependent on anal sphincter function and rectal compliance. If the rectum is diseased from Crohn's proctitis, rectal compliance and storage capability are reduced, causing fecal urgency, soilage, and incontinence. Prior anal surgery and fistulas can also impair sphincter function.

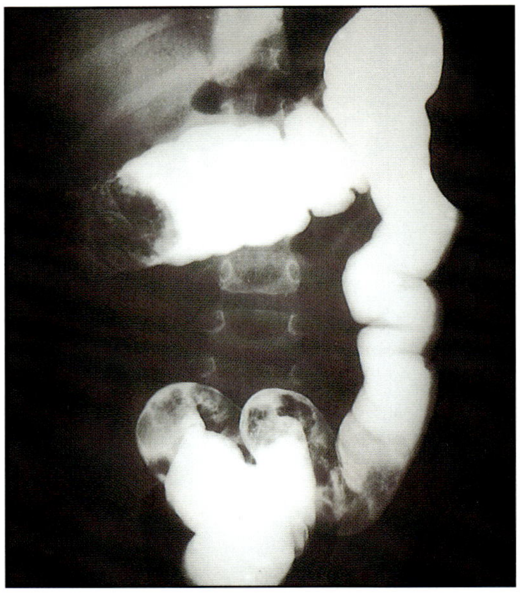

FIGURE 4–8.

Intussusception of the proximal transverse colon on barium enema. This patient presented with intermittent abdominal pain, diarrhea, and fecal incontinence. Fecal incontinence is secondary to the bowel spasm and liquid stool that "overcomes" the anal sphincter. Patients with a weakened or shortened anal sphincter may become incontinent only to liquid stool.

DIAGNOSTIC METHODS

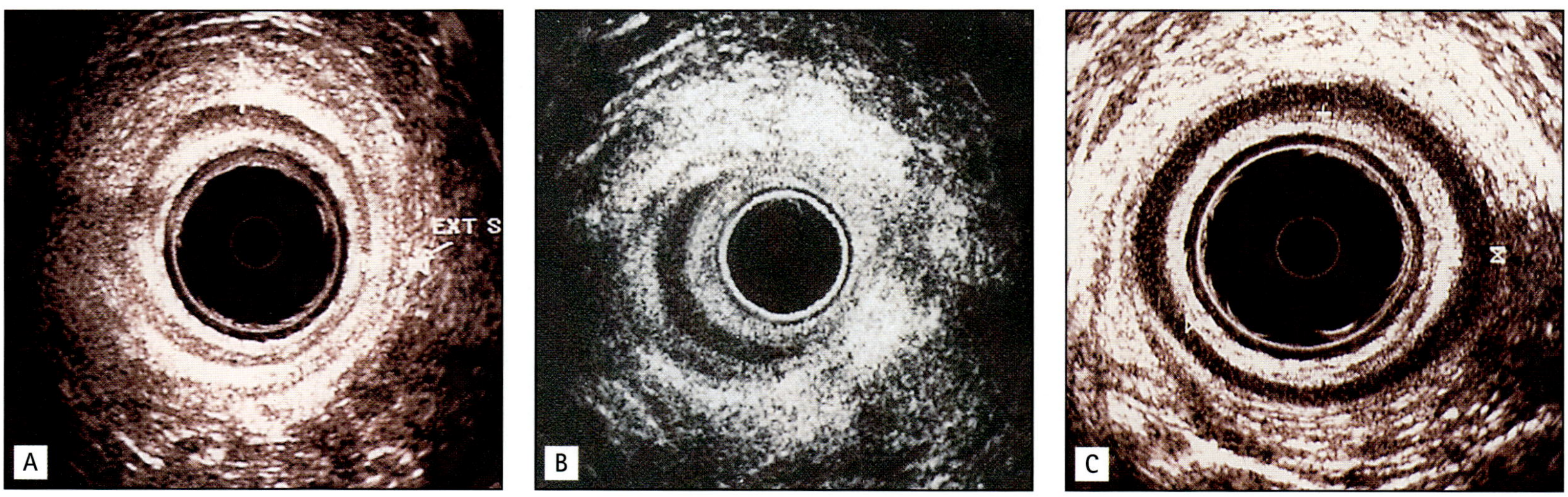

FIGURE 4–9.

Anal ultrasound. **A**, Anal ultrasound has significantly enhanced the ability to delineate defects of both the internal and external anal sphincters. The internal anal sphincter is visible as a hypoechoic circle and external anal sphincter is seen as a hyperechoic circle. Scarred areas have a homogeneous, gray appearance. **B**, With the patient lying on her left side, a defect in both the internal and external anal sphincters is seen at the 3 o'clock position. This injury is the result of a difficult vaginal delivery. **C**, With the vagina again at the 3 o'clock position, there is an intact internal anal sphincter and a defect in the external anal sphincter.

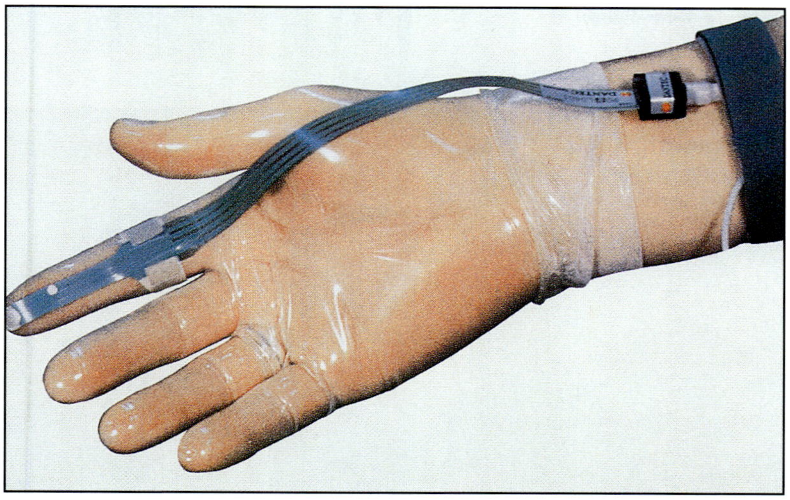

FIGURE 4-10.

St. Mark's electrode. Neurophsyiologic testing for evaluation of fecal incontinence can include pudendal nerve terminal motor latencies (PNTML) and needle electromyography. Pictured is a St. Mark's electrode used to stimulate the pudendal nerve at the level of the ischial spine, transrectally or transvaginally, and to record the response at the anal sphincter. This test evaluates the neuromuscular function of the anal sphincter. Prolonged PNTML can be found in patients with idiopathic fecal incontinence and after vaginal delivery or pelvic surgery. Pudendal neuropathy may predict continence after surgeries for rectal prolapse and sphincter lacerations. Laurberg *et al*, [8] noted 8 of 10 patients with normal PNTML had excellent or good results after a sphincteroplasty and only 1 of 9 patients with abnormal PNTML had good results after a sphincteroplasty for obstetric trauma.

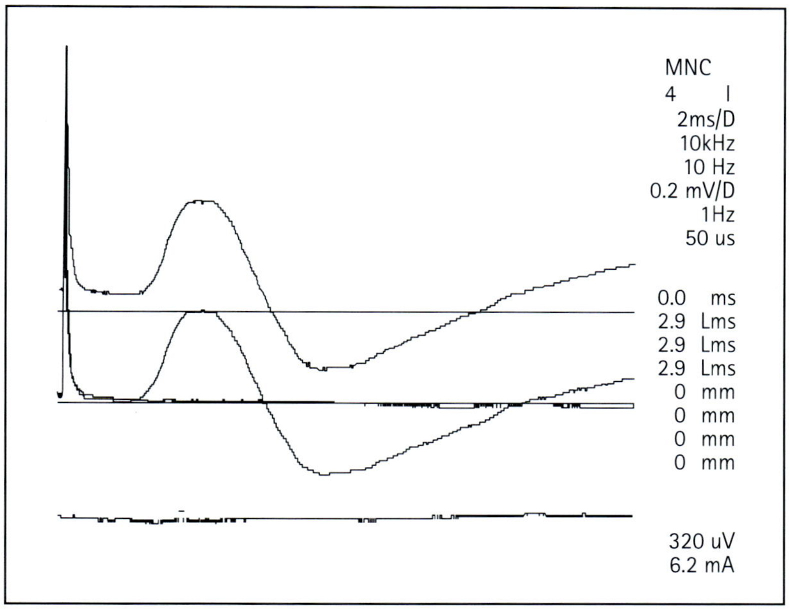

FIGURE 4-11.

Pudendal nerve terminal motor latencies (PNTML). Normal bilateral PNTML have been shown to be 2.0 ± 0.2 ms. The latency response is measured from the onset of the stimulus to the onset of the response in the external anal sphincter. A normal PNTML is the measurement of the fastest response of the pudendal nerve and does not necessarily mean the entire nerve is normal. Neither does an abnormal latency indicate abnormal muscle function. A damaged nerve can heal and reinnervate the muscle, and although the PNTML may be slightly prolonged, the muscle functions normally.

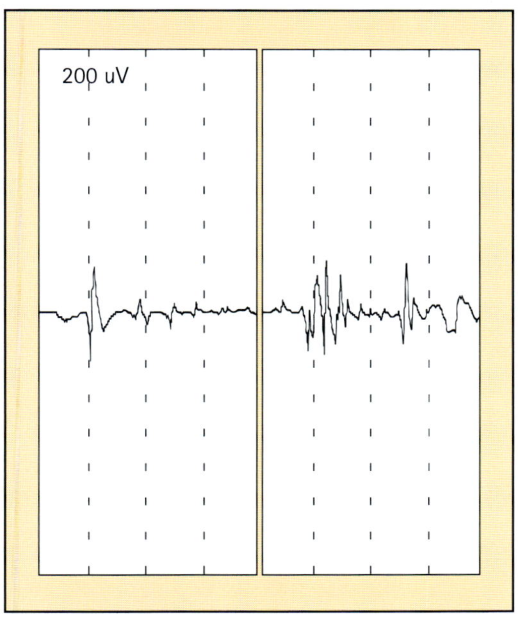

FIGURE 4-12.

Sphincter electromyography (EMG). Single-fiber EMG may be used to investigate the external anal sphincter. On the left half of the diagram is a normal single-fiber EMG tracing of a single muscle fiber, firing in a time-locked manner as a constituent of a motor unit. A motor unit consists of the anterior horn cell, its axon and branches, and the muscle fibers it supplies. Each motor unit potential will have a characteristic amplitude, duration, and characteristic shape of electrical response. The waveform on the right reflects several muscle fiber action potentials as a result of "grouping" from reinervation resulting in several fibers belonging to a motor unit. Counting several fields estimates the fiber density which is increased in neurogenic and myopathic conditions. EMG mapping of the sphincter requires multiple insertions around the anal sphincter to detect areas of scarring or gaps in the muscle.

A. MANOMETRY

Test	Sphincter Characteristics
Longitudinal resting pullout	Length
	Maximum average pressure
	Pressure volume
	Cross-sectional asymmetry
Station squeeze	Voluntary augmentation
	Fatigue
	Rest vs. squeeze cross-section
Motility	Slow wave
	Ultraslow wave
Balloon reflex	Rectal-anal inhibitory reflex
	Rectal-anal excitatory reflex

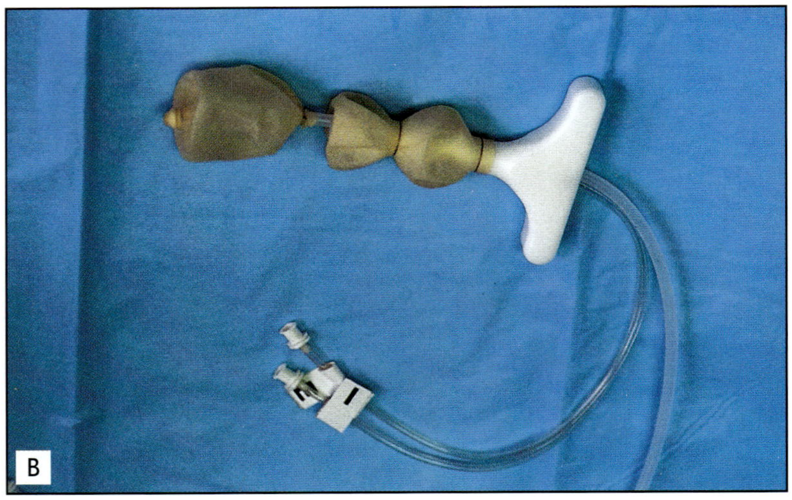

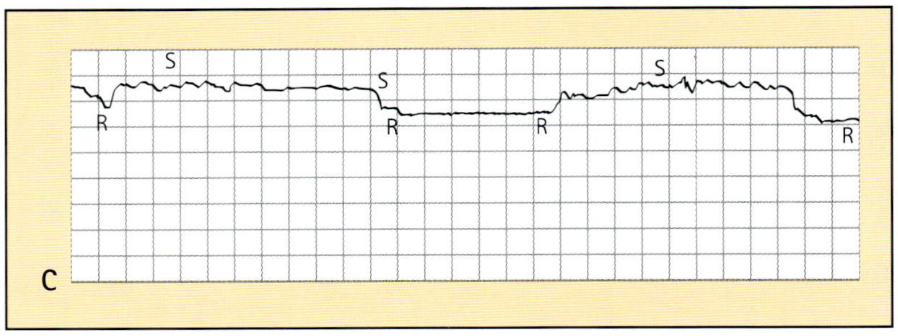

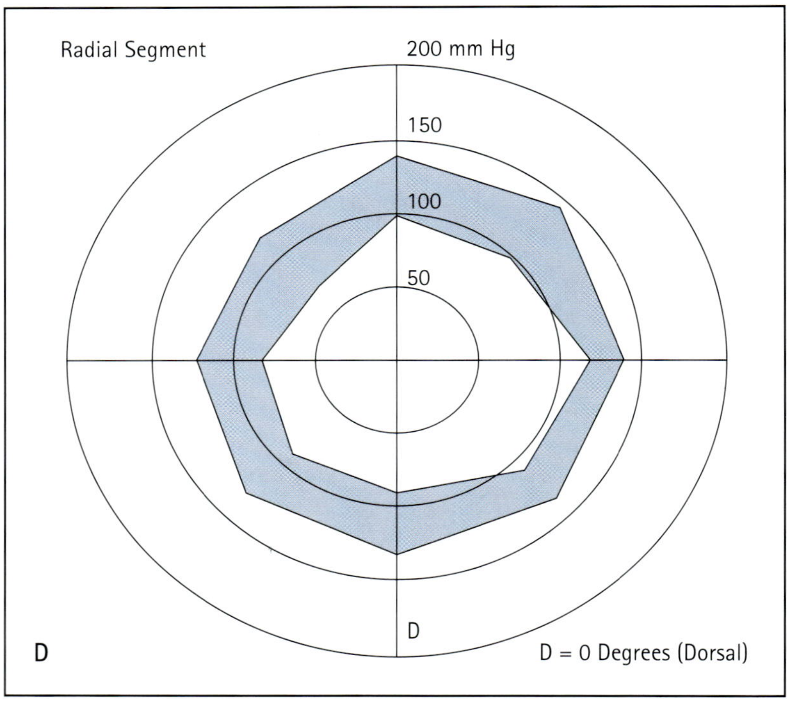

FIGURE 4-13.

Anal manometry. **A**,There are many different types and methods for performing anal manometry. Essentially a balloon or probe is inserted into the rectum and a pressure transducer relays information to a recorder or computer. Important manometric parameters include sphincter length, resting and squeeze pressures, anal canal sensation, compliance, and the presence of the anorectal inhibitory reflex. **B**, A double-balloon manometry device with third distention balloon in the rectum. The top balloon is inserted to the level of the rectum. Filling of the top balloon assesses rectal compliance, sensation, and the rectoanal inhibitory reflex. The middle balloon records the pressures in the internal anal sphincter, and the outer balloon records those in the external anal sphincter. **C**, Anal manometry can determine the baseline resting pressure of the anal canal (*R*) and the squeeze pressure (*S*). The internal anal sphincter contributes 80% of the resting pressure. Voluntary contraction or squeezing of the external anal sphincter should double the resting pressures [9]. **D**, Perfusion anal manometry. A radial cross-section of the resting or squeeze pressures can be obtained using an eight-channel water profusion probe that records pressures radially around the anal canal. The pressures are sent to a computer that analyzes the data and develops the model. A sphincter defect at the 12 o'clock position would cause a loss of pressure in that position and asymmetry of the diagram.

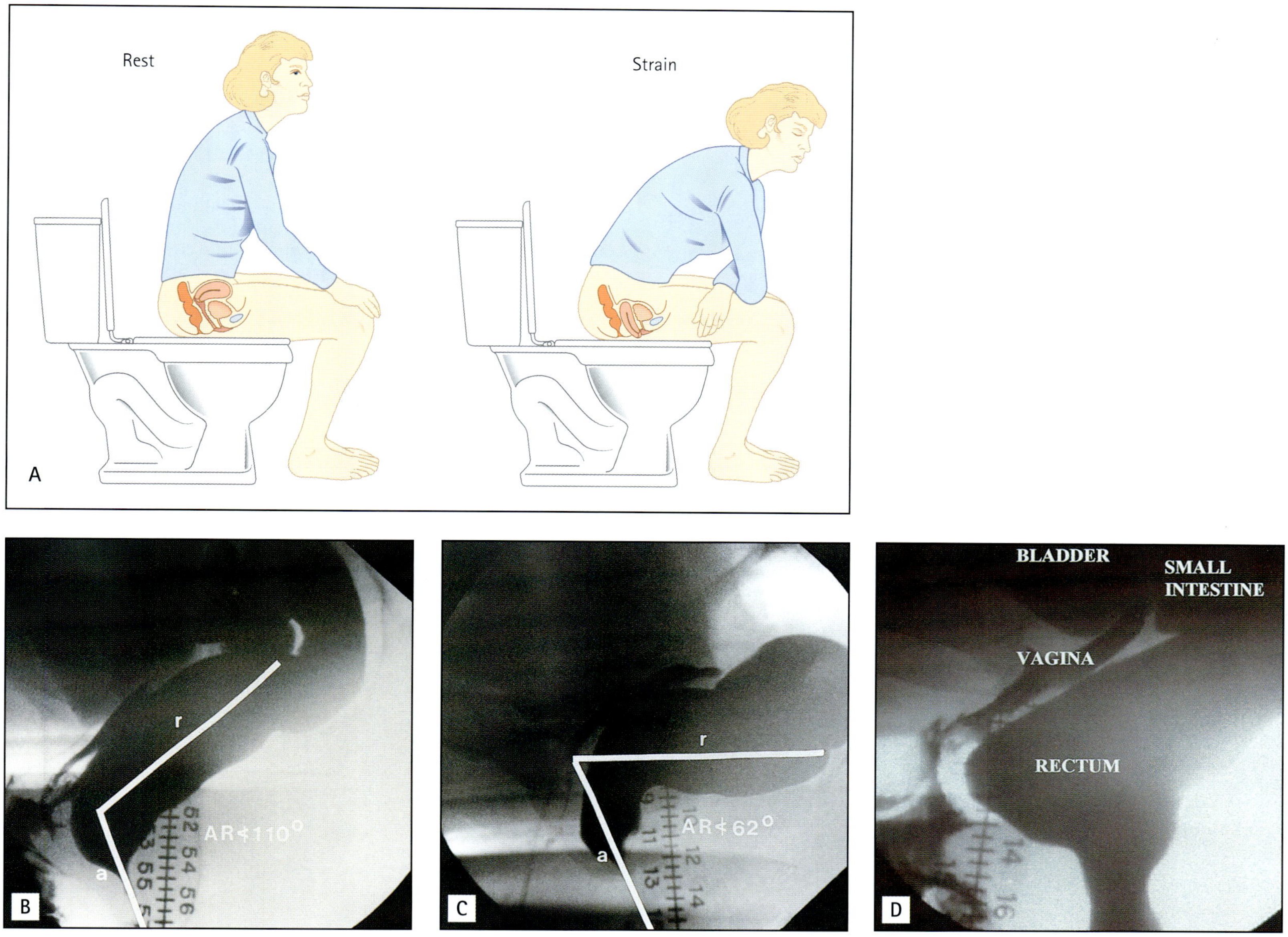

FIGURE 4–14.

Defecography. **A**, Defecography is used in the evaluation of defecation disorders, including constipation and fecal incontinence, as well as in the evaluation of pelvic organ prolapse. Barium paste is inserted into the rectum, the small bowel is opacified by oral contrast, and the vagina and bladder may also be highlighted using barium paste and liquid contrast. The patient sits on a radioluscent commode and is asked to squeeze her pelvic floor, to relax her pelvic floor, and to evacuate her bowels. Fluoroscopy is used to record the dynamic activity of the bowel and pelvic organs. Defecography is used to identify rectal prolapse, internal rectal intussusception, or rectocele. In general, it is not a first-line test in evaluating fecal incontinence. **B** and **C**, The anorectal angle, as measured on these defecographies, was once thought to be predictive of pelvic floor function and useful in evaluating fecal incontinence. Although some studies show that incontinent patients have a more obtuse angle at rest, during straining, and during voluntary contraction of the sphincter, the overlap with results from normal, control patients is too great for diagnostic significance. **D**, Defecography showing a large rectocele. Rectoceles can trap stool at the time of defecation that occasionally evacuates without sensation, causing fecal soiling. Fecal impaction can work similarly from chronic distention of the rectum leading to relaxation of the internal anal sphincter, loss of resting tone, and stool leakage.

REFERENCES

1. Lee RA, Madoff RD, Pemberton J, Fleshman J: Panel presentation: current understanding of anal continence/incontinence. *J Pelvic Surg* 1998, 4:115–125.
2. Madoff RD, Willams JG, Caushau PF: Fecal incontinence. *N Engl J Med* 1992, 326:1002–1007.
3. Kamm MA: Obstetric damage and fecal incontinence. *Lancet* 1994, 344:730–733.
4. Jackson SI, Weber AM, Hull TL, *et al.*: Fecal incontinence in women with urinary incontinence and pelvic organ prolapse. *Obstet Gynecol* 1997, 89:423–427.
5. Sultan AH, Kamm MA, Hudson CN, *et al.*: Anal-sphincter disruption during vaginal delivery. *N Engl J Med* 1993, 329:1905–1911.
6. Keating JP, Stewert PJ, Eyers AA, *et al.*: Are special investigations of value in the management of patients with fecal incontinence? *Dis Colon Rectum* 1997, 40:896–901.
7. Snooks SJ, Henry MM, Swash M: Anorectal incontinence and rectal prolapse: differential assessment of the innervation of the puborectalis and external anal sphincter muscles. *Gut* 1985, 26:470–476.
8. Laurberg S, Swash SJ, Henry MM: Delayed external sphincter repair for obstetric tear. *Br J Surg* 1988, 75:786–788.
9. Pemberton JH, Kelly KA: Achieving enteric continence: principles and applications. *Mayo Clin Proc* 1986, 61:586–599.

CHAPTER 5

Diagnostic Evaluation of Pelvic Organ Prolapse

Linda Brubaker

Traditionally, the diagnostic evaluation of pelvic organ prolapse has been limited to physical examination. Current teaching emphasizes the importance of assessing the maximum protrusion before recommending surgical correction. The recently adopted quantification system has special importance for surgeons who research and report surgical outcomes. Imaging modalities, such as fluoroscopy and magnetic resonance imaging, offer additional diagnostic information. This chapter highlights common findings on physical examination and demonstrates visceral abnormalities seen by four-contrast fluoroscopy of the pelvic floor. Unusual postoperative findings, including foreign body complications, may markedly alter topography and visceral function.

ASSESSMENT OF VAGINAL TOPOGRAPHY

DIAGNOSTIC EVALUATION TOOLS

Physical Examination

Screening neurologic examination (S2–4)

Speculum examination and age appropriate cancer screening

Bimanual examination

- Visceral support
- Muscle strength and symmetry

Pelvic Floor Fluoroscopy (four contrast)

Bladder

Vagina

Small bowel

Large bowel

FIGURE 5-1.

Diagnostic evaluation tools. The physical examination is the single most essential evaluation tool. Assessment should include a screening neurologic examination, standard gynecologic speculum and bimanual examination, and determination of symmetry and strength of levator ani muscles. The maximum extent of the pelvic organ prolapse should be verified by the patient. The standing, straining position is most helpful. Pelvic floor fluoroscopy is a useful adjunct, especially when assessing visceral position and function of the rectum.

ANTERIOR VAGINAL WALL

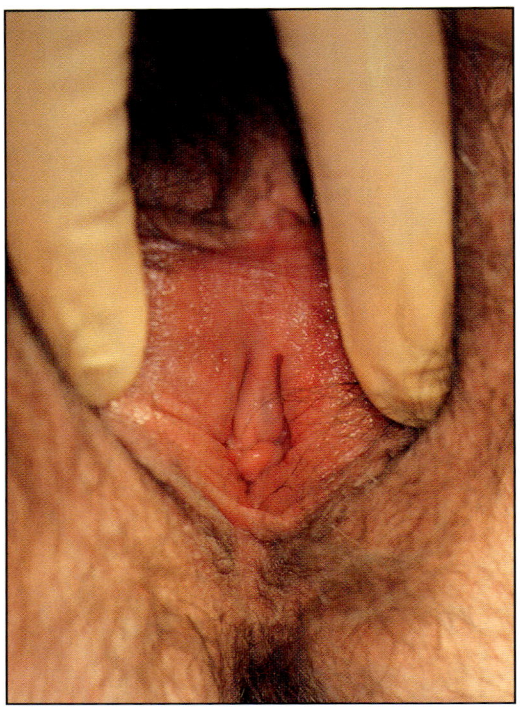

FIGURE 5-2.

Nulliparous. The normal anterior vaginal wall is rugous with lateral attachments to the pelvic sidewall at the arcus tendineous fasciae pelvis. The corresponding vaginal topography of this attachment is the lateral sulci and 10 and 2 o'clock (patient in dorsal lithotomy position). The urethrovesical junction is about 3 cm proximal to the hymen. This corresponds with point Aa in the quantified evaluation scheme (*see* Figures 5-14 and 5-15). The external urethral meatus and urethrovesical junction should be stable with a limited range of motion during strain and cough.

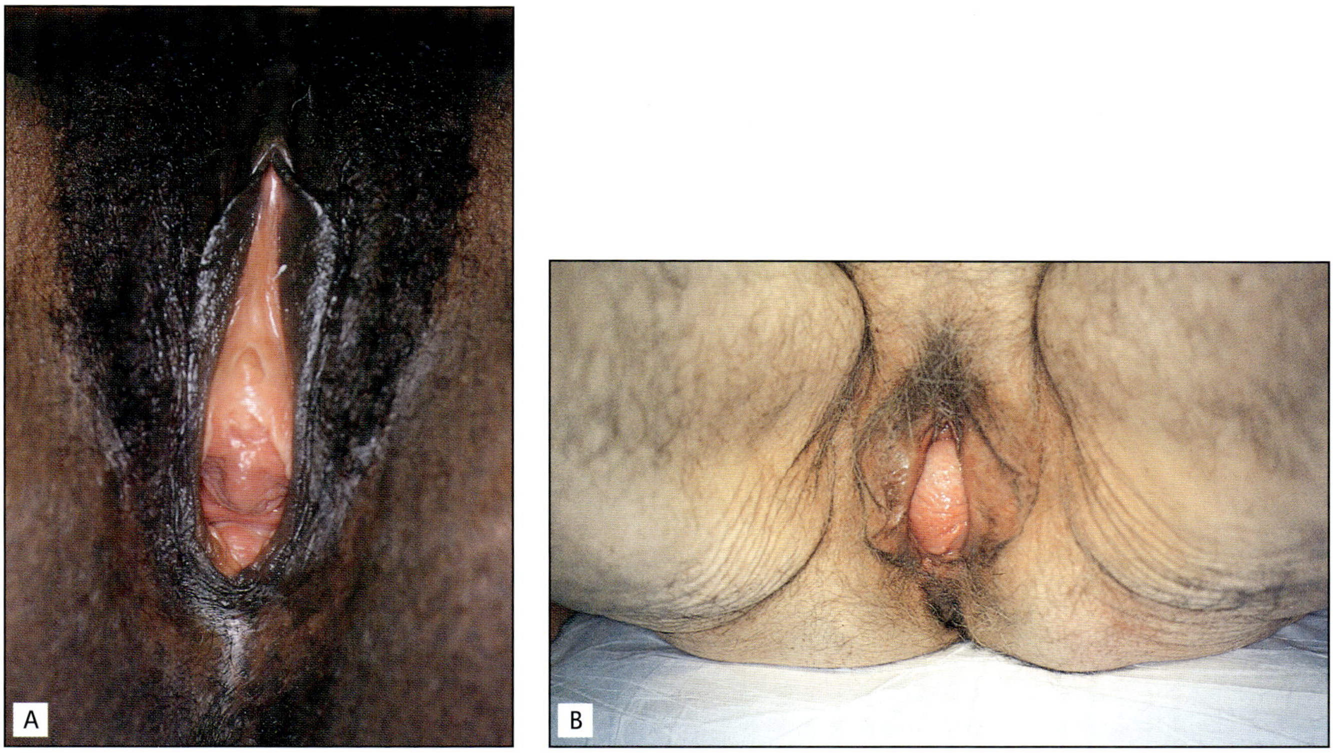

FIGURE 5-3.

Parous. **A**, After vaginal delivery, the anterior vaginal wall commonly has altered topography. These changes can include loss of one or both lateral attachments, also called the paravaginal defect. This picture demonstrates the unilateral/bilateral loss of the lateral attachment. **B**, Other topographic changes may include loss of midline support. There may be less stability of the urethrovesical junction and external urethral meatus, although this is neither symptomatic nor clinically relevant in many women. Despite marked parity-induced alterations of the vaginal topography, the woman may remain asymptomatic.

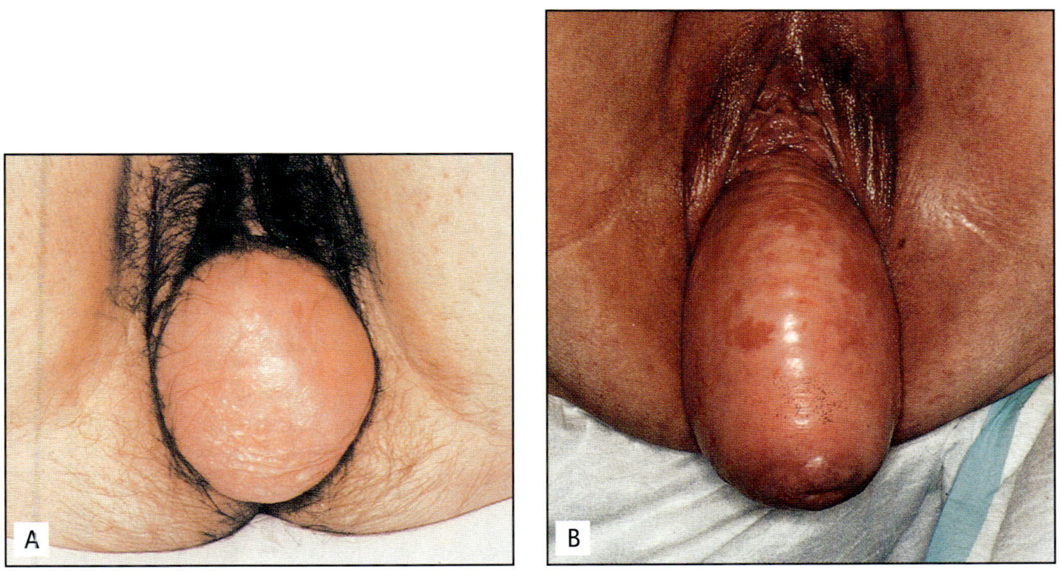

FIGURE 5-4.

Abnormal. **A**, Stage 3 pelvic organ prolapse. Minor topographic changes may progress and cause the anterior vaginal wall to protrude beyond the hymen. With continued progression of the anterior wall, there may be difficulty assessing the anatomic components that have contributed to this process. In general, once the anterior wall is more than 1 cm beyond the hymen, there is an increased likelihood of a lateral detachment (paravaginal defect, unilateral or bilateral). **B**, Stage 4 pelvic organ prolapse. Major anatomic alterations include complete loss of anterior wall support. Without speculum or bimanual examination, a loss of lateral detachment can be diagnosed, because the sites that would be normally attached are completely outside the body. Complete loss of anterior wall support always coexists with apical support abnormalities.

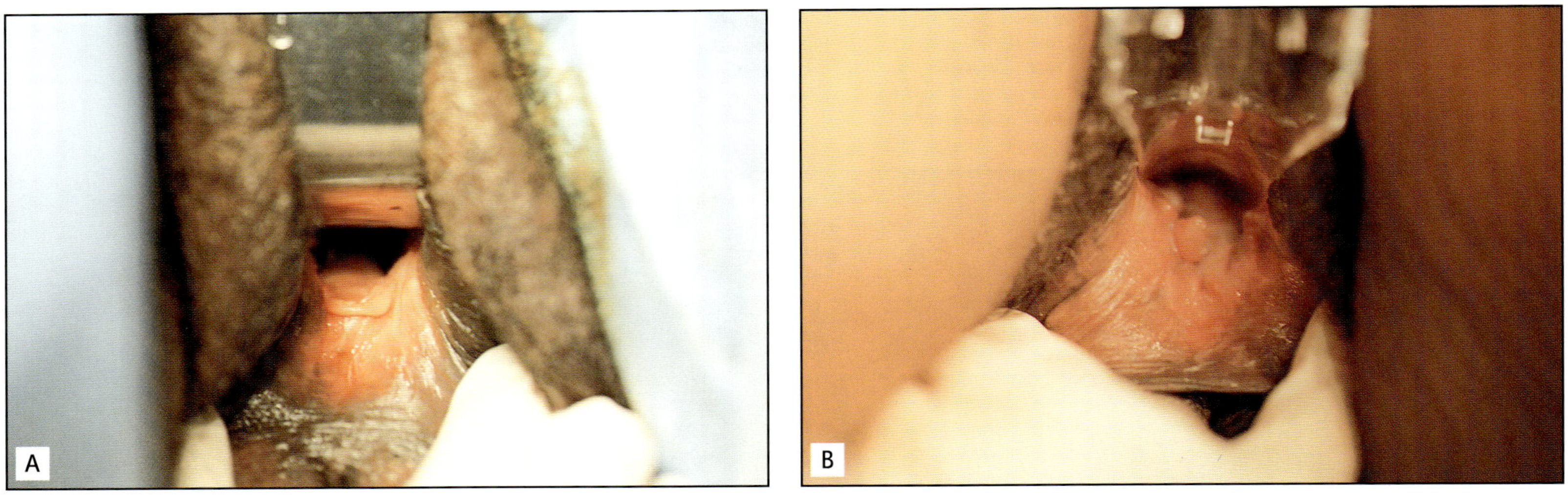

FIGURE 5-5.

Nulliparous and parous. **A**, The normal posterior vaginal wall is rugous with a firm distal attachment to the perineal body. There is a limited range of motion of the posterior wall during rectovaginal examination due to the rectovaginal fascia, which is firmly and broadly attached to the perineal body. **B**, Parous—posterior vaginal wall of a vaginally parous woman typically shows a greater range of motion during rectovaginal examination. Asymptomatic distal protrusion is common. The levator muscle strength and integrity can be digitally palpated in the posterolateral aspect of the vagina. Muscle plication during rectocele repair or perineal body reconstruction is associated with postoperative dyspareunia in some women.

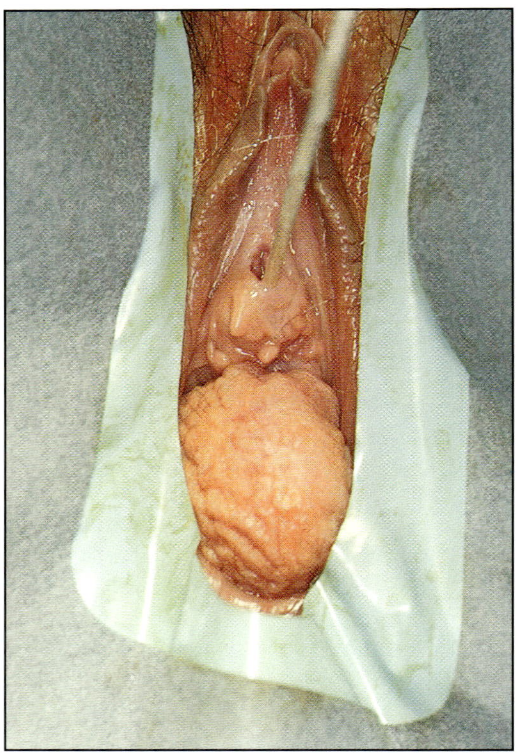

FIGURE 5-6.

Abnormal (stage 3 pelvic organ prolapse). The posterior vaginal wall may lose its support superiorly (at the upper vagina) and demonstrate prolapse beyond the hymen. The normal rugosity of this posterior wall is generally believed to represent the presence of the rectovaginal fascia, which is composed of smooth muscle and modified connective tissue.

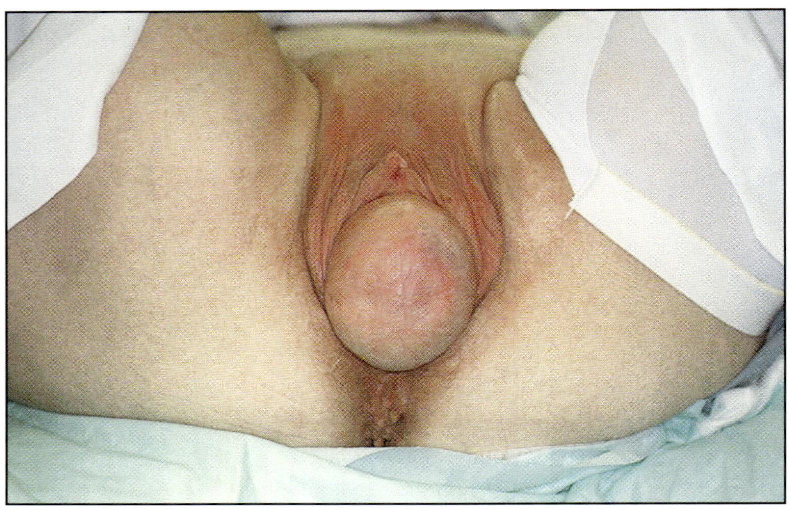

FIGURE 5-7.

Abnormal (stage 4 pelvic organ prolapse). The anatomic support of the entire posterior vaginal wall may be lost, resulting in complete eversion of the posterior vaginal wall (commonly exists with a complete vaginal vault prolapse). Beginning at the hymen, the entire posterior wall is everted. Although a rectocele may be present, about 30% of patients with this topography do not have fluoroscopic evidence for rectocele formation.

It is desirable to consider apical prolapse as the primary problem because the uterus is essentially an innocent passenger in the process of support loss. Removal of the uterus without restoring apical support may achieve a suboptimal surgical outcome. The normal apical structures (see Chapter 1) are no longer effective. The evaluation of apical support must distinguish whether or not there is cervical elongation. In cases of cervical elongation, the initial finding of cervical protrusion may be mistaken for uterine prolapse. This is best assessed in the standing, straining position.

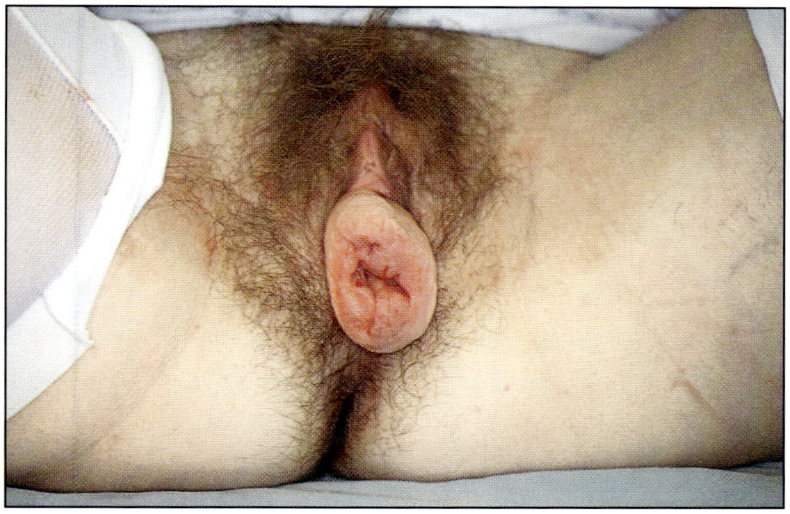

FIGURE 5-8.
Uterus present (stage 3 pelvic organ prolapse). The normal-sized uterus is present. Due to a loss of uterosacral integrity, the uterus has descended several centimeters below the hymen. Standing, straining evaluation is essential to demonstrate additional components of this prolapse. Although the primary support loss is apical, the clinician must assess the anterior and posterior walls as well. Hysterectomy must be accompanied by adequate apical support measures beyond simple attachment of elongated uterosacral ligament pedicles to the cuff. As discussed in the subsequent treatment chapters, the use of uterosacral ligaments for apical support requires shortening and reinforcement of these structures. If these ligaments are surgically inadequate, alternative apical support procedures must be performed.

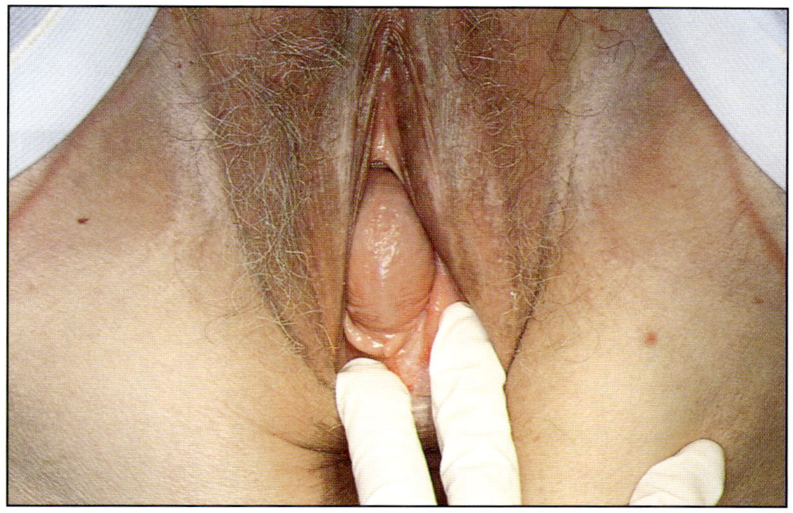

FIGURE 5-9.
Uterus absent (stage 3 pelvic organ prolapse). Vaginal vault prolapse may follow removal of the prolapsed uterus unless the apical support is addressed. Repair efforts that are directed at the anterior and posterior walls will not solve the primary problem of apical support loss in these patients. The apical support loss can be suspected by a history of prolapse developing shortly after hysterectomy for prolapse. Additionally, the apical loss can be visualized during a straining, speculum examination as the speculum is withdrawn slowly from the upper third of the vagina.

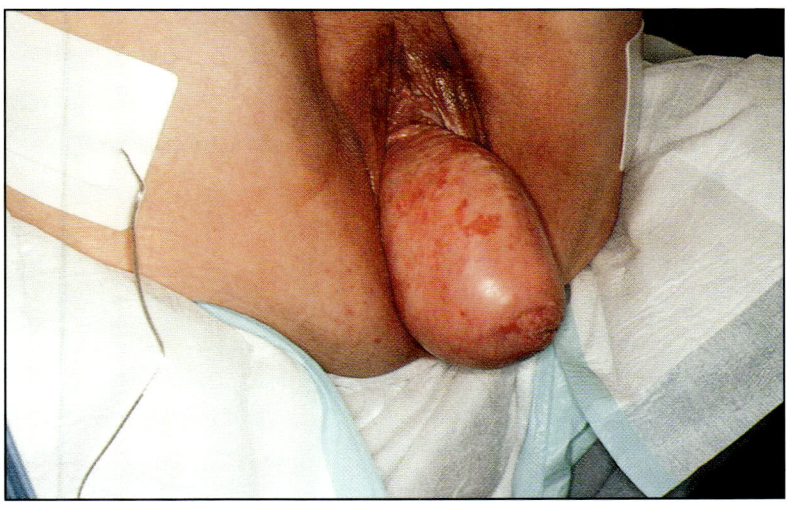

FIGURE 5-10.
Uterus present (stage 4 pelvic organ prolapse). This postmenopausal woman presents with complete lack of vaginal support. The 40-g uterus has descended well outside the body because there has been complete failure of the normal support structures of the vagina. When complete eversion is present in the supine position, it is not necessary to examine the patient in the standing, staining position because all vaginal points are maximally everted at rest.

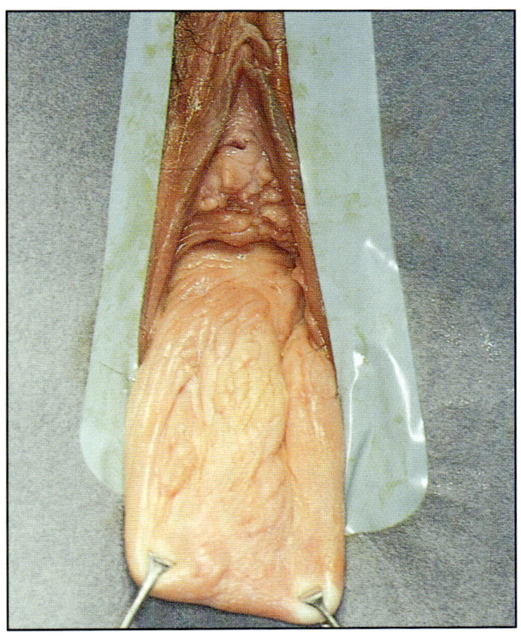

FIGURE 5-11.
Uterus absent (stage 4 pelvic organ prolapse). Hysterectomy (for stage 4 pelvic organ prolapse) without effective treatment of the apical loss will result in persistent prolapse, as demonstrated in this patient. Anatomically, it is important to recognize that the patient in Figure 5-10 and this patient both have apical failures. The major difference is the presence or absence of the uterus.

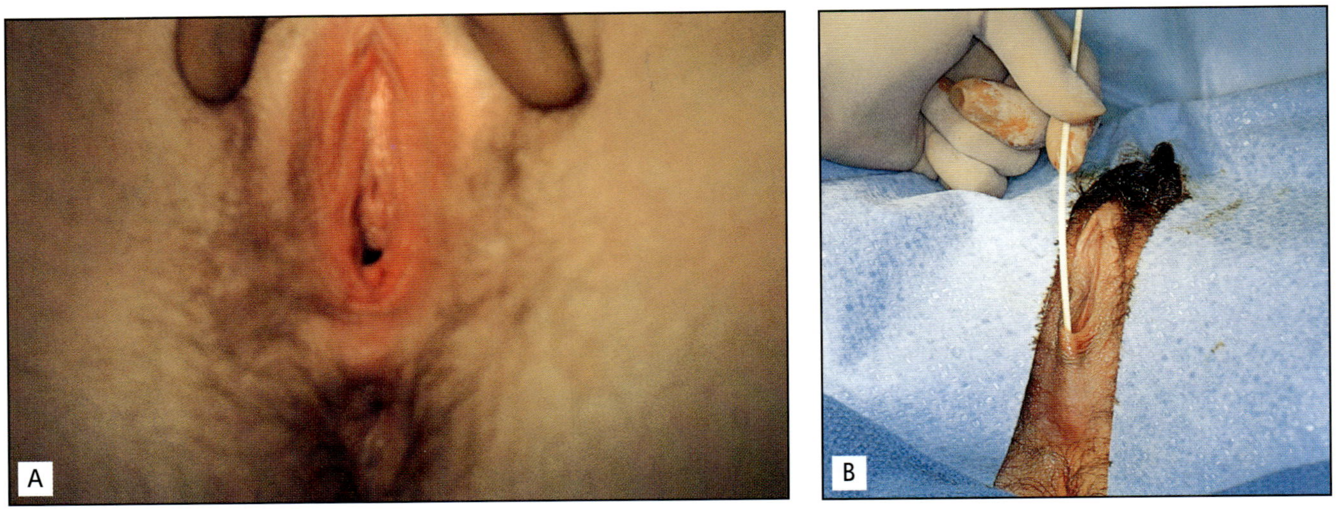

FIGURE 5-12.
Perineal body/genital hiatus. **A**, The closure of the genital hiatus is facilitated by the levator ani muscle complex. When this muscle group is poorly functioning, a widened vaginal opening may be apparent. This may or may not coexist with a small perineal body of poor integrity. Many nulliparous women have perineal body lengths of 2 to 3 cm. The function of the muscle group is certainly more important than the length of the perineal body. However, the importance of rectovaginal fascial attachment to the perineal body is critical for optimal defecation. **B**, A surgically lengthened perineal body is often a surgeon's goal during reconstruction. Preoperatively, the perineal body must be palpated carefully for strength and integrity. A surgically created bridge of skin may mask recurrent or persistent pelvic organ prolapse. This patient reported postoperative dyspareunia and a pelvic pressure consistent with the prolapsing viscera, which were held in by this band of perineal skin.

PELVIC ORGAN PROLAPSE—METHODS OF RECORDING

Systems of Grading	Advantages	Disadvantages
POP-Q[1]	Most quantitative Demonstrated reproducibility Suited for research and outcome measures	Not widely adopted Not intuitive for many clinicians Limited in descriptions of anatomic site Limited in ability to describe anterior and posterior walls
Baden Halfway System [2]	Clinically used Describes apical loss well Easy to use and understand	Pools data into four categorical groups Limited usefulness for research Reproducibility not known
Grades (0/1–3/4) [3]	Most well known Easy	Poorly described Reproducibility poor Inadequate for outcomes research
Stages (0/1–4) [3]	Easy	Poorly described Reproducibility poor Inadequate for outcomes research

FIGURE 5-13.
Pelvic organ prolapse—methods of recording. Multiple methods for describing the severity of pelvic organ prolapse have been reported. Each system has it's aspects of clinical utility and limitations. Each physician must select and adhere to his or her preferred system. Objective outcomes of surgical results are best achieved with a quantified system such as the POP-Q [1].

SITES OF POP-Q

Description		Range of Possible Values
Anterior wall		
Aa	Single point 3 cm in from hymen	-3 to +3
Ab	Using segment from 3 cm in (Aa) to apex, describes position of most distal point of anterior wall	-3 to + total vaginal length
Fosterior Wall		
Pa	Single point 3 cm in from hymen	-3 to +3
Pb	Using segment from 3 cm in (Pa) to apex, describes position of most distal point of anterior wall	-3 to + total vaginal length
Apex		
C	Position of apex when prolapse at maximum protrusion	
D	If uterus present, position posterior fornix (helpful in determining extent of cervical elongation)	
Total vaginal length (to cuff or cervix)		

FIGURE 5-14.

Sites of POP-Q. The specific sites of the POP-Q examination become more familiar with frequent use. These points are particularly helpful in recording the surgical outcomes in an objective manner. The conditions of the examination (patient position, use of strain, recording instrument) should be identical before and after surgery to obtain a meaningful comparison of any change.

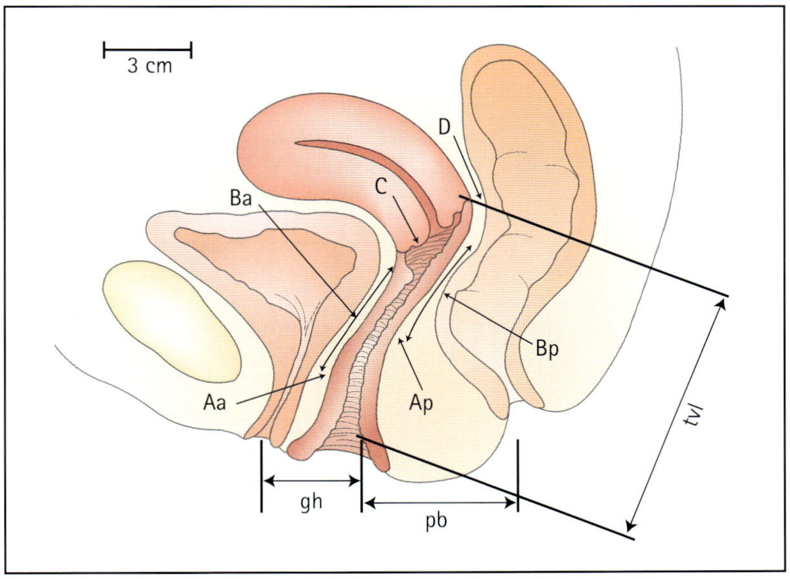

FIGURE 5-15.

Diagram of the POP-Q sites. This figure illustrates the anatomic positions of the POP-Q sites [1].

Pcint Aa Anterior wall	Point Ba Anterior wall	Point C Cervix or cuff
Cenital hiatus	Perineal body	Total vaginal length
Point Ap posterior wall	Point Bp posterior wall	Point D posterior fornix

FIGURE 5-16.

Recording the POP-Q—numeric form. This figure shows a simple method of recording the POP-Q values in an office chart. Although this method is convenient, each clinician may develop a method most suited to her or his situation.

Pelvic Floor Fluoroscopy

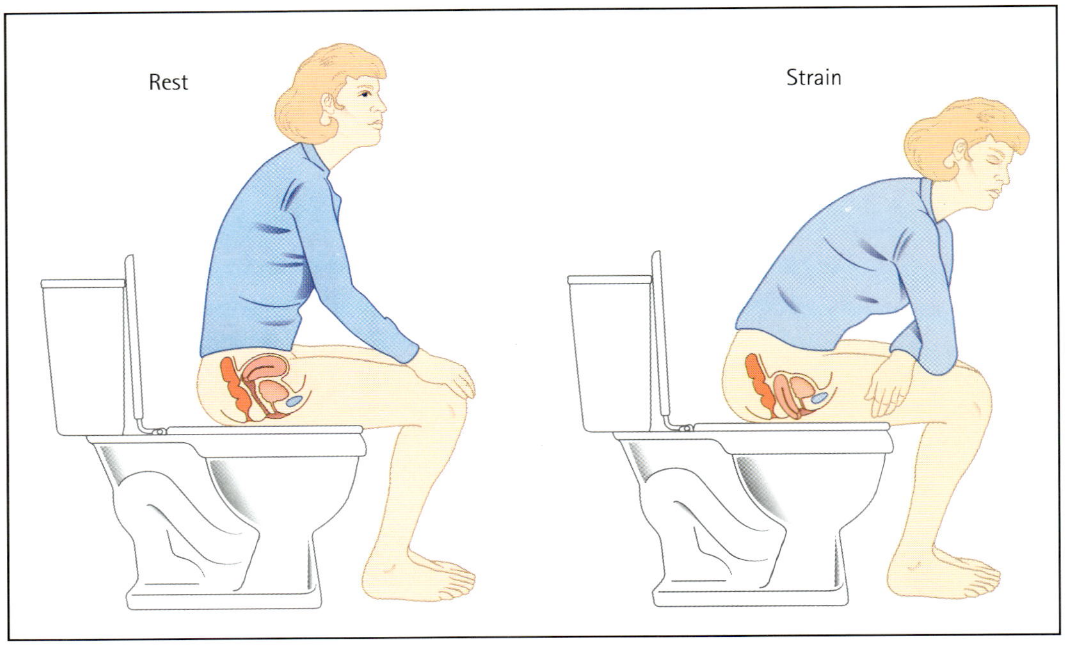

FIGURE 5-17.
Commode. Defecating cystoproctography is one of the terms used for fluoroscopic, dynamic imaging of the pelvic viscera. This technique can be performed using opacification of a single viscera or all four relevant pelvic viscera (bladder, vaginal, small bowel, and large bowel). This adjunct to physical examination provides additional information about visceral function and support. Technical aspects have been described elsewhere [4,5]. The pelvis is imaged in the lateral, seated position. Simulated defecation efforts promote maximal protrusion of the prolapsed structures.

The patient is seated on a radiolucent commode. After contrast administration, defecation of the rectal contrast occurs. Abnormalities such as an open anal canal before defecation may be important clues to undiscovered fecal incontinence. Serial lateral images are obtained throughout the defecation process. This degree of strain maximizes the prolapse, frequently beyond what was visible during standard physical examination.

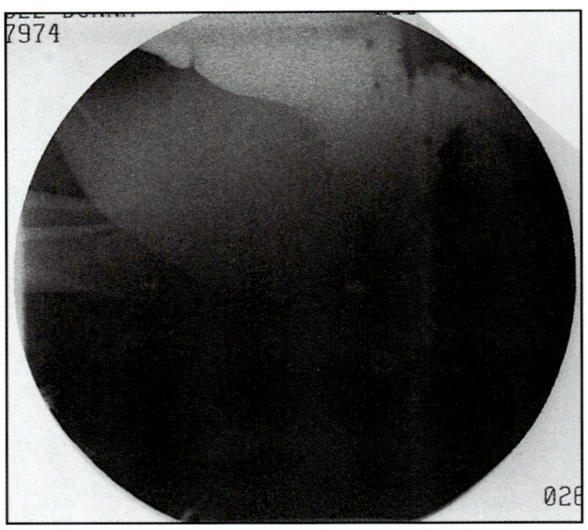

FIGURE 5-18.
Normal bladder/urethrovesical junction (UVJ) position. The well-supported UVJ is demonstrated with reference to the symphysis pubis in an asymptomatic woman. Small "beaking" at the UVJ is inconsequential and does not represent sphincteric dysfunction. The urethrovesical angle is no longer considered an important diagnostic aid for either function or anatomic assessment.

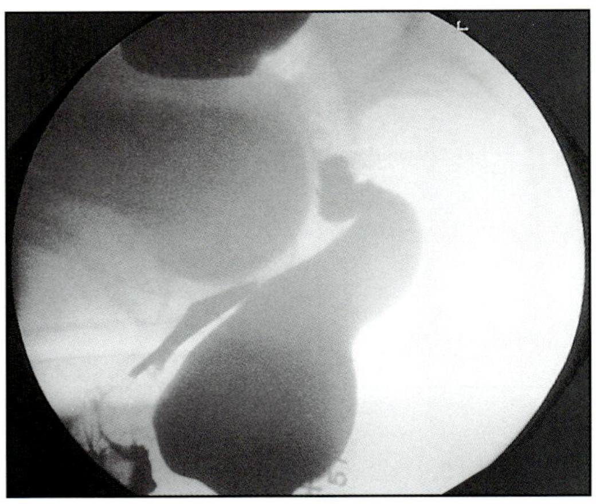

FIGURE 5-19.
Bladder neck support after urethropexy. After Burch urethropexy, the bladder neck has high support, although the more proximal portion of the bladder is less well supported.

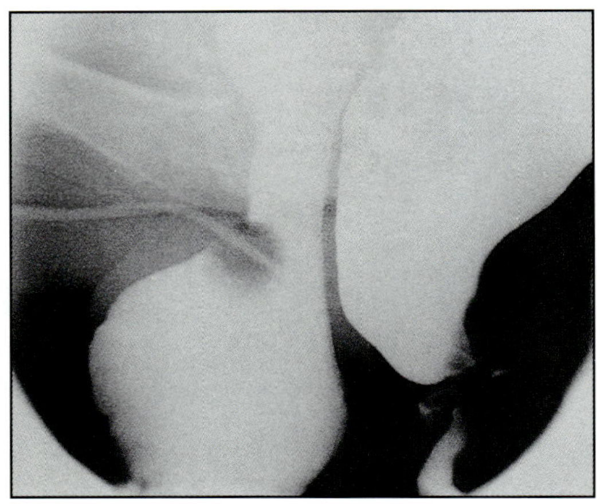

FIGURE 5-20.
Bladder prolapse. This image demonstrates complete loss of bladder support. The Foley bulb estimates the position of the urethrovesical junction. At the completion of defecation, only the bladder was in an abnormal position. There was no rectocele or enterocele. The physical examination was consistent with stage 4 pelvic organ prolapse (complete vaginal vault eversion). This image demonstrates the importance of combining the topographic findings with the visceral abnormalities, which are confirmed with imaging modalities.

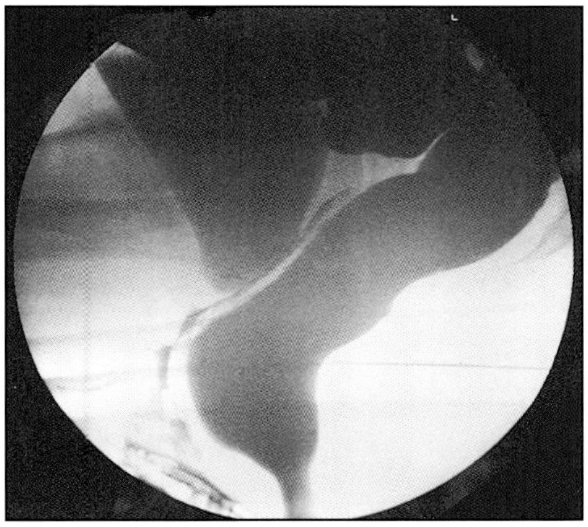

FIGURE 5-21.

Normal rectal emptying. During defecation, there is a protrusion of the anterior rectal wall into the posterior vaginal wall. This normal "range of motion" is not well understood or quantified as yet. No rectocele is diagnosed when the anterior rectal protrusion is transient and there is complete, spontaneous rectal emptying. A great deal of overlap occurs between "normal" and "abnormal" and these studies must be interpreted with caution.

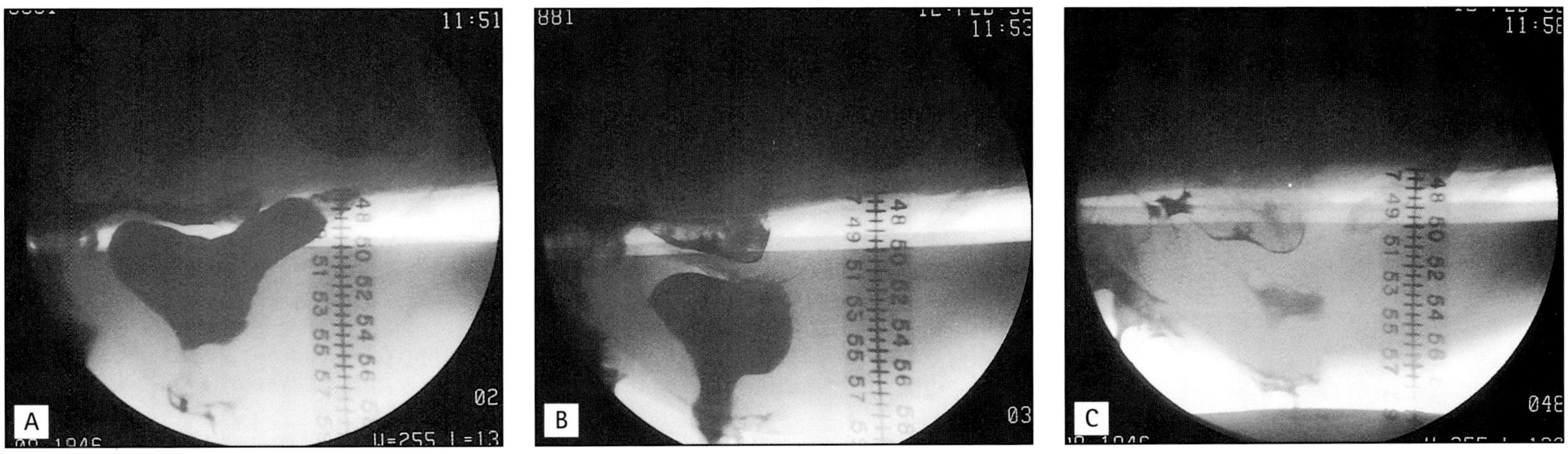

FIGURE 5-22.

Transient "rectocele" formation. This series of images (**A–C**) demonstrates rectal protrusion (3.5 cm) during the study. However, the rectum empties completely and spontaneously by the end of the study.

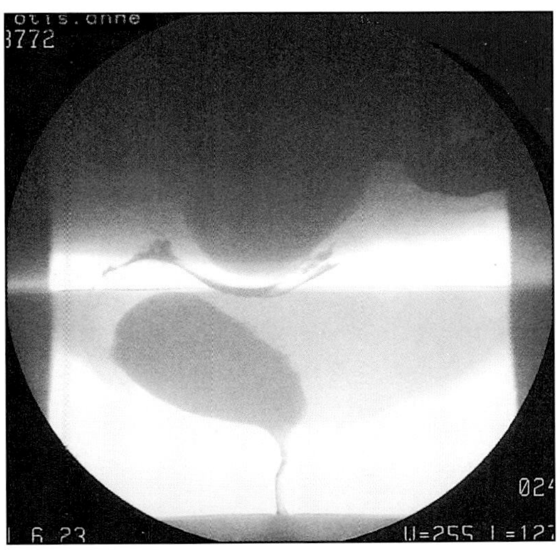

FIGURE 5-23.

Retaining rectocele. This image demonstrates a large rectal protrusion that persists and appears to trap contrast at the end of spontaneous defecation. This distal abnormality is the most common appearance of a rectocele on fluoroscopy. The distal location is typical for the initial presentation of a rectocele, whereas previously operated rectoceles may be located more proximally.

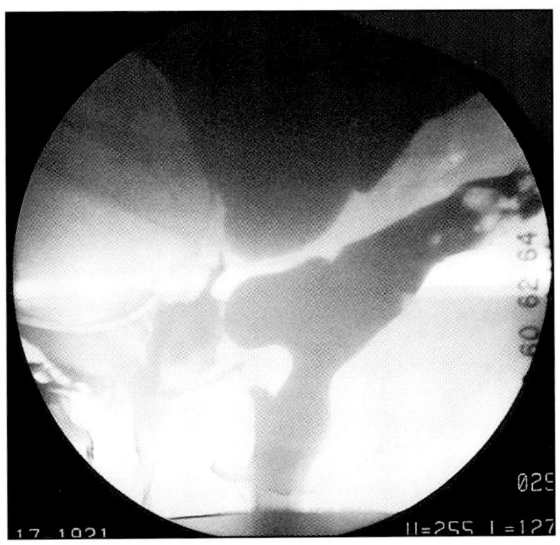

FIGURE 5-24.

Abnormal position of rectocele (post-colporrhaphy). This image demonstrates the more proximal position of a recurrent rectocele after posterior colporrhaphy. The plication of the levator complex can be seen distally. Proximal to this plication, the area of lesser strength protrudes over the plicated muscles. The patient reported persistent difficult defecation with the need to manually assist her defecation.

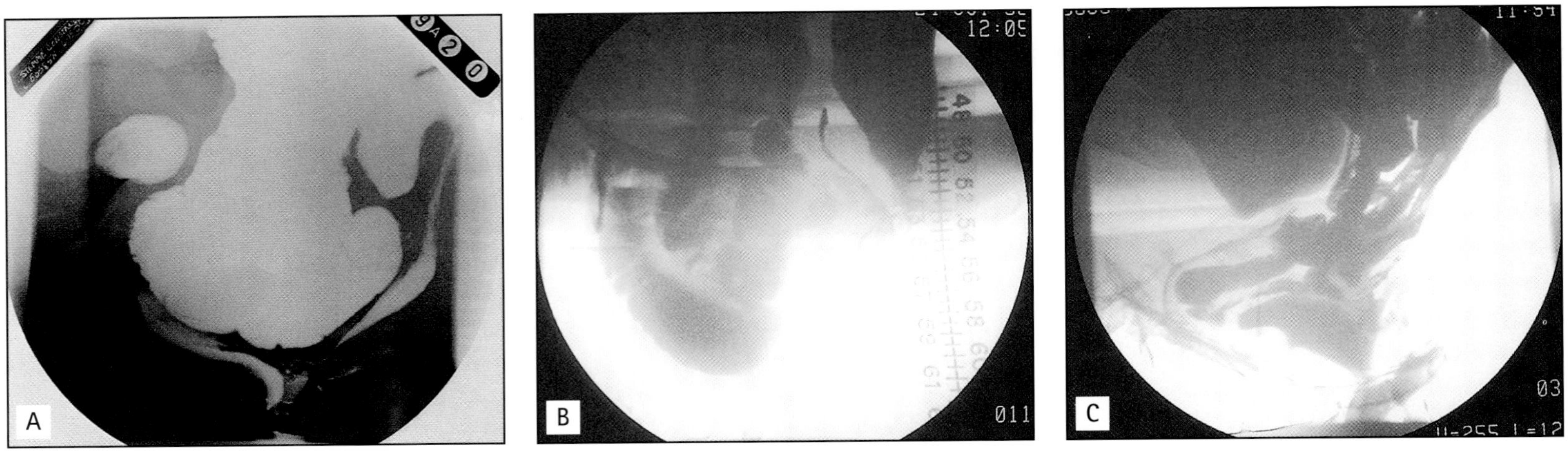

FIGURE 5-25.

Enterocele. **A**, Small bowel loops are seen posterior to the vagina in the absence of any rectocele formation. This image clarifies the visceral position when the posterior vaginal wall protrudes, causing the clinician to suspect rectocele. Likewise the bladder is adequately supported. Topographically, this patient had recurrent apical prolapse following vaginal hysterectomy for uterine prolapse. **B**, Enterocele, uterus present. This image demonstrates the abnormal small bowel position in a woman who clinically presents with uterine prolapse. The small bowel is abnormally located in the majority of such patients. In this patient, the enterocele is anterior to the uterus. **C**, Enterocele after sacrospinous ligament suspension. This patient had undergone vaginal hysterectomy with sacrospinous ligament suspension for uterine prolapse. Her rapidly recurrent posterior vaginal wall prolapse was assumed to be rectocele formation, although this image clarifies the situation. Here a loop of small bowel has passed through the purse-string cul-de-plasty stitch that was placed at the time of the original surgery.

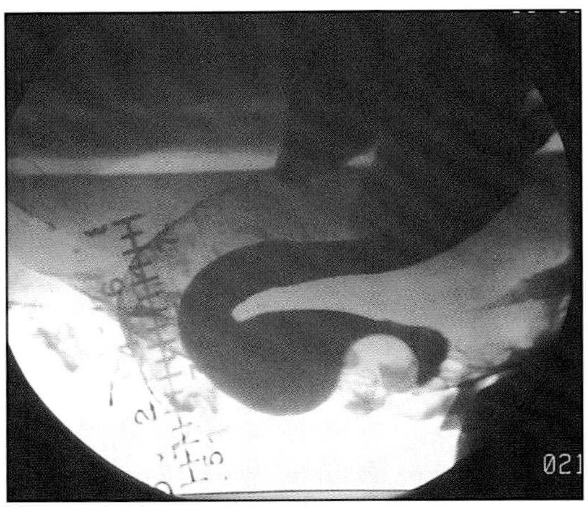

FIGURE 5-26.

Sigmoidocele. Less commonly, posterior wall or apical prolapse can be caused by redundant rectosigmoid. The optimal surgical management of this finding remains under study.

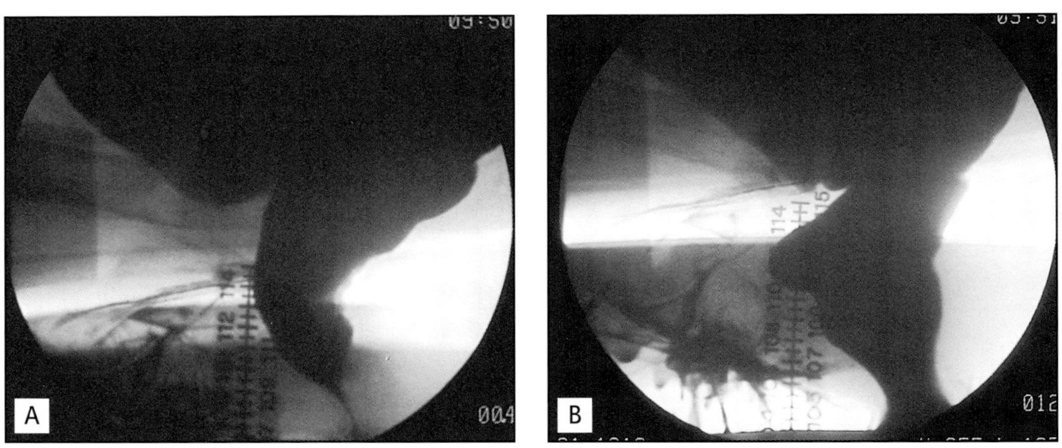

FIGURE 5-27.

Enterocele with rectocele. These photographs (**A–D**) demonstrate an apparently retaining rectocele that ultimately empties after maximal protrusion of the large enterocele. Although the patient may not report defecation difficulties, isolated enterocele repair may unmask rectocele symptoms.

(*Continued on next page*)

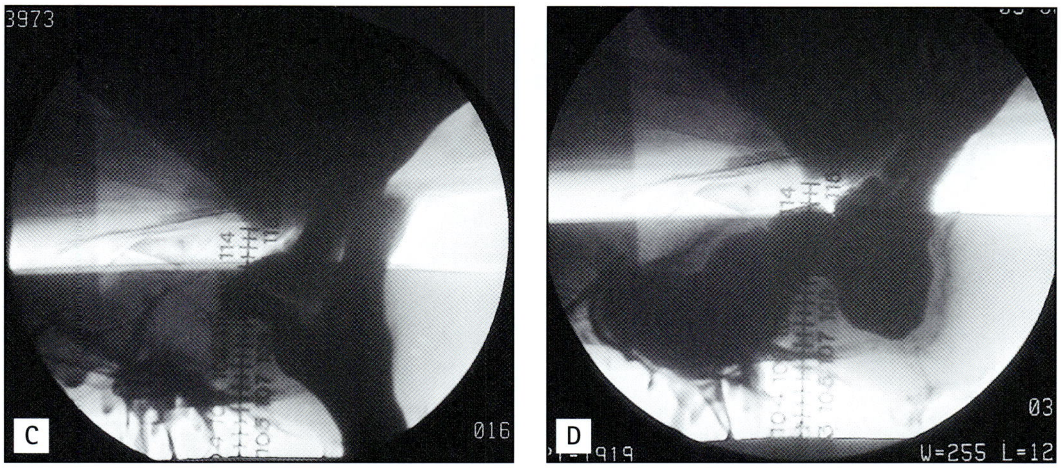

FIGURE 5-27. *(Continued)*
Thus, this possibility may warrant consideration if such symptoms have a new onset after reconstructive procedures.

OTHER PROLAPSES

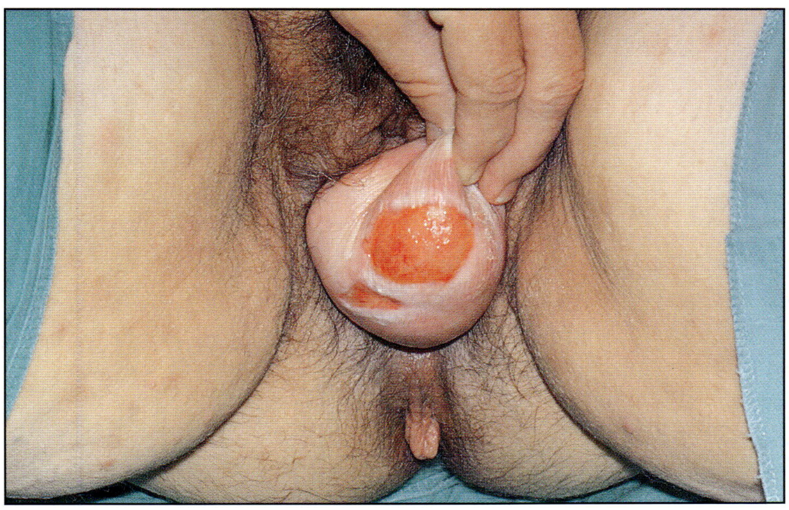

FIGURE 5-28.
Chronic ulceration of long-standing vaginal prolapse. This patient was told that she did not require surgical repair of her posthysterectomy prolapse because she was no longer sexually active. She sought care when she experienced increasing vaginal bleeding. The chronic ulceration should prompt evaluation for vaginal neoplasia. Experts consider these patients to be at increased risk for vaginal evisceration.

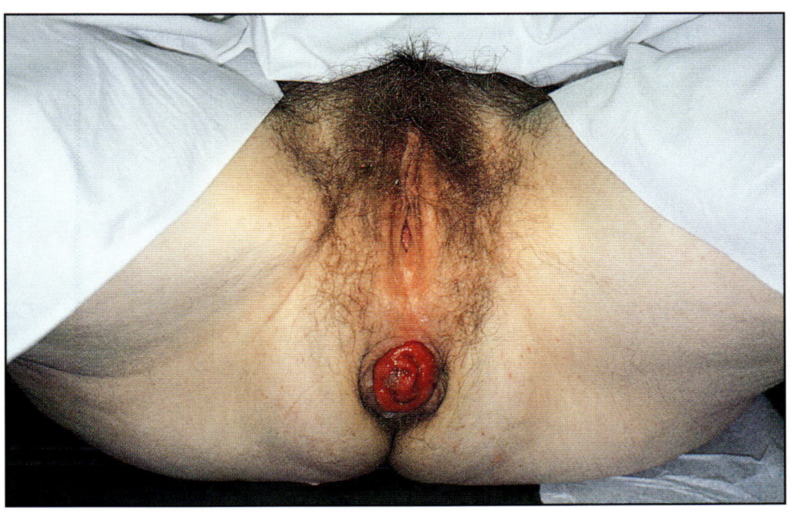

FIGURE 5-29.
Rectal prolapse. The report of hemorrhoids should prompt evaluation of defecation habits and careful anorectal examination. This patient believed her rectal prolapse was severe hemorrhoids. Although she did have hemorrhoids in the typical locations, they were very small. The rectal prolapse extended about 4 cm outside her anal skin and became increasingly difficult to replace, prompting her to consult a physician.

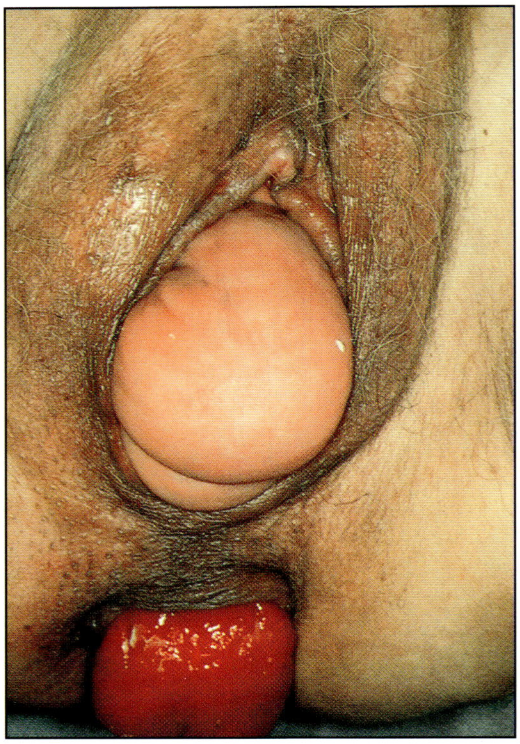

FIGURE 5-30.

Coexisting rectal and vaginal prolapse. Rectal and vaginal prolapse can coexist, albeit uncommonly. Simultaneous repair procedures can be accomplished, relieving the patient of both conditions with an adequate surgical outcome.

RECURRENT PROLAPSE/SURGICAL COMPLICATIONS

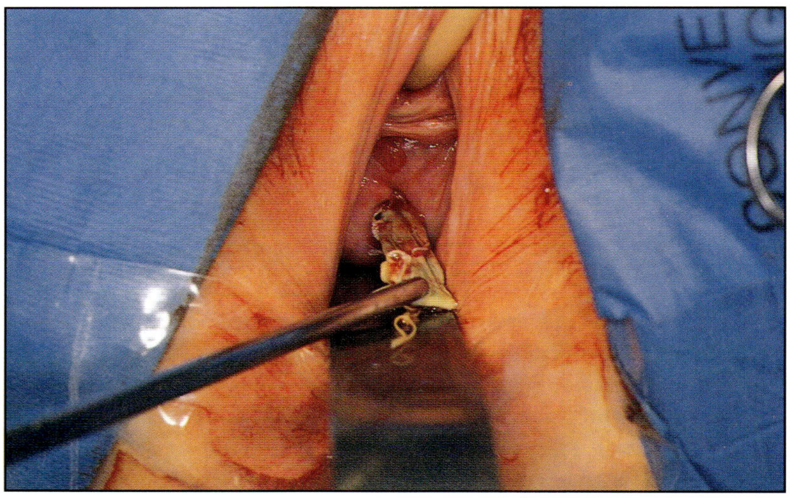

FIGURE 5-31.

Foreign body complications. The use of foreign bodies, either sutures or mesh, is common in the treatment of pelvic organ prolapse. The consultant may be faced with patients with an unsatisfactory or complicated surgical course. It is helpful to have an awareness of foreign body complications that can be detected during the physical examination. The previously placed sacrocolpopexy graft has eroded into the markedly shortened vagina in three places. Patients typically present with chronic, foul-smelling vaginal discharge.

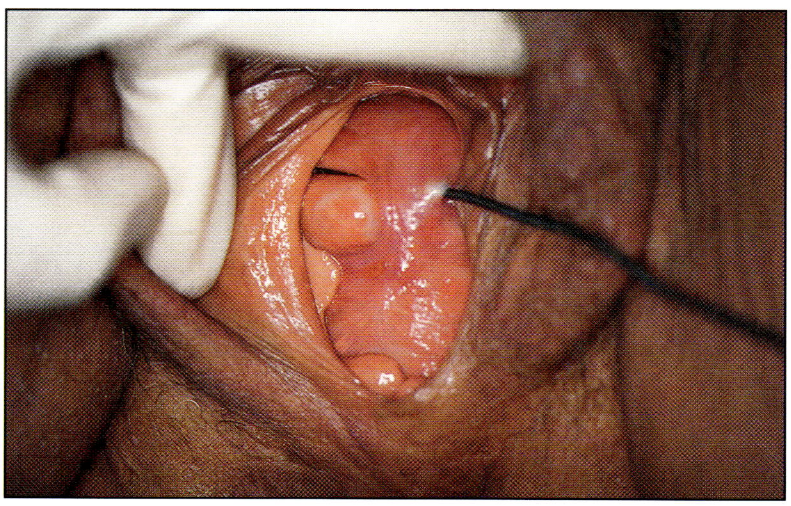

FIGURE 5-32.

Loss of vaginal length after colporrhaphy. This patient had recurrent pelvic organ prolapse that was treated with a series of three anterior and posterior colporrhaphies. Her chief complaint of pelvic pressure persisted. The vaginal length had been reduced to 4 cm with a markedly reduced caliber and pliability.

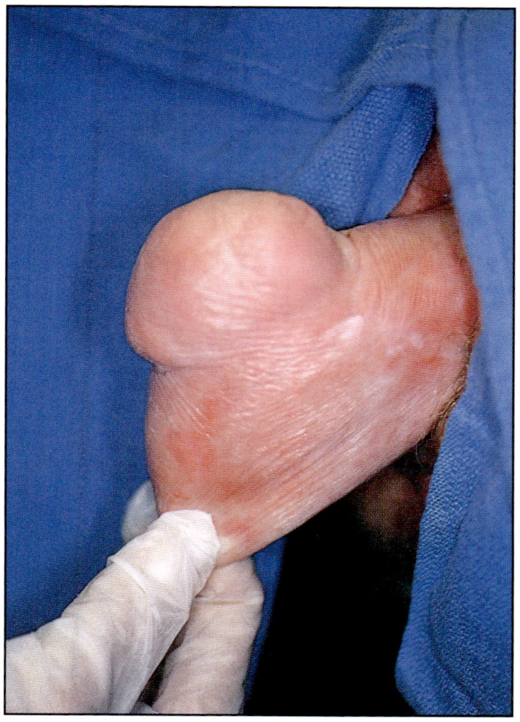

FIGURE 5-33.
Recurrent prolapse. This patient presented with pelvic organ prolapse after a transvaginal paravaginal with sacrospinous ligament suspension performed for posthysterectomy vaginal vault prolapse. The unusual midline defect may have resulted from an undetected midline defect preoperatively, which was exacerbated by lateral attachments.

REFERENCES

1. Bump RC, Mattiasson A, Bø K, *et al.*: The standardization of terminology of female pelvic organ prolapse and pelvic floor dysfunction. *Am J Obstet Gynecol* 1996, 175:10–17.
2. Baden WF, Walker T: *Surgical Repair of Vaginal Defects*. Philadelphia: JB Lippincott; 1992.
3. Brubaker L, Norton P: Current clinical nomenclature for description of pelvic organ prolapse. *J Pelvic Surg* 1996, 2:257–259.
4. Kelvin FM, Maglinte DDT, Benson JT: Evacuation proctography (defecography): an aid to the investigation of pelvic floor disorders. *Obstet Gynecol* 1994, 83:307–314.
5. Brubaker L, Saclarides T, eds: *The Female Pelvic Floor: Disorders of Function and Support*. Philadelphia: FA Davis; 1996.

CHAPTER 6

Treatment of Urinary Incontinence

Jeffrey Cornella

Millions of Americans can benefit from interventions directed at the management of urinary incontinence. The approach to the incontinent patient requires an understanding of genitourinary pathophysiology, pelvic anatomy, and neurology, balanced with astute clinical acumen. It is important to understand the limitations of urodynamic testing and the benefits of behavioral intervention. Medical treatment may be used in the care of the incontinent patient, but patient education is also a key component of management, with attention directed especially toward quality of life considerations. Patients with incontinence often have chronic symptoms that must be addressed over the long-term.

DETERMINATION OF URINARY INCONTINENCE

GENERAL ASSESSMENT

A. MANAGEMENT OF URINARY INCONTINENCE

Behavioral
Pharmacologic
Surgical

B. MANAGEMENT OF SUI

History and physical examination
Simple office bladder filling
Residual urine determination

C. MEDICAL CONDITIONS

Diabetes
Pulmonary disease
Neurologic disorders
Medications

FIGURE 6-1.

Categories of management. **A**, The three categories of management of female urinary incontinence are behavioral, pharmacologic, and surgical. To use the modalities appropriately, the practitioner must have a strong knowledge of pelvic floor pathophysiology and the limitations of laboratory assessment. **B**, Management of stress urinary incontinence (SUI) requires clinical decisions. The initial office visit allows careful historical review and objective examination of pelvic support. Simple bladder filling and residual urine determination are significantly beneficial in assessing parameters of basic bladder function in the majority of instances. Clinical decisions are affected by the impact of the incontinence on the patient's lifestyle and previous treatments and surgical procedures. Symptoms may not accurately predict objective findings. **C**, Relevant medical conditions in the patient's medical history should be reviewed for entities that may affect the bladder, such as neurologic processes, environmental exposures, and diseases that compromise the bladder or put additional stresses on the pelvic floor. Previously used unsuccessful medications may be successful when used at different dosages or when combined with timed voiding.

PHYSICAL EXAMINATION AND DIAGNOSIS

A. SUPINE PHYSICAL EXAMINATION

Deep tendon reflexes
Neurologic examination
POP Q evaluation
Bimanual examination of the pelvis

B. STANDING PHYSICAL EXAMINATION

Stress testing
Examination of prolapse
Evaluation of perineal descent

FIGURE 6-2.

Supine and standing examinations. **A**, The pelvic floor examination varies and is related to position and the amount of force placed on the tissues. It is important to assess tissue integrity, neurologic support (S2–4), ability to contract the circumvaginal musculature, pelvic organ support, urethrovesical junction support, and the absence of pathology on bimanual examination. **B**, Perineal descent is evaluated with straining in both the supine and standing positions. In the standing position a digital examination of the vagina allows assessment of apex and vaginal wall descent, which may vary compared to the supine position. POP Q — pelvic organ prolapse quantification.

A. COMPARISON OF SIMPLE OFFICE FILLING AND MULTICHANNEL TESTING

Sensitivity	88.1%
Specificity	77%
Positive predictive value	82%

B. OFFICE DIAGNOSIS OF DETRUSOR INSTABILITY

Sensitivity	64%
Specificity	86.8%
Positive predictive value	83.3%

C. SIMPLE OFFICE CYSTOGRAM

Residual urine determination
Simple bladder filling
Measurement of sensation and maximum capacity
Standing and supine stress test

FIGURE 6-3.

Bladder filling. **A**, The value of simple office bladder filling tends to be underestimated and multichannel urodynamics overestimated by many practitioners. Wall and colleagues [1] have shown office filling to be a valuable component of patient assessment with a positive predictive value of 82% for genuine stress incontinence (GSI). **B**, Wall noted that the demonstration of urge incontinence during simple bladder filling is a reliable predictor of detrusor instability, but its absence is less reliable in excluding detrusor overactivity. The negative predictive value for detrusor instability was 70.2%. **C**, In a simple office cystogram, residual urine determination is accomplished by ultrasound or with the filling catheter. The bladder is filled under gravity and subjective sensation of first desire, fullness, and strong desire are recorded. Stress testing follows with and without prolapse reduction in the supine and standing positions. Rises in the fluid meniscus suggestive of possible bladder contractions are recorded. Urinalysis and urine cultures are performed.

CLINICAL DIAGNOSIS OF SUI

Predominant complaint: SUI
Positive stress test
Residual volume: < 50 ml
Functional bladder capacity: > 400 cc

FIGURE 6-4.

Criteria for clinical diagnosis. Videla and Wall also investigated simple criteria that correlate with the diagnosis of stress urinary incontinence (SUI). Criteria were evaluated in 652 women presenting for evaluation of lower urinary tract complaints. If these four criteria were met, SUI was confirmed in 94% of such patients. In 15% of patients with stress incontinence, detrusor instability was also demonstrated [2].

Algorithms and Education

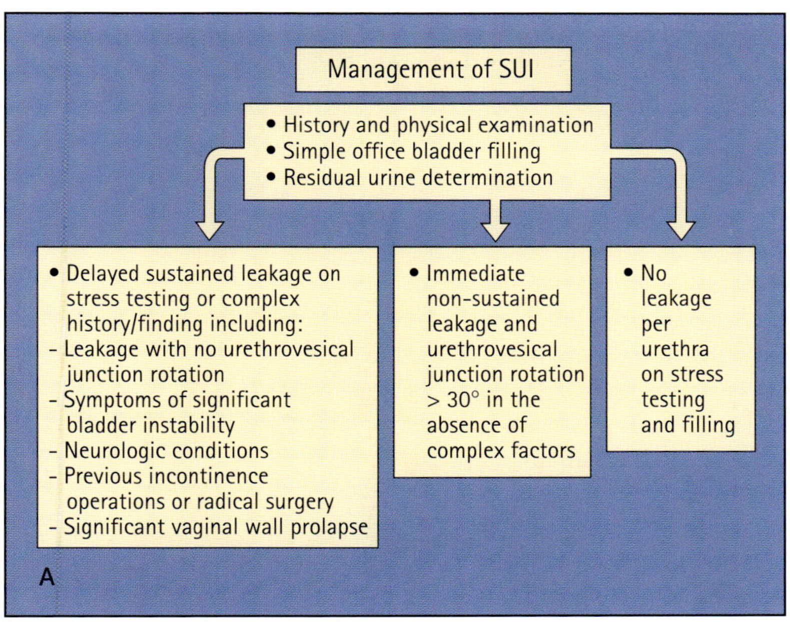

FIGURE 6-5.

Management algorithms. **A**, On initial evaluation, patients can be categorized as having complex incontinence, simple incontinence, or no evidence of incontinence. This allows use of a management algorithm [3].

(*Continued on next page*)

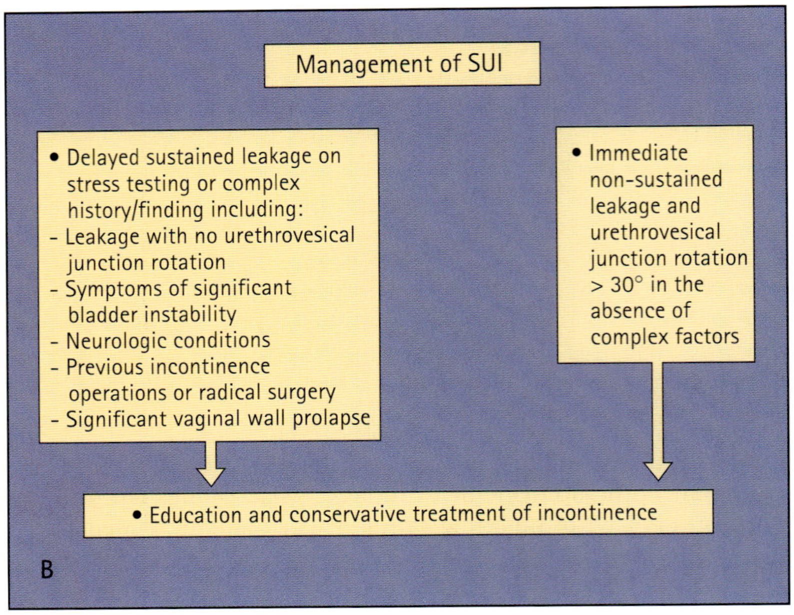

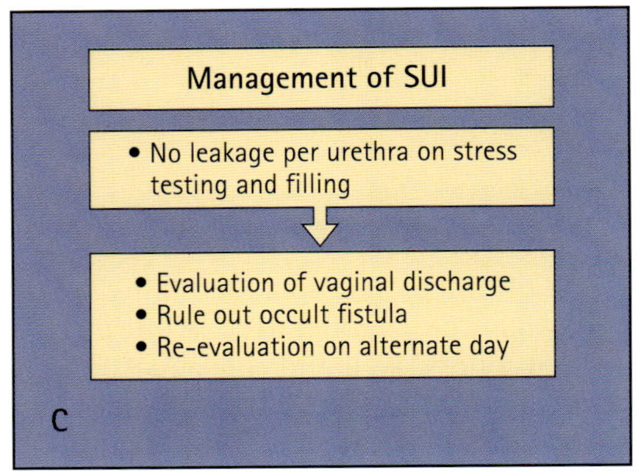

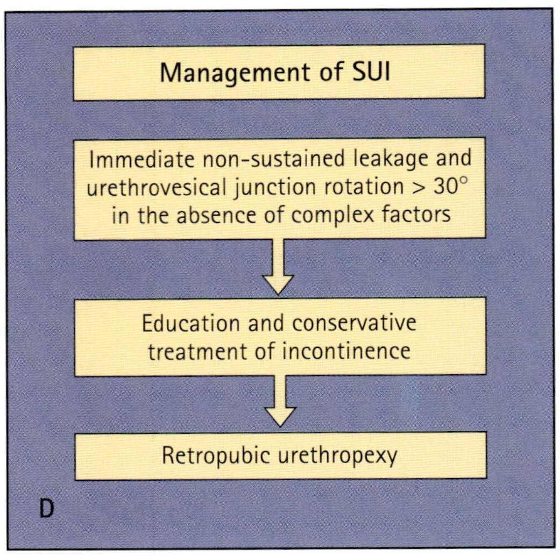

FIGURE 6-5. *(Continued)*

B, Patents who demonstrate urinary incontinence benefit from education and behavioral management. A trial of conservative treatment may be considered before additional evaluation. **C**, If no leakage of urine is noted at the time of office assessment and testing, consider vaginal discharge as a possibility, especially if the history of urinary incontinence is mild. **D**, The majority of patients with primary stress urinary incontinence (SUI) will be in this category.

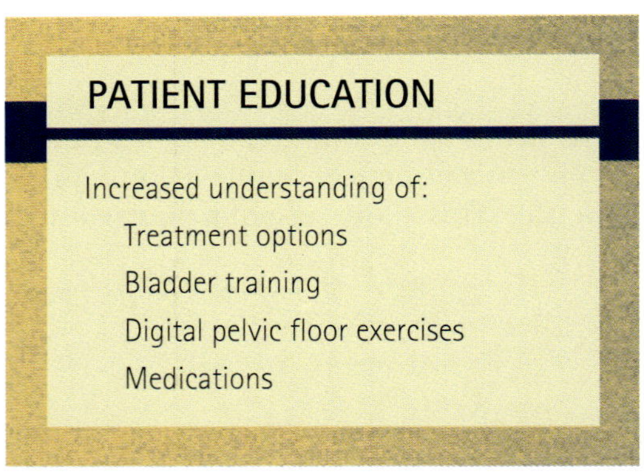

FIGURE 6-6.

Patient education. An office educator or nurse can accomplish patient education if a classroom option is not available. Education allows better participation by the patient in the decision-making process. It also facilitates treatment because the patient receives reinforcement of management principles that may aid in motivation. The patient may also have the opportunity to meet others with urinary incontinence.

BEHAVIORAL TREATMENT

BEHAVIORAL THERAPY

Timed voiding/prompted voiding

Bladder retraining

Pelvic muscle rehabilitation

FIGURE 6-7.

Behavioral therapy. Behavioral treatments benefit most individuals and do not compromise future treatment options. If patients have physical or mental limitations, a caregiver may be required for toileting assistance (scheduled voiding/habit training). Cognitive ability and motivation are highly important when using bladder retraining and pelvic muscle rehabilitation. Behavioral treatments often benefit patients choosing pharmacologic and surgical options as well.

A. PELVIC MUSCLE REHABILITATION

Pelvic muscle exercises

Pelvic floor biofeedback

Functional electrical stimulation

Vaginal cones

B. LONG-TERM EFFECT 5 YEARS AFTER CESSATION

Significant increase in incontinence measured by pad test at 5 years

75% showed no leakage on stress testing

C. MULTIMEASUREMENT BIOFEEDBACK

Used in conjunction with PME and bladder retraining

Stresses avoidance of co-muscular contraction

Increases response when compared to verbal feedback alone

D. FUNCTIONAL ELECTRICAL STIMULATION

Results of randomized controlled trials are conflicting

Pelvic floor exercises should be the first choice of treatment

Studies with optimal stimulation parameters needed

FIGURE 6-8.

Pelvic muscle rehabilitation. **A**, The specific effects of Kegel exercises or pelvic muscle exercises on lower urinary muscle function are not well understood. Kegel exercises may be helpful both in instances of stress and urge incontinence. The literature suggests that if exercises are appropriately performed with multiple interaction follow-up, that much higher response rates may be achieved. Other methods of pelvic floor rehabilitation such as cones and functional electrical stimulation may facilitate teaching Kegel exercises and do not appear to have objective benefits aside from the actual exercises [4,5]. **B**, The weaker the urethra, the less effective Kegel exercises may be in treating urinary stress incontinence. Patients lose muscle and nerve function each year of their lives with a tendency to exhibit further decreases in urethral pressure. The results of this study [6] showed a significant increase in leakage assessed by pad test and leakage index. Other variables such as visible leakage, social activity index, and satisfaction rates demonstrated stable results. **C**, The addition of biofeedback increases the response rates of pelvic floor exercises. Multimeasurement biofeedback allows feedback of bladder pressure, rectal pressure, and external anal sphincter function. When compared to verbal-digital feedback alone, multimeasurement feedback allowed improvement in strength and selective control of pelvic muscles. The multiple biofeedback group demonstrated a reduction of 75.9% incontinence when compared to verbal feedback (51%) [7]. **D**, Bo reviewed the literature on randomized-controlled trials of functional electrical stimulation. Nine studies evaluated the effect of electrical stimulation on stress loss and one on urge incontinence. Only three studies had sufficient sample size to enable a conclusion. Two studies demonstrated a negative effect and one a positive effect [4]. PME—pelvic muscle exercises.

PHARMACOLOGIC TREATMENT

PHARMACOLOGIC

Class	Drug	Dosage, mg
Anticholinergic	Hyoscyamine	0.125–0.25 qid
	Propantheline	7.5–30 tid– qid
Antispasmodic	Oxybutynin	2.5 bid–10 qid
	Oxybutynin XL	5 qd – 10 qd
Antimuscarinic	Tolterodine	1–2 bid
Tricyclic	Imipramine	10–25 qd–tid

FIGURE 6-9.

Common drugs for the treatment of urgency incontinence. α-Agonist agents such as phenylpropanolamine may be used for patients with stress incontinence.

TOLTERODINE

Features	Study	Urodynamic Outcome Measures	Compared to Placebo
Muscarinic receptor antagonist Dose dependent inhibition: Bladder contractility (DD 01) Less affinity for parotid receptors (3-fold) Clinically equivalent to oxybutynin	306 patients Randomized to 3 groups Placebo 1 mg bid 2 mg bid	First desire to void Volume at first bladder contraction Maximum capacity Max Pdet	Significant reduction: voids/day Increased: mean voided volume Significant improvement: FDV Significant increase: threshold volume

FIGURE 6-10.

Tolterodine. Tolterodine is a muscarinic receptor antagonist recently approved for treatment of urinary frequency and incontinence. It is metabolized in the liver, forming an active metabolite, a 5-hydroxymethyl derivative. Both tolterodine and the derivative show high affinity for muscarinic receptors and low affinity for other receptors or calcium channels. The drug is contraindicated in patients with urinary retention, gastric retention, or uncontrolled narrow-angle glaucoma [8]. Millard performed a phase III study to determine the clinical and urodynamic efficacy of the drug and to monitor the safety/adverse event profile in patients with bladder overactivity. Frequency-volume charts were taken at 2, 4, 8, and 12 weeks [9]. The main outcome measures were number of voids/day, number of incontinence episodes/day, and the mean volume voided per micturition. In comparison to placebo, both the 1- and the 2-mg doses of tolterodine were associated with a significant reduction in voids per day and an increase in mean voided volume and first desire to void (FDV). The majority of patients treated with tolterodine are begun on 2 mg twice daily. Max Pdet—maximum detrusor pressure.

RECTAL OXYBUTYNIN

Clinical Features	Effect	Oral, min	Rectal, min	Rectal administration results
N-desethyl oxybutynin	Detection	15	Gradual	Steady state levels in excess of oral which last < 12 h
Metabolic levels 6 times parent drug	Peak	45	240	Reduction in metabolite
20 volunteer students	Metabolite	15	Slow	Reduced side effects
Multiple blood samples: Comparing 5 mg oral group with 5 mg rectal group (open, cross-over)	Metabolite peak	60	Slow	
Symptom questionnaires				
Gas chromotography blood levels				

FIGURE 6-11.

Oxybutynin. Patients who cannot tolerate oral anticholinergic medication may benefit from intravesical or intrarectal administration. Intravesical administration has been used in children with myelodysplasia and adult female patients with neurogenic bladder. Winkler and Sand described rectal oxybutynin suppositories for patients unable to tolerate the oral medication. Nine of 25 women (36%) had a greater than 50% overall subjective improvement. Collas noted that antimuscarinic activity of oxybutynin is a property of both the drug and its metabolite [10–12]. The drug was rapidly absorbed after oral administration, detectable after 15 minutes with a peak level at 45 minutes, followed by a rapid decline. The metabolite was detectable at 15 minutes and reached a peak at 60 minutes with a less rapid decline. Absorption was gradual after rectal administration, slowing at 80 minutes, with a maximum at 240 minutes and a relatively constant concentration (mean 1.17 ng/mL lasting for at least 12 hours). This level was higher than that maintained after oral administration (P <0.05). Production of the metabolite was much slower. After rectal administration, fewer subjects reported side effects with a late onset and a decreased severity (P <0.05). [12]

URGENCY

Medications and the Elderly	Significant associations (P <.05)	Neither urgency or incontinence associate with
85% of elderly east Boston residents	Anticholinergics	Tricyclics
Home interviews	Antipsychotics	β- and α- blockers
Medication reviews	Sedative/hypnotics	β- and α- agonists
Associations equal for urgency and urinary incontinence	Loop diuretics	Calcium blockers, antihistamines
	Choline/lecithin	Thiazide diuretics
	Drugs	

FIGURE 6-12.

Drug use and the elderly. Kirschner-Hermanns and coworkers evaluated the association between medication usage and incontinence/urgency in older adults. Eighty-five percent of all elderly East Boston residents (n = 3754) agreed to participate. Participants were interviewed in their homes regarding demographic characteristics, medical conditions, and urinary symptoms. A physician reviewed all drugs. Associations between drug usage and urgency/urinary incontinence were assessed using odds ratios [13].

Associations for each drug were similar for both urgency and urge incontinence. Neither urgency nor incontinence associated with any of the listed drugs. Associations did not differ by sex, although they were stronger in men than women for antipsychotics, pure anticholinergics, and sedatives. Loop diuretics and antipsychotics were particularly problematic for people over the age of 75 [13].

SURGICAL TREATMENT

COLPORRHAPHY

SURGICAL TREATMENT OF GSUI

Anterior Colporrhaphy vs Burch	Modified Anterior Colporrhaphy
Most studies	Consistent Good Success (Beck)
Nonrandomized	Objective cure rate at 2 years
Retrospective/prospective	91% delayed absorbed
Some objective results	"Vaginal retropubic urethropexy"
	Plication periurethral "fascia"
	Elevation/fixation UVJ retropubic position

FIGURE 6-13.
Surgical anterior colporrhaphy. Anterior colporrhaphy should be considered a plastic procedure and not a primary operation for incontinence. The majority of studies have been retrospective with limited objective testing. Beck and coworkers reported a 25-year experience with 519 anterior colporrhaphy procedures [14]. GSUI—genuine stress urinary incontinence; UVJ—urethrovesical junction.

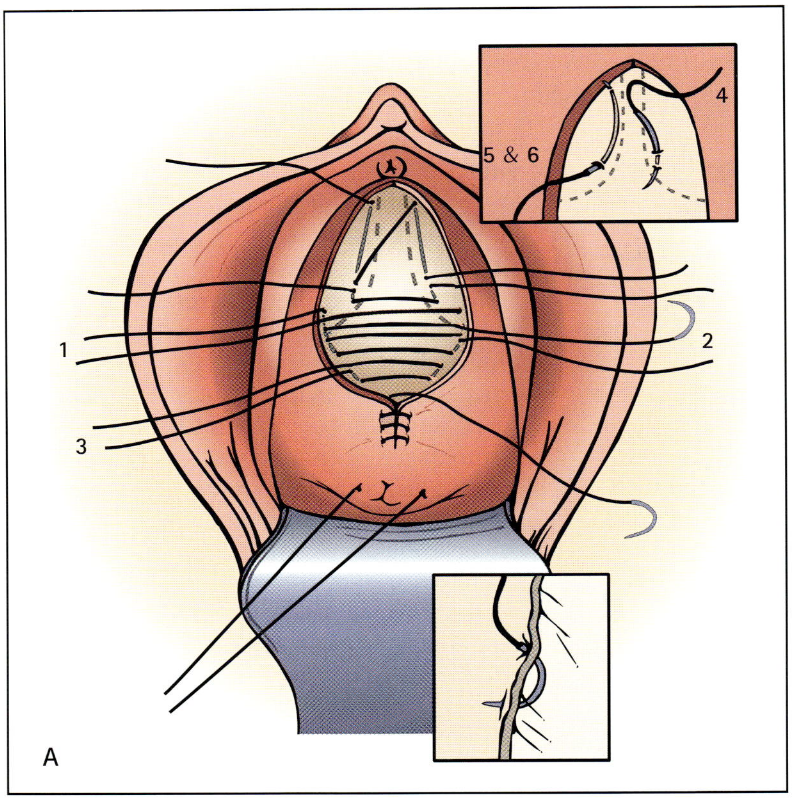

FIGURE 6-14.
Technique of anterior colporrhaphy as described by Beck and colleagues [14]. **A**, Placement of no. 1 chromic catgut, vertical mattress sutures (*1, 2,* and *3*) plicating the fascia under the bladder base with long axis of the needle parallel to the fascial surface (*bottom insert*). Figure-of-eight no. 1 polyglycolic sutures (*5* and *6*) are inserted into the pubocervical fascia, scratching the back of the symphysis pubis with long axis of the needle held at right angles to the fascial surface (*top insert*).

(*Continued on next page*)

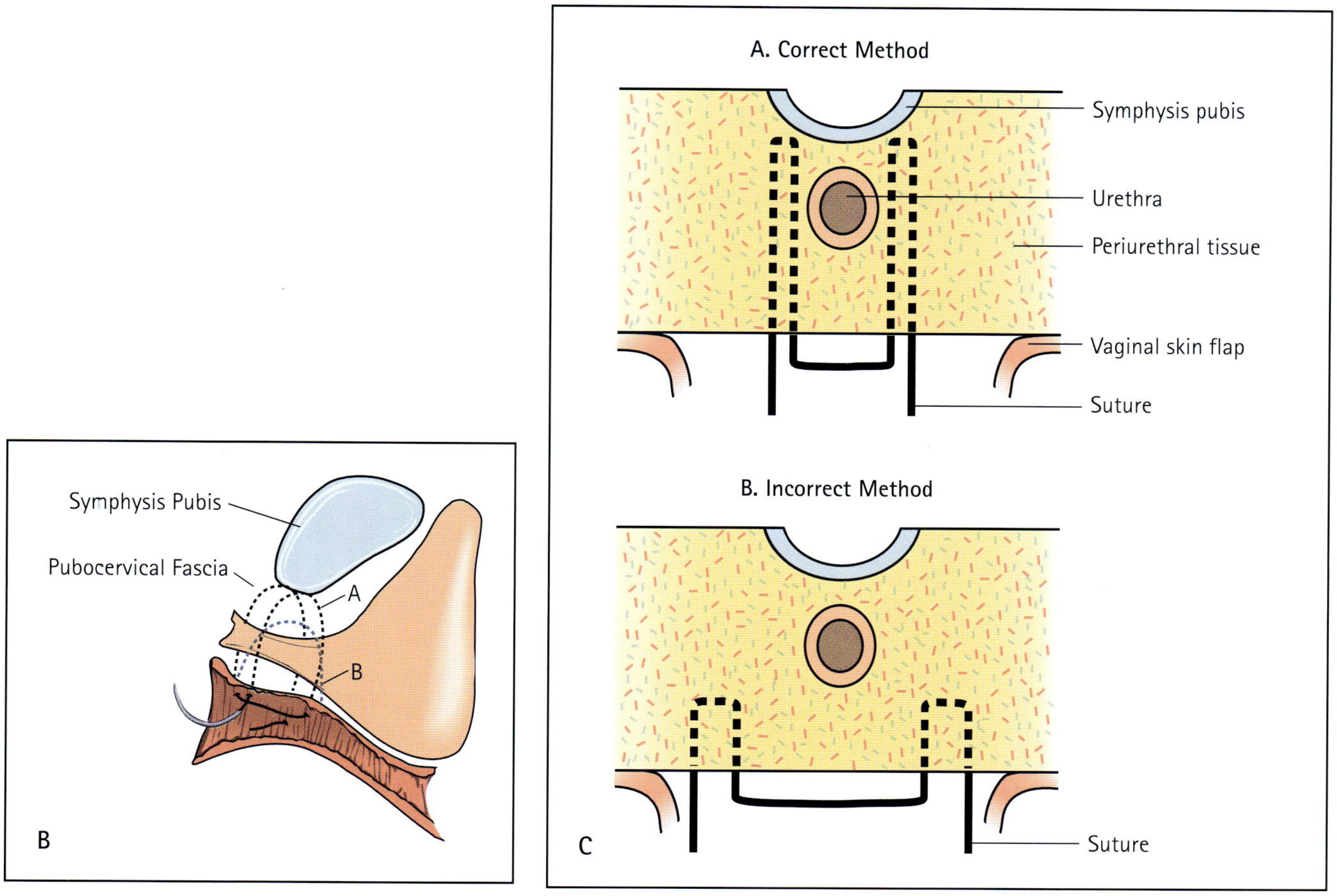

FIGURE 6-14. *(Continued)*

B, Suture *A* shows proper depth and placement of figure-of-eight suture in the pubocervical fascia lateral to and close to the urethra. When tied, the suture plicates the fascia lateral to and under the urethra, elevating it. Suture *B* illustrates improper placement with respect to depth and direction. **C**, Diagram illustrates correct (*A*) and incorrect (*B*) placement of sutures under and around the urethra. Correct placement of deep sutures close to the urethra tightens and elevates the urethra, whereas incorrect placement (too shallow and remote from the urethra) might correct prolapse, but produces minimal urethral tightening and elevation. (*From* Beck *et al.* [14]; with permission from the American College of Obstetricians and Gynecologists.)

BURCH RETROPUBIC URETHROPEXY

Types
- 5–10 year follow-up
  - Cure rate: 78–89%
- Modified anterior colporrhaphy
  - Cure rate: 31–37%

Herbertsson
- 72 patients
- 8–12 year objective follow-up
- Surgical cure: 90.3%
- Mean age: 46.2
- 31/38 patients continent with incompetent bladder neck

Stanton
- 109 patients
- 10–20 year follow-up
- Cure rate: 69%
- De Novo DI: 14.7%
- Postoperative voiding difficulty: 22%

Kjolhede
- 98% return-rate questionnaire
- 232 of 243 patients
- Subjective cure: 63%
- Improvement: 27%
- Voiding symptoms prevalent in failures

Feyereisl
- Postoperative urodynamic studies: 5–10 years
- 87 patients
  - Cure 81.6%
  - Failure 18.4%
- 52.8% patients with prior history of incontinence operation
- No significant voiding dysfunction described
- Patients with > prolapse excluded

FIGURE 6-15.
Long-term studies. The Burch procedure is noted to have a higher cure rate in several long-term studies. Herbertsson and Iosif noted that bladder neck competence is not necessary for postoperative continence because the bladder neck was noted to open in 38 patients of whom 31 were continent. Urodynamic studies were accomplished 10 years after retropubic urethropexy in 72 women. Herbertsson placed four permanent sutures on each side of the urethra. Stress testing was accomplished with 300 cc within the bladder [15]. A 10- to 20-year follow-up of Burch colposuspension in 109 patients found that although 22% of the patients reported subjective voiding difficulty, objective evidence was not permanent (4 patients did require urethrotomy) [16]. This study evaluated the importance of different preoperative estimates and postoperative complications on the outcome of Burch colposuspension with respect to urinary incontinence [17]. Long-term clinical and urodynamic outcome at 5 to10 years showed that the cured group had increased urethral functional length, closure pressure at rest, and pressure transmission [18]. DI—detrusor instability; GI—gastrointestinal.

A. BURCH: PROSPECTIVE/RANDOMIZED

5 year postoperative objective testing	Percent
Anterior colposcopy	37
Modified Pereyra	43
Burch	82

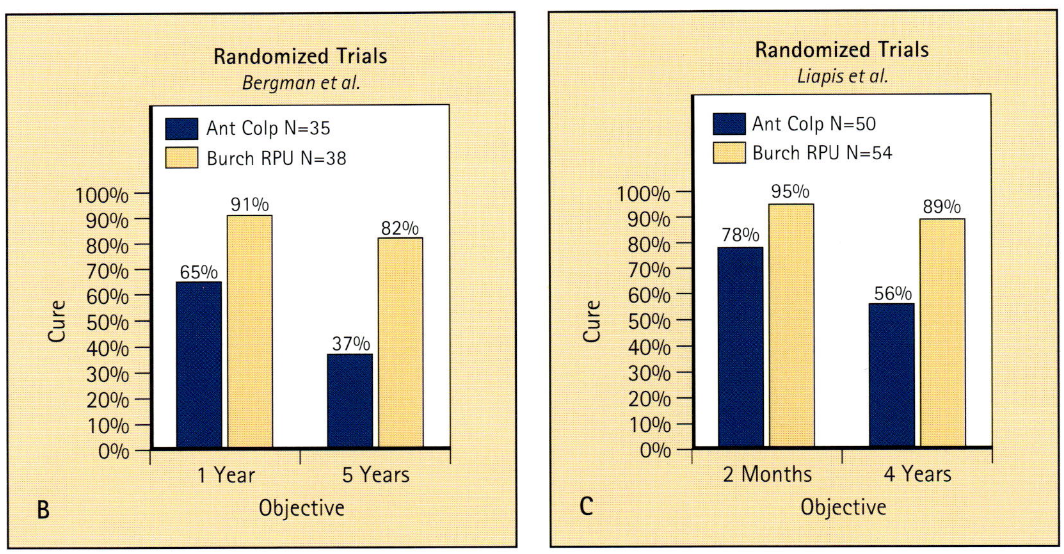

FIGURE 6-16.
Randomized trials. **A**, Bergman and Elia compared the long-term results of the Kelly plication, modified Pereyra needle suspension, and the Burch retropubic urethropexy (RPU). Multiple studies have now established the higher failure rate of the needle suspension in comparison to the Burch procedure [19]. **B**, This graph compares anterior colporrhaphy (Ant Colp) and the Burch RPU [19]. **C**, Liapis and colleagues assessed 170 women with genuine stress incontinence after three alternate procedures, the Marshall-Marchetti-Krantz (MMK) procedure, the Burch procedure, and anterior colporrhaphy. The patients were examined clinically and urodynamically 2 and 60 months after operation. There was no statistical difference in cure at 2 months, but as noted in the graph, a significant difference is noted at 60 months. The MMK procedure had a 67% cure rate at 60 months [20].

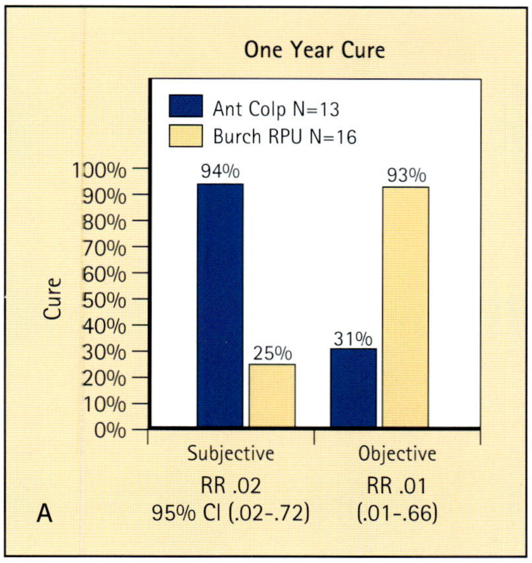

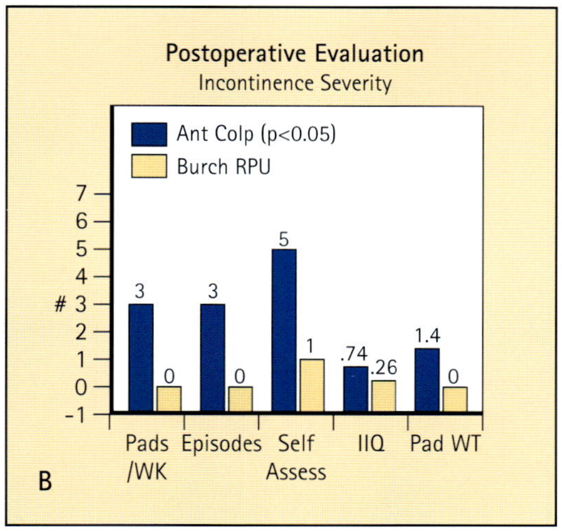

FIGURE 6-17.

Prospective study. **A**, Kammerer and coworkers prospectively compared the anterior colporrhaphy (Ant Colp) and Burch retropubic urethropexy (RPU). **B**, The procedures were compared in terms of incontinence severity. (Personal communication; slides reprinted with permission of Dr. Dorothy Kammerer-Doak.)

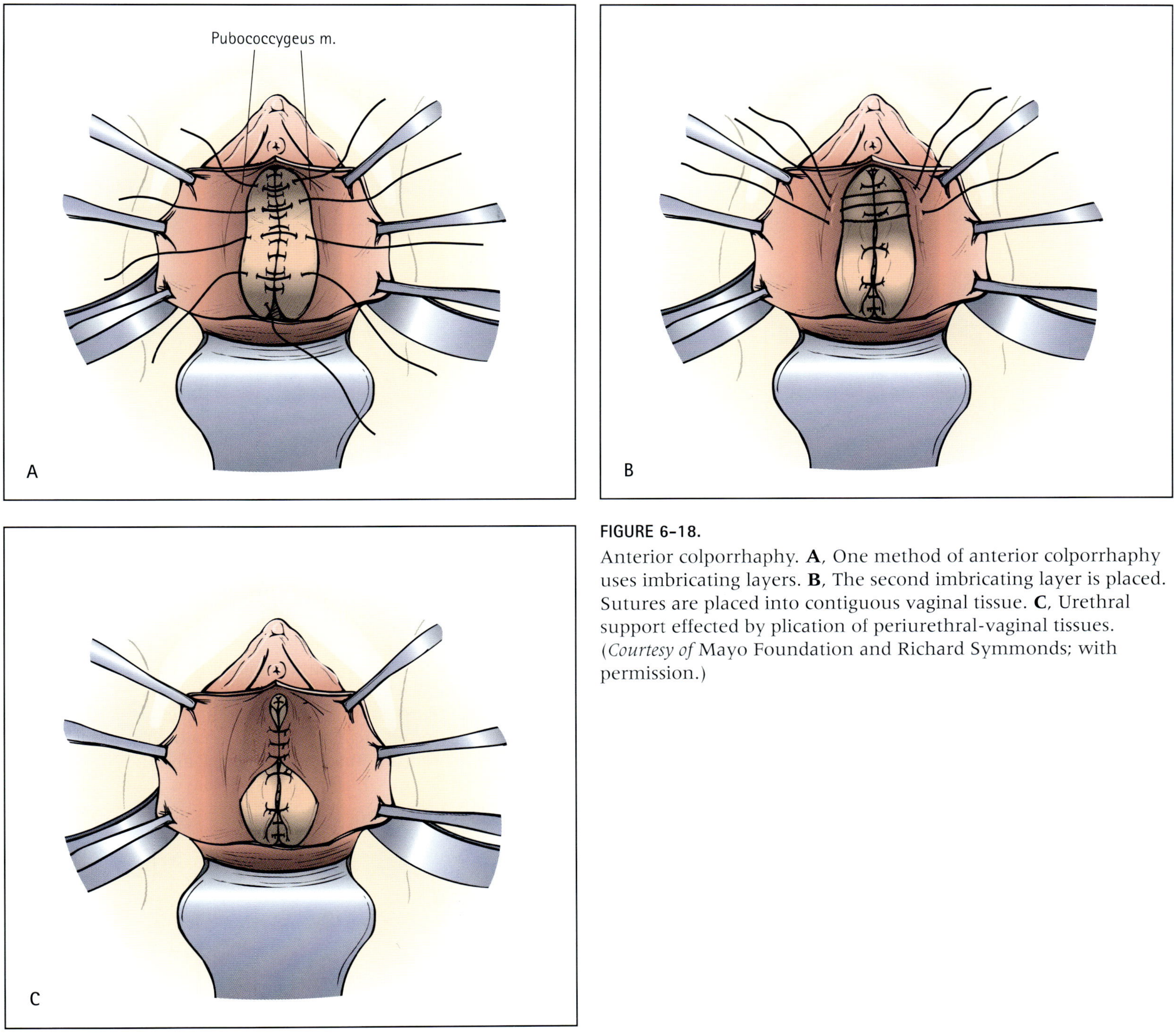

FIGURE 6-18.

Anterior colporrhaphy. **A**, One method of anterior colporrhaphy uses imbricating layers. **B**, The second imbricating layer is placed. Sutures are placed into contiguous vaginal tissue. **C**, Urethral support effected by plication of periurethral-vaginal tissues. (*Courtesy of* Mayo Foundation and Richard Symmonds; with permission.)

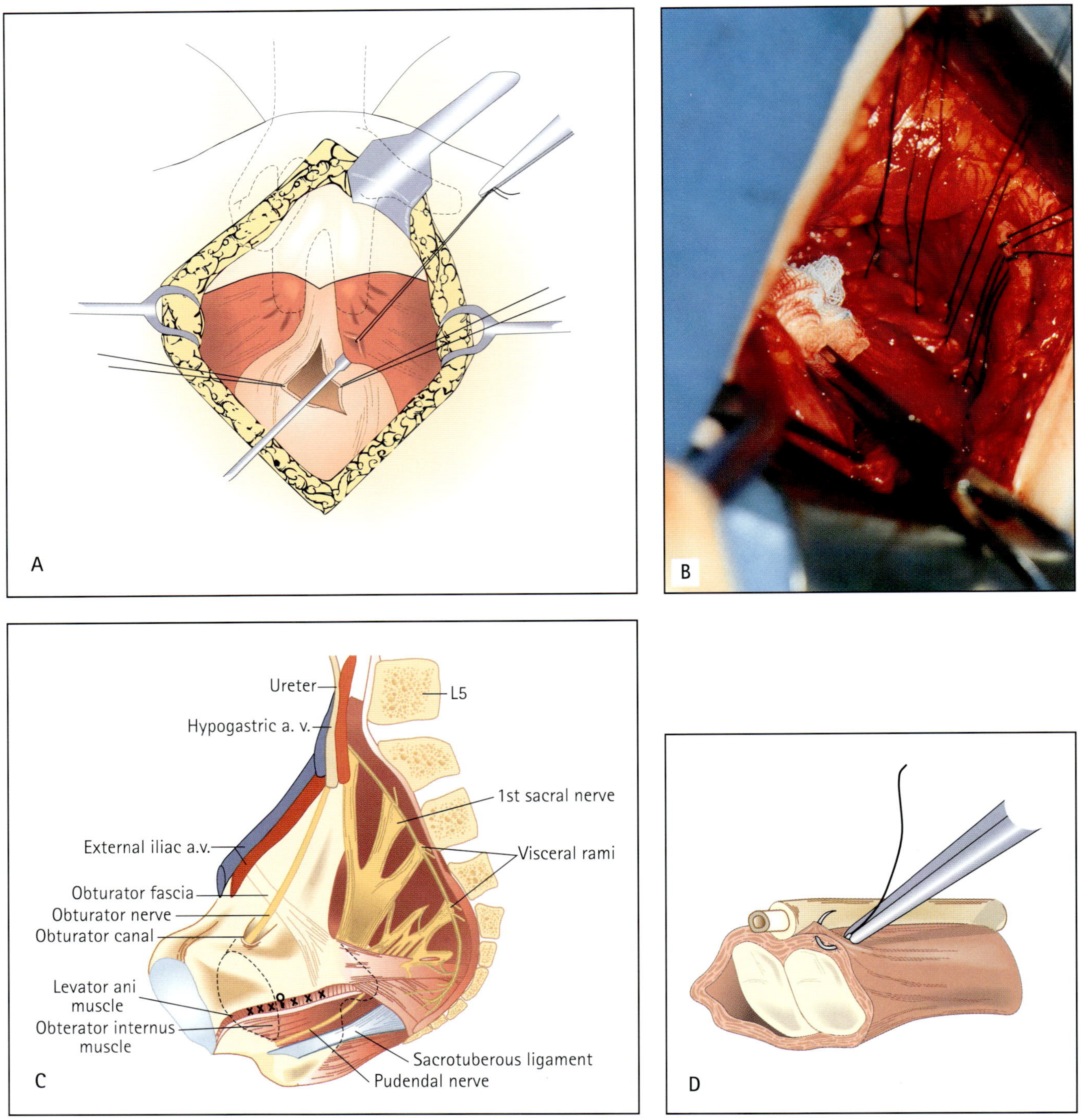

FIGURE 6–19.

Burch retropubic urethropexy. **A**, The bladder is opened to allow precise suture placement and in addition subsequent suprapubic catheterization. All suture strands are brought through Cooper's ligament with the second strand passing a second time. (*Courtesy of* Mayo Foundation and Richard Symmonds; with permission.) The urethrovesical junction is stabilized, not elevated. The horizontal angle of the urethra is measured before suture tying to ensure an angle of 0° to -10°. **B**, Photograph of Burch and paravaginal sutures in situ before tying. The tissues are stabilized rather than elevated. (*Courtesy of* Mayo Foundation and Jeffrey L. Cornella.) **C**, Diagram of paravaginal defect repair suture line along obturator internus muscle (*Courtesy of* Dr. Harvey T. Huddleston; with permission). **D**, Permanent sutures take double bites 4 mm lateral and in a perpendicular orientation to the urethra. This applies to both the Burch urethropexy and the Marshall-Marchetti-Krantz procedure. (*Courtesy of* Mayo Foundation and Raymond A. Lee.)

Marshall-Marchetti-Krantz Procedure

A. MARSHALL-MARCHETTI-KRANTZ

Urinary Stress Incontinence 1960–75
- 227 patients
  - Primary MMK: 91% cured/improved
- 322 patients
  - Recurrent incontinence
  - Average 2.3 previous incontinence operations per patient
  - 90% cured/improved

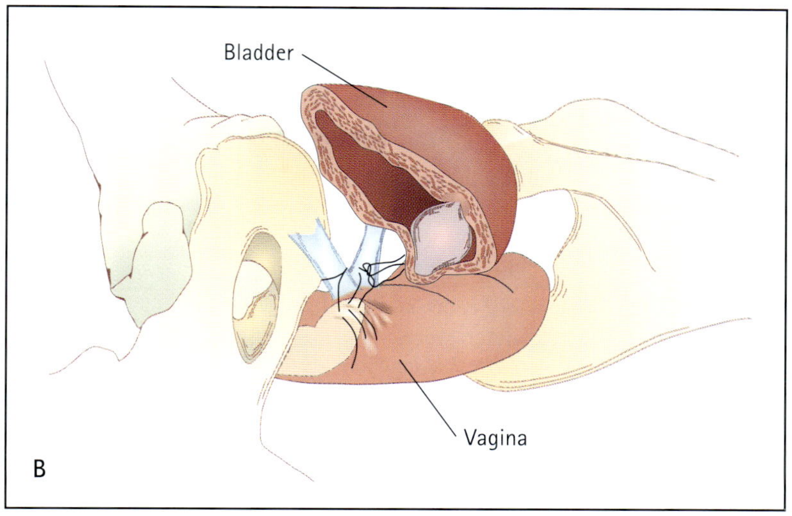

FIGURE 6-20.

Modified Marshall-Marchetti-Krantz (MMK) procedure. **A**, At the Mayo Clinic from January 1960 through December 1975, 673 patients underwent a modification of the MMK procedure. Patients were followed 2 to 16 years. The MMK is a safe and effective operation [21]. **B**, This modification of the MMK procedure attaches the tissues surrounding the urethrovesical junction to the most inferior aspect of the midline cartilage. (*Courtesy of* Mayo Foundation and Raymond A. Lee.)

Treatment of Complex Urinary Incontinence

Cystometrography

A. MANAGEMENT OF SUI

Delayed sustained leakage on stress testing or complex history/findings including:
- Leakage with no urethrovesical junction rotation
- Symptoms of significant bladder instability
- Neurologic conditions
- Previous incontinence operations or radical surgery
- Urinary retention or low bladder capacity
- Significant vaginal wall prolapse

B

Management of SUI

Cystometrogram

↓

Group 1: Significant bladder instability and/or an advanced neurologic process that precludes operation
Group 2: No evidence of significant detrusor instability and no urethral junction descent on examination
Group 3: No evidence of significant detrusor instability; urethrovesical junction descent is present
Group 4: Urinary retention on previous testing with or without detrusor instability (cystourethroscopy only in select patients)

C

Management of SUI

Group 1: Significant bladder instability and/or an advanced neurologic process that precludes operation

↓

Conservative treatment program (cystourethroscopy only in select patients)

FIGURE 6-21.

Cystometrography. Patients with complex urinary incontinence (**A**) can be divided into four groups after a cystometrogram. **B**, These four groups have significant differences in potential management. Groups two and three should undergo cystoscopic examination. **C**, Patients in group 1 do not require cystoscopy unless other indications are present such as abnormal cytology, pyuria, hematuria, or previous incontinence surgery. Nonoperative patients in group 1 are treated with conservative measures [3].

(*Continued on next page*)

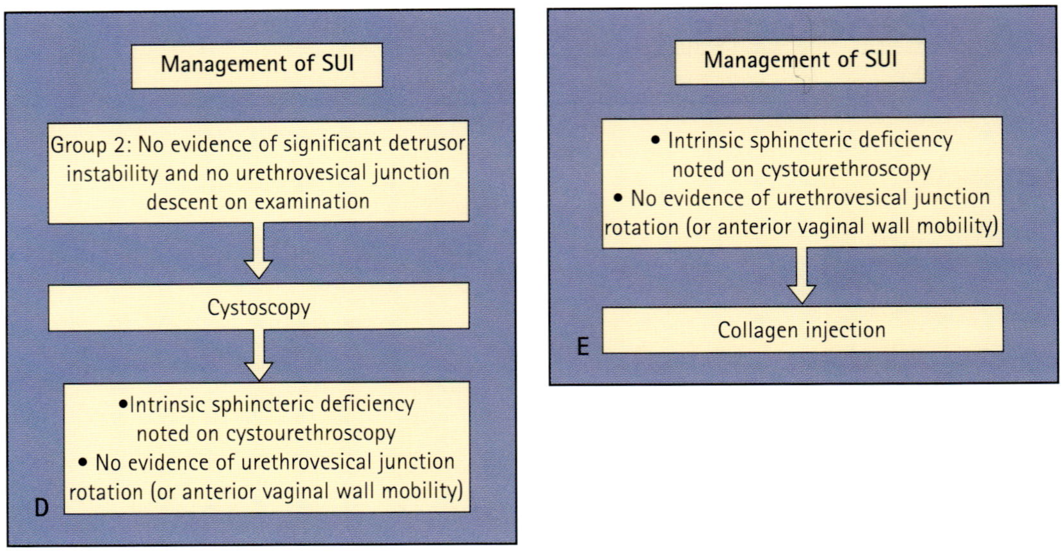

FIGURE 6-21. *(Continued)*

D, The bladder neck is examined to confirm the lack of urethrovesical junction descent and for urethral flaccidity or scarification. Most patients with intrinsic sphincteric deficiency do not have any abnormal appearance to the urethrovesical junction on cystourethroscopy. **E**, If the patient has no urethrovesical junction descent, significant stress incontinence, and a lack of severe detrusor instability, collagen injection is a consideration.

Collagen Injection

INTRINSIC SPHINCTERIC DEFICIENCY

ISD is a functional definition, there do not exist any anatomic factors or laboratory parameters that allow the diagnosis, either in combination or as a solitary factor.

A combination of urethral anatomic and physiologic factors which fail to prevent stress urinary incontinence despite the presence or potential achievement of complete urethrovesical junction support.

FIGURE 6-22.

Intrinsic sphincteric deficiency (ISD). Collagen injection is used to treat ISD. The functional definition of ISD is stress incontinence in the absence of a detrusor contraction despite nonrotation or fixation of the urethrovesical junction.

A. INTRINSIC SPHINCTERIC DEFICIENCY

Viscoelastic properties
Integrity of striated muscle support
Optimal neurologic innervation
Urethral vascularity
Rhabdosphincter integrity
Mucosal surface tension

B. SINGLE CONDITIONS THAT ARE NOT ISD

Low urethral pressure
Open bladder neck
Distal sphincteric compromise
Low pressure transmission

C. NONHISTORICAL FACTORS SUGGESTIVE OF ISD

Lack of UVJ rotation in presence of GSI
Abdominal leak point pressure < 60 cm
Fixed UVJ on cystoscopy with GSI
Scarified urethra

FIGURE 6-23.

Criteria for intrinsic sphincteric deficiency (ISD). **A**, Although any single (or currently combination of) factor (s) does not define ISD, loss of these factors contributes to the potential for its development. **B**, It is important not to be confused by the literature. There is no single factor or defined combination of factors that makes the diagnosis of ISD [22]. **C**, These nonhistorical factors are suggestive of, but not diagnostic for, ISD. GSI—genuine stress incontinence; UVJ—urethrovesical junction

URETHRAL FUNCTION

Urethral muscle thickness (25 cadavers)

- Striated muscle becomes thinner and then absent at the vaginal side of the urethra with age
- 4/7 women over age 70: No posterior muscle
  - Individuals age < 30 had significant muscle present

FIGURE 6-24.

Muscular damage. This study gives an example of the type of muscular damage that may contribute to intrinsic sphincter deficiency. The urethra and its surrounding tissues were removed en bloc from 25 cadavers aged 19 months to 80 years of age. A midsagittal section and cross sections from the midurethra were used for the analysis. Aging brings a high risk of sustaining loss of the striated urogenital sphincter muscle along the vaginal (dorsal) side of the urethra [23].

COLLAGEN

Glutaraldehyde cross-linked (GAX) collagen (bovine dermal collagen, cross-linked with glutaraldehyde, suspended in phosphate-buffered NS)

- 95% type I collagen
- < 5% type III collagen

FIGURE 6-25.

Collagen material. The collagen injected into the urethra is different from that used by plastic surgeons for cosmetic surgery. A skin test is required to rule out sensitivity. The collagen can be injected periurethrally or transurethrally; each is accomplished during cystoscopic visualization of the urethrovesical junction. NS—normal saline.

COLLAGEN INJECTION

- Nonmobile urethrovesical junction
- Stress urinary incontinence
- Absence of moderate to severe DI
- Adequate bladder capacity
- Leak point pressure < 100

FIGURE 6-26.

Criteria. It is important to recognize that most patients with incontinence may not fit the criteria for injection of collagen that were originally established. The criteria for periurethral injection are listed. DI—detrusor instability.

COLLAGEN INJECTION STUDIES

Study 1

187 women (mean age: 63)

- 23% cure (42 patients) (22 month follow-up)
- 52% improved (97 patients)
- 25% failed (47 patients)

No relationship to age or pretreatment severity of incontinence

Study 2

No difference in outcome related to UVJ mobility

2 month cure probability of dryness at 3 years was 46%

Study 3

MRI after injection

32 women at median 12 months

Neither volume or position of retained collagen was predictive of clinical outcome

Volume of injected material strongly correlated with retained volume in successful and failed patients

Study 4

111 women

Paraurethral injections

Postinjection urodynamics, minimum 2 year follow-up

25% cured

40% improved

No predictive factors of success were found

FIGURE 6-27.

Outcome studies. A study addressed the selection parameters and duration of response in the use of collagen injections. A total of 187 women with a mean age of 64 years underwent injection. Treatment outcome was determined by individual change in incontinence grade [24]. The follow-up was a mean of 21 months. No difference in outcome was seen in relation to patient age or pretreatment grade of incontinence. In a separate study involving 337 patients injected with collagen, Stothers and coworkers noted a 12.6% incidence of de novo urinary urgency incontinence. The urinary retention rate was 1.9% (transient retention) [25]. Neither volume nor position of collagen is predictive of clinical outcome. In addition, Kim showed that urodynamic and endoscopic findings do not predict long-term success after collagen injection [26,27]. Another study determined the medium-term outcome in 111 women after collagen injection [28]. UVJ—urethrovesical junction.

Cystourethroscopy

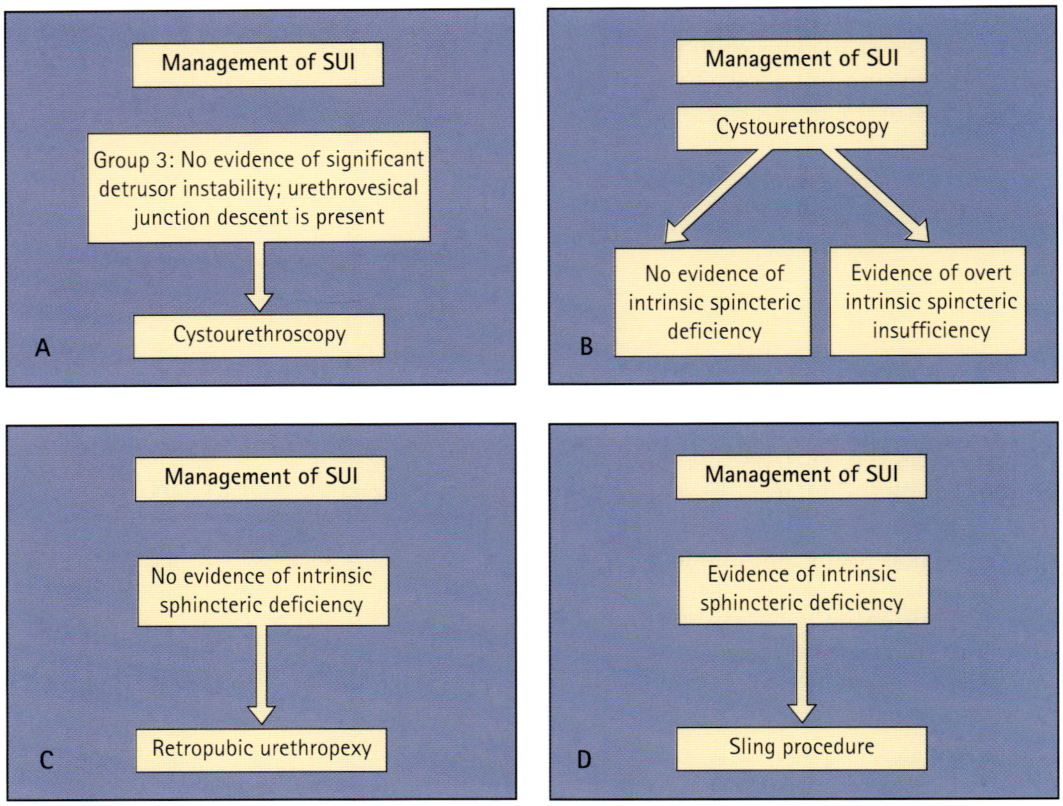

FIGURE 6-28.

Group 3. **A**, The majority of patients who have complex urinary incontinence have criteria that place them into this group, most commonly previous operations for incontinence. **B**, Group 3 is further divided into those with and without a strong suspicion of intrinsic sphincteric deficiency (ISD). **C**,Those without evidence of ISD are treated with retropubic urethropexy. The cure rate in the urethropexy group remains high [21]. **D**, Patients with high suspicion of ISD or who have clinical factors, which predispose to failure (weak tissues, history of multiple operations for incontinence, chronic straining and coughing), receive a pubovaginal sling procedure.

Sling Procedure

A. PUBOVAGINAL SLING INDICATIONS

The increased morbidity of sling procedures is such that its exclusive use as a primary incontinence operation is not indicated

Multioperated patient

Suspected ISD

Combined procedures
- Vesicovaginal fistula
- Urethral destruction
- Augmentation ileocystoplasty

B. MORBIDITY

Increase dissection with penetration of urogenital diaphragm
- Neurogenic damage
- Increased potential for bleeding/voiding dysfunction

Material risk

Autologous
- Requirement for additional dissection

Synthetic
- Risk of erosion and removal

C. SUMMARY

Important part of the surgeon's armamentarium

Durable, brings strength to repair

Risk of increased morbidity and voiding dysfunction

Synthetic materials should be a second choice as sling material

FIGURE 6-29.

Indications and outcomes. **A**, Possible indications for the pubovaginal sling procedure. Considering the long-term studies that show success of Burch urethropexy over 10 to 20 years, the sling procedure should not become the first-line procedure for routine urinary incontinence in women. **B**, Increased dissection and thus morbidity are seen with the sling procedure. Synthetic material has a small but significant risk of erosion [29]. **C**, The pubovaginal sling involves an inverted U-shaped vaginal incision, plication of endopelvic fascia over the bladder, penetration of the urogenital diaphragm, and overlapping placement at the urethrovesical junction. The sling should be placed with no tension or if possible an angle of 0° to the horizontal on cotton-swab testing to decrease the incidence of voiding dysfunction.

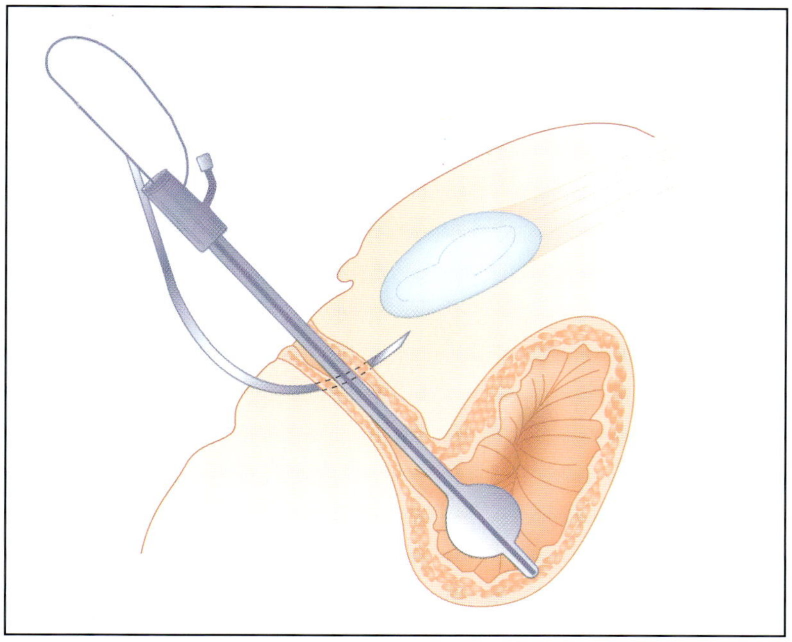

FIGURE 6-30.

A new surgical technique for treating female stress incontinence, the "tension-free vaginal tape", has been devised by Ulmsten [30]. The technique involves the use of a non-disposable metal handle to which two plastic disposable 5-6 mm needles attached to a plastic sheath covered with prolene gauze, is inserted into a 1.5 cm long midline suburethral vaginal incision starting 0.5 cm from the urethral meatus. The needles are passed paraurethrally to exit small abdominal insicions, making a "U" shape sling around the mid urethra. The abdominal ends of the tape are not fixed, but cut with scissors below the skin surface. The sling is loosely placed, without elevation, around the urethra.

The procedure is performed on an out-patient basis under local anesthesia. An 84% two year cure rate is reported and no rejection or infection occured. The technique allows sling placement by a vaginal route, incorporates sling material covered by a plastic sheath, and is placed without tension in the *mid urethra*.

An ongoing Scandinavian multicenter study encompassing 500 patients is in process, and long-term results wil be necessary before the ultimate value of this procedure is established.

TREATMENT OF URINARY RETENTION

Management of SUI

Group 4: Urinary retention on previous testing with or without detrusor instability (cystourethroscopy only in select patients)

- Consideration of intermittent self catheterization
- Consider other testing/intervention
- Treatment

A

B. OVERFLOW INCONTINENCE

Self-intermittent catheterization

α-blockers for urethral relaxation

Patients with severe De Novo DI and retention from overcorrection

Consideration of RPU takedown

FIGURE 6-31.

Group 4. **A**, Patients who have urinary retention are usually treated with self-intermittent catheterization. Urinary retention may predispose to overflow incontinence, which is not treated pharmacologically with anticholinergic medications. **B**, α-Adrenergic blockers may warrant trial in patients with urinary retention because a small percentage of patients will respond. Sacral nerve stimulation may also be considered in select patients. Patients may also develop detrusor instability from overcorrection at the time of incontinence operation. Patients with non-obstructive retention may not be candidates for sacral neuromodualtion (see chapter 2).

DE NOVO DETRUSOR INSTABILITY

No objective Stress Incontinence

Medical management

Behavioral management

Future reassessment

Overcorrected UVJ with or without obstruction

High residual urine with overflow

FIGURE 6-32.

De novo detrusor instability. Patients may have de novo detrusor instability after surgery. These patients are managed medically. Investigation should rule out urinary retention or evidence of foreign material in the bladder. The urethral angle to the horizontal should be measured. If patients have overcorrection, a takedown procedure may be cautiously considered. A percentage of patients may be considered for takedown of the incontinence operation who require self-intermittent catheterization or who experience significant detrusor instability in the presence of a high negative angle of the urethra to the horizontal (overcorrection). The outcome is not completely predictable and patients should be counseled in this regard. A percentage of patients will be dry and experience return of voiding, a percentage will continue to experience detrusor instability despite improved voiding, a percentage will continue to experience retention, a percentage will manifest recurrent stress incontinence after takedown, and a combination of these manifestations may also be seen. UVJ—urethrovesical junction.

RPU TAKEDOWN

Voiding Dysfunction Following Cystourethropexy
- Dysfunctional voiding: 15 patients
- Resolution of bladder instability: 13/13 patients
- Continence: 13/15 patients
- Resolution of CISC: 6/7 patients

FIGURE 6-33.
Takedown procedure. Webster and Kreder reported a series of retropubic urethropexy (RPU) takedown procedures that were followed by paravaginal defect repair in 15 patients. All patients had evidence of overcorrection and dysfunctional voiding [31]. CISC—clean intermittent self-catheterization.

A. RECURRENT/PERSISTENT URINARY INCONTINENCE

Continence
- Vaginolevator support
- Neurophysiologic support
- Absence of detrusor instability
- External sphincter support
- Compliance
- Viscoelastic/collagen urethral support

B. RECURRENT INCONTINENCE

Does the patient have urethrovesical junction rotation?
Does the patient have intrinsic sphincteric deficiency?
Does the patient have a low capacity?
Does the patient have objective stress and/or urgency incontinence?
Does the patient have a neurologic deficit?

C. UNRECOGNIZED DETRUSOR INSTABILITY WITH LOW-CAPACITY BLADDER

Medical management
Intravesical oxybutynin
Sacral nerve stimulation
Urologic consultation for augmentation or diversion (severe cases)

FIGURE 6-34.
Recurrent incontinence. **A**, Patients who present with recurrent incontinence usually have a combination of factors responsible for the sphincteric incompetence. Factors that aid continence are listed. **B**, The following questions are pertinent and reflect the management algorithm. Patients with recurrent incontinence are evaluated using the complex category. **C**, A small percentage of patients with recurrent incontinence may have had an unrecognized low-capacity bladder with severe detrusor instability before operation. Management considerations are listed.

LOW-PRESSURE URETHRA: BURCH COLPOSUSPENSION

Pressure	Failure Rate, %
> 20 cm H_2O	18
< 20 cm H_2oO	54

Significant independent risk factor for women under 50 years?

FIGURE 6-35.
Low-pressure urethra. The arbitrary designation of low-pressure urethra should not determine the type of incontinence operation used. This initial study may not have considered the amount of urethrovesical junction descent. A more recent randomized, prospective study by Sand and colleagues randomized 37 patients with low urethral pressure to sling procedures versus Burch procedures. The cure rate in the two groups was essentially commensurate on objective studies at 3 months (100%, sling; 90%, Burch). All 14 patients having the sling procedure and 16 of 17 having the Burch procedure were subjectively cured at 1 year [32,33].

REFERENCES

1. Wall LL, Wiskind AK, Taylor PA: Simple bladder filling with a cough stress test compared with subtracted cystometry for the diagnosis of urinary incontinence. *Am J Obstet Gynecol* 1994, 171:1477–1479.
2. Videla FL, Wall LL: Stress incontinence diagnosed without multichannel urodynamic studies. *Obstet Gynecol* 1998, 91:965–968.
3. Cornella JL, Magrina JF: An algorithm for the management of urinary stress incontinence. *Int Urogynecol J* 1996, 7:221–226.
4. Bo K: Effect of electrical stimulation on stress and urge urinary incontinence. *Acta Obstet Gynecol Scand* 1998, 168:3–11.
5. Luber KM, Wolde-Tsadik G: Efficacy of functional electrical stimulation in treating genuine stress incontinence: a randomized clinical trial. *Neurourol Urodyn* 1997, 16:543–551.
6. Bo K, Talset T. Long-term effect of pelvic floor muscle exercise 5 years after cessation of organized training. *Obstet Gynecol* 1996, 87:261–265.
7. Burgio KL, Robinson JC, Engel BT: The role of biofeedback in Kegel exercise training for stress urinary incontinence. *Am J Obstet Gynecol* 1986, 154:58–64.
8. Abrams P, Freeman R, Anderstrom C, Mattiasson A: Tolterodine, a new antimuscarinic agent: as effective but better tolerated than oxybutynin in patients with overactive bladder. *Br J Urol* 1998, 81:801–810.
9. Millard R, Moore K, Tuttle J: Treatment of detrusor instability. *Neurourol Urodyn* 1997, 16:343–344.
10. Buyse G, Verpoorten C, Casaer P: Intravesical application of a stable oxybutynin solution improves therapeutic compliance and acceptance in children with neurogenic bladder dysfunction. *J Urol* 1998, 160:1084–1087.
11. Winkler HA, Sand PK: Treatment of detrusor instability with oxybutynin rectal suppositories. *Int Urogynecol J* 1998, 9:100–102.
12. Collas D, Malone-Lee JG: The pharmacokinetic properties of rectal oxybutynin—a possible alternative to intravesical administration. *Neurourol Urodyn* 1997, 16:346–347.
13. Kirschner-Hermanns R, Scherr P, Resnick NM: Relationship of medication use to urinary urgency and incontinence in the elderly: a population-based study. *Neurourol Urodyn* 1997, 16:437–438.
14. Beck RP, McCormick S, Nordstrom L: A 25-year experience with 519 anterior colporrhaphy procedures. *Obstet Gynecol* 1991, 78:1011–1018.
15. Herbertsson G, Iosif CS: Surgical results and urodynamic studies 10 years after retropubic colpourethrocystopexy. *Acta Obstet Gynecol Scand* 1993, 72:298–301.
16. Alcalay M, Monga A, Stanton SL: Burch colposuspension: a 10-20 year follow up. *Br J Obstet Gynecol* 1995, 102:740–745.
17. Kjolhede P, Ryden G: Prognostic factors and long-term results of the Burch colposuspension. *Acta Obstet Gynecol Scand* 1994, 73:642–647.
18. Feyereisl J, Dreher E, Haenggi W, *et al I>.: Long-term results after Burch colposuspension.* Am J Obstet Gynecol *1994, 171:647–652.*
19. Bergman A, Elia G: Three surgical procedures for genuine stress incontinence: five-year follow-up of a prospective randomized study. *Am J Obstet Gynecol* 1995, 173:66–71.
20. Liapis AE, Asimiadis V, Loghis CD, *et al.*: A randomized prospective study of three operative methods for genuine stress incontinence. *J Gynecol Surg* 1996, 12:7–13.
21. Lee RA, Symmonds RE, Goldstein RA: Surgical complications of modified Marshall-Marchetti-Krantz procedure for urinary incontinence. *Obstet Gynecol* 1979, 53:447–450.
22. Cornella JL: Intrinsic sphincteric deficiency: a clinical opinion. *AUGS Quarterly* 1995, 13:2–3.
23. Perucchini D, DeLancey JOL, Ashton Miller JA: Regional striated muscle loss in the female urethra: where is the striated muscle vulnerable? *Neurourol Urodyn* 1997, 16:407–408.
24. Herschorn S, Radomski SB: Collagen injections for genuine stress urinary incontinence: patient selection and durability. *Int Urogynecol J* 1997, 8:18–24.
25. Stothers L, Goldenberg SL, Leone EF: Complications of periurethral collagen injection for stress urinary incontinence. *J Urol* 1998, 159:806–807.
26. Carr LK, Herschorn S, Leonhardt C: Magnetic resonance imaging after intraurethral collagen injected for stress urinary incontinence. *J Urol* 1996, 155:1253–1255.
27. Kim YH, Kattan MW, Boone TB: Correlation of urodynamic results and urethral coaptation with success after transurethral collagen injection. *Urology* 1997, 50:941–948.
28. Swami S, Batista JE, Abrams P: Collagen for female genuine stress incontinence after a minimum 2-year follow-up *Br J Urol* 1997, 80:757–761.
29. Tanagho EA: Urinary stress incontinence: surgical treatment (editorial). *Int Urogynecol J* 1998, 9:1–2.
30. Ulmsten U, Henriksson L, Johnson P, *et al.*: An ambulatory surgical procedure under local anesthetic for teatment of female urinary incontinence. *Int. Urogynecol J* 1996, 7:81–86.
31. Webster GD, Kreder KJ: Voiding dysfunction following cystourethropexy: its evaluation and management. *J Urol* 1990, 144:670–673.
32. Sand PK, Bowen LW, Panganiban R, Ostergard DR: The low pressure urethra as a factor in failed retropubic urethropexy. *Obstet Gynecol* 1987, 69:399–402.
33. Culligan PJ, Winkler HA, Sand PK: A prospective randomized study of modified Burch retropubic urethropexy and suburethral sling for genuine stress incontinence and low pressure urethra. Proceedings of the 19th Annual Meeting of the American Urogynecologic Society, 1998, Washington, DC.

CHAPTER 7

Treatment of Fecal Incontinence

J. Scott Pittman

The hope for successful management of fecal incontinence depends on the clinician's thorough understanding of normal pelvic anatomy and function. This understanding will guide the clinician in obtaining the appropriate diagnostic tests to identify the etiology of symptoms and thus treat the problem appropriately.

Continence is not fully understood, but depends on bowel consistency and frequency; intact myenteric reflexes and autonomic, sensory, and motor nerves; and pelvic anatomy. If only one of these factors is abnormal, compensation can occur so that there may be no noticeable or significant symptoms. If one or more of the factors is sufficiently compromised, the person can become incontinent. Incontinence may be very mild and hardly noticeable or it may be severe and lead to a confined life-style.

A detailed history is necessary to determine the degree of incontinence. This is important because the severity of symptoms dictates the aggressiveness of management. If a patient has a major sphincter abnormality, but no fecal incontinence, then treatment is not warranted. If a patient has very severe symptoms, which significantly affect her life-style and mental state, then even risky or experimental surgery might be in order. The detailed history is also necessary to help identify the causative factors (*i.e.*, childbirth). This will guide the physical examination or ancillary testing to help identify a specific anatomic or functional abnormality (*i.e.*, sphincter defect) resulting in optimal treatment (*i.e.*, sphincteroplasty) and continence.

The options for treatment of fecal incontinence are the focus of discussion.

ALGORITHMS FOR EVALUATION AND TREATMENT OF FECAL INCONTINENCE

FACTORS CONTRIBUTING TO FECAL INCONTINENCE

- Functional
  - Irritable bowel syndrome
  - Diarrhea (*ie*, malabsorption, endocrine disorder, upper intestinal disease, food intolerance)
  - Constipation impaction
- Diet
- Medications (*ie*, laxatives)
- Proctitis/colitis
  - Infectious
  - Idiopathic (ulcerative colitis, Crohn's disease)
- Polyp/cancer
- Diverticulitis/volvulus
- Neurologic (*ie*, diabetes, trauma, spinal defects, multiple sclerosis)
- Pelvic defects
  - Enterocele
  - Rectocele
  - Enterogenital fistula
  - Rectal intussusception/prolapse
- Anal outlet defects
  - Birth defects (*ie*, anal atresia, imperforate anus)
  - Traumatic delivery
  - Iatrogenic (fistulotomy, sphincterotomy, hemorrhoidectomy, mucosal ectropion)

FIGURE 7-1.

Factors contributing to fecal incontinence. Multiple factors may contribute to fecal incontinence. A thorough history and physical examination will often identify these factors and lead to an appropriate diagnosis and treatment plan.

TESTS FOR EVALUATION OF FECAL INCONTINENCE

- Anoscopy
- Rigid sigmoidoscopy
- Vaginoscopy
- Flexible sigmoidoscopy
- Air contrast barium enema
- Endoanal ultrasound
- Electrodiagnostic testing
  - Pudendal nerve terminal motor latency (PNTML)
  - Needle electromyography
- Manometry
- Dynamic voiding cystoproctogram

FIGURE 7-2.

Tests for evaluation of fecal incontinence. In addition to the history and physical examination, appropriate testing is necessary to identify the causative factors for fecal incontinence. A knowledge of the appropriate use of these tests is important so that information obtained will lead to appropriate decision-making regarding diagnosis and treatment for fecal incontinence.

NONSURGICAL TREATMENT OF FECAL INCONTINENCE

- Manipulation of stool consistency
  - Diet—high fiber, fiber supplements, fluids
  - Medication—Imodium, Lomotil
- Kegal exercises
- Bowel training regimen
  - Regular periodic suppositories or enemas
  - Digital stimulation
- Biofeedback
  - Electromyography—sensory, topical, stimulatory
  - Manometry—sensory, pressure
- Anal plug

FIGURE 7–3.

Nonsurgical treatment of fecal incontinence. Functional fecal incontinence, with no history of sphincter trauma and no major sphincter deformity, can be treated very successfully by nonsurgical means, even in patients with major fecal incontinence. The first line of management is to encourage and educate the patient to eat a high-fiber diet with plenty of fluids and fiber supplements as needed. This is helpful and sometimes all that is required. The fiber with the fluids tends to make the bowels more consistent, regular, and predictable, allowing for an easier and more complete fecal evacuation. In patients who tend to have more loose or frequent bowel movements, the addition of Imodium or Lomotil as indicated can decrease the bowel frequency to a more manageable level. Kegel sphincter strengthening exercises are also recommended as a first-line treatment. Patients are instructed to practice contracting the anal sphincter and holding it in that state for a count to 10, for a series of 10 times, several times per day. They are encouraged to try to do this routinely whether it is while sitting down for meals or while driving to and from regular activities, such as work. The more often a person performs that exercise, the more successful it will be. It may take several weeks to accomplish noticeable improvement.

A bowel training regimen may be beneficial when the initial measures are unsuccessful. Initially, daily suppositories, glycerin or bisacodyl, or enemas, are given the same hour every morning. Ideally, these measures are administered 15 to 20 minutes after breakfast to take advantage of the gastrocolic reflex. Lower abdominal massage can be performed at the same time. As the bowels become more predictable, the frequency of this type of stimulation can be decreased. In patients with spinal cord injuries, digital stimulation is performed to accomplish the same purpose by stimulating a rectocolic evacuation reflex.

If the above measures are unsuccessful or if the patient is not a candidate for a sphincteroplasty, or a sphincteroplasty has failed, then different types of biofeedback have about a 70% success rate [1]. Sensory biofeedback can be accomplished with an electromyographic electrode or a distal rectal balloon by applying either increasing electrical current or increasing the volume of water, respectively, to train the patients to recognize these stimuli at lower levels of current or water volume. Biofeedback trains the patient to recognize the presence of rectal contents at a lower threshold. This allows the patient more time to voluntarily contract the sphincter or head toward the bathroom and avoid an episode of incontinence.

Sphincter motor function can be trained electrically or manometrically by placing topical electrical leads in the anal region or a manometry catheter in the anal canal to pick up electrical activity or pressure responses to sphincter contraction. The electrical activity reading or pressure measurement is the feedback that the patients see to gauge their success. These measures have been successful, but not as successful in patients with a pudendal neuropathy. In those patients with no or minimal sphincter activity, electrical stimulation to the muscle at gradually increasing levels to accomplish a tetanizing stimulus to the sphincter has also led to improved symptoms [2].

The anal plug has been reported to be successful in some patients, but that device has not been widely used [3].

SURGICAL MANAGEMENT OF FECAL INCONTINENCE
Anal sphincteroplasty
Levatorplasty
Posterior anal repair
Total pelvic floor repair
Anal encirclement procedures
Foreign material encirclement
Graciloplasty—stimulated or unstimulated
Gluteoplasty
Artificial anal sphincter
Colostomy
Sacral spinal nerve stimulation

FIGURE 7-4.

Surgical management of fecal incontinence. In the discussion of the surgical management options, except for the colostomy, the strategy is to improve the function of the sphincter mechanism. The anal sphincteroplasty is by far the most frequently used and most successful of the procedures for treating fecal incontinence. Therefore, this procedure needs to be considered in great detail. It is most successful in treating clearly identified sphincter defects in those without a neuropathy. As with any of the surgical procedures, a thorough bowel preparation with an antegrade colonic lavage prep, antibiotics the night before surgery, and intravenous antibiotics preoperatively are in order. An approximating technique for a sphincteroplasty will be described. An overlapping sphincter technique has been championed, but it has no proven higher success and requires excessive dissection and traction on the muscle. The anterior obstetric injury is the most common location, but the approximation technique can be used in any quadrant. Each of these procedures will be considered individually. The anal encirclement procedures may be considered when there is a nonfunctioning anal sphincter with a patulent anal canal. These procedures have low to modest success with a noticeable risk. Some of these procedures are still in the development phase.

Another development has been the application of electrostimulation to the sacral spinal nerves for the control of fecal incontinence. There is more experience with this technique for the treatment of urinary incontinence. So far, with limited experience, there has been noticeable success [4].

Fecal incontinence can be a terrible problem, but appropriate treatment can bring marked improvement in a person's life-style and function.

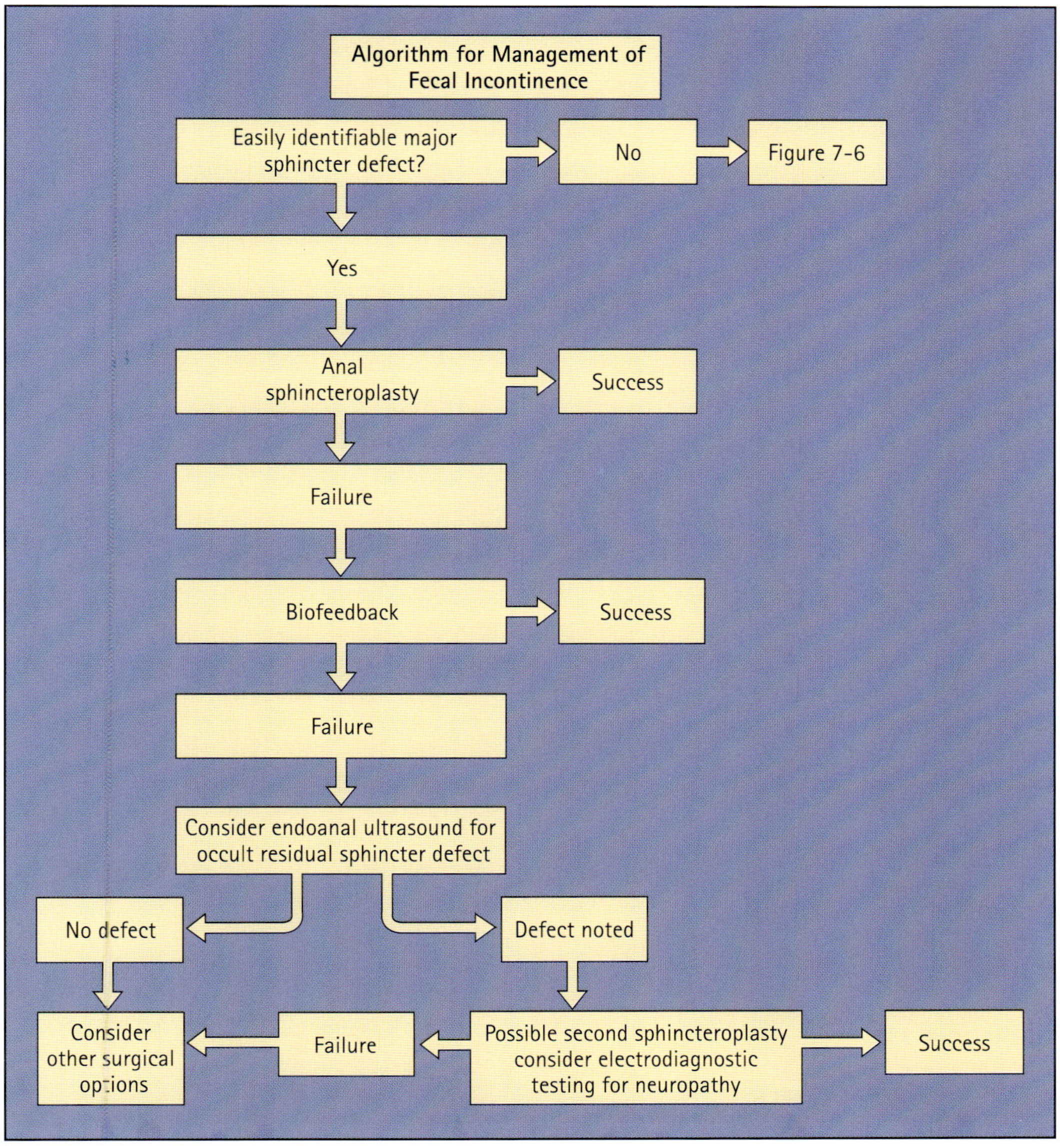

FIGURE 7-5.

Algorithm for management of fecal incontinence. This algorithm uses basic concepts and follows a logical progression. A few key clinical points lead to a logical flow. These are the identification of a major or minor sphincter defect and identification of contractile or noncontractile sphincter muscle. This algorithm assumes that the patient has significant symptoms that have not responded to dietary manipulation, Kegel exercises, or bowel regimens. It also assumes that the patient has had an appropriate and thorough evaluation that has revealed no major proximal intestinal cause. It should be noted that the role of manometry is not routinely helpful in clinical decision-making, although it may be helpful in identifying patients who would benefit from anorectal sensory biofeedback. It can also be useful for clinical documentation or trials.

The most common scenario is seen in the first portion of this algorithm in a patient identified with a sphincter defect. Treatment consists of a sphincteroplasty, which yields an 80% success rate [5]. If failure occurs or the results are not completely acceptable, biofeedback may contribute to improvement of the patient's symptoms [6]. Endoanal ultrasound has been shown to identify occult sphincter defects that may benefit from further surgical management [7]. However, endoanal ultrasound has a notable rate of falsely abnormal tests [8]. In certain clinical situations, anal electrodiagnostic testing can be helpful in predicting surgical outcome. For example, if a patient is found to have a pudendal neuropathy one might expect a lower success rate from sphincteroplasty. However, this may not preclude success from surgery [7] if an anatomic sphincter defect is documented. When these measures have failed, other surgical options can be considered, including anal encirclement procedures or a colostomy.

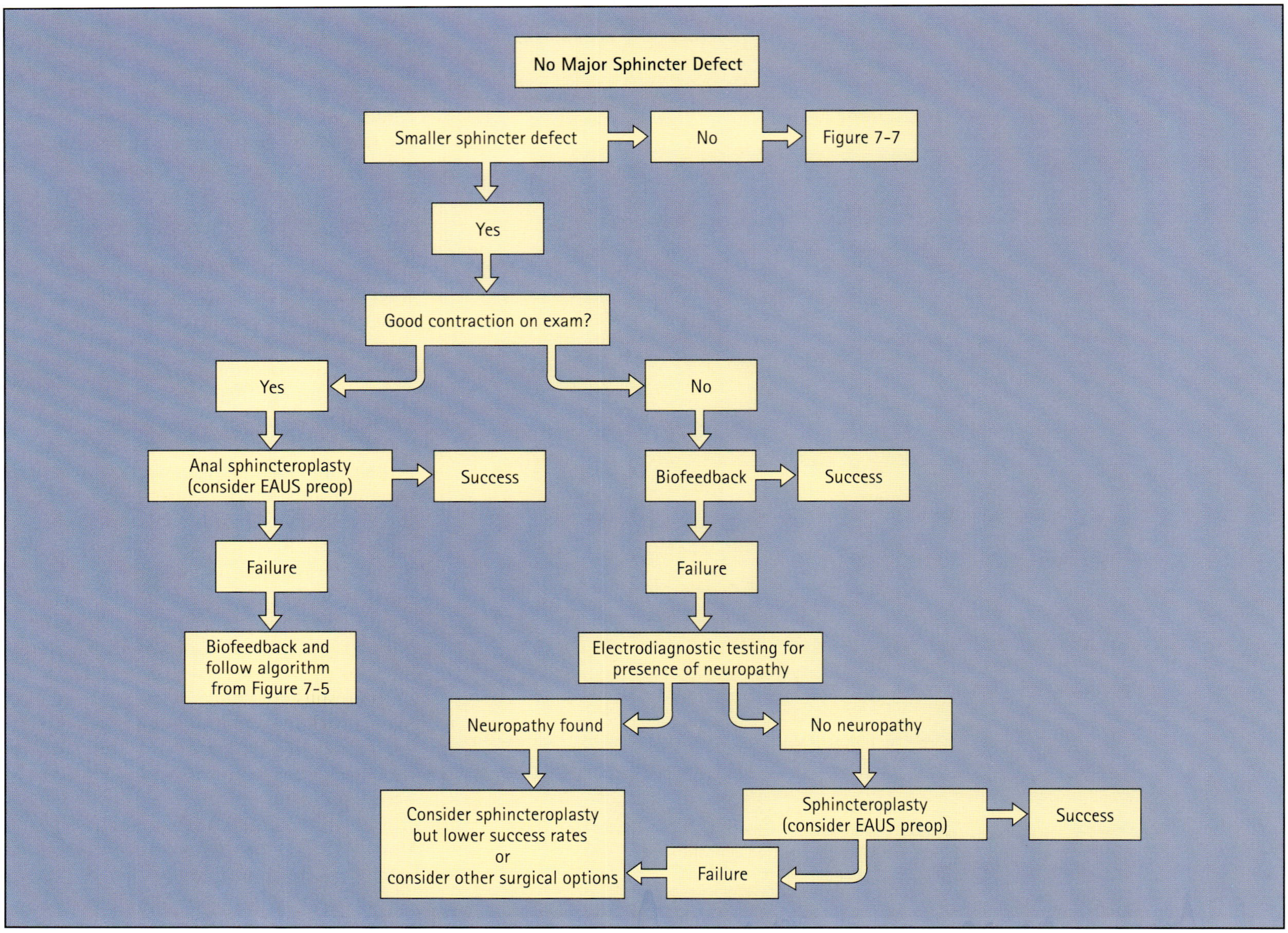

FIGURE 7-6.

Fecal incontinence algorithm with no major sphincter defect. In the presence of a minor sphincter defect with good sphincter contraction on physical examination, a sphincteroplasty would be reasonable. In this situation it may be helpful to map the sphincter with a preoperative anal ultrasound. If sphincteroplasty fails, then biofeedback could be considered following the algorithm in Figure 7-5. In a patient with a minor defect with poor contraction, biofeedback should be the initial line of management. Certainly, one needs to be thinking that this patient may have a neuropathy, and if biofeedback fails, testing for a neuropathy would be in order. Again, in the presence of a neuropathy, one might expect a lower chance of success. If a neuropathy is found, depending on multiple clinical circumstances, one might go on to consider other surgical options. EAUS—endoanal ultrasound.

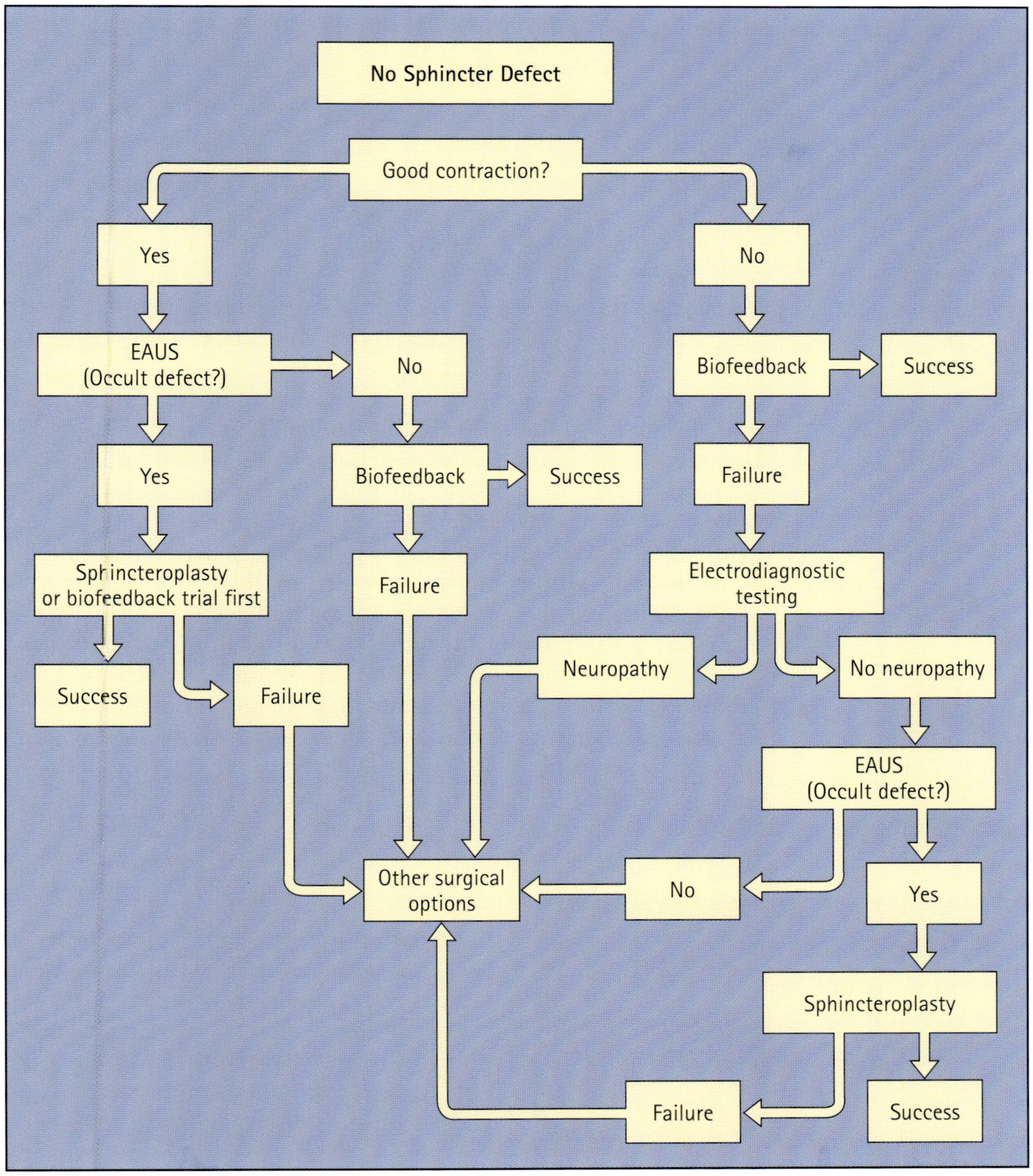

FIGURE 7-7.

Fecal incontinence algorithm with no sphincter defect. In a patient with no identifiable sphincter defect on examination with good contraction, an endoanal ultrasound (EAUS) would be reasonable to help identify an occult sphincter defect that might benefit from a sphincteroplasty. In that circumstance, a trial of biofeedback could be considered and, if unsuccessful, a sphincteroplasty could be performed if one was found to have satisfactory sphincter anatomy, satisfactory contraction, and still have incontinence. In this circumstance, manometry and electrodiagnostic testing could be considered and may help in directing a course of biofeedback. If a person should have satisfactory anatomy or a minor defect but no contraction of the sphincter, then a neuropathy is likely. If this patient is postpartum, a waiting period for up to 1 year is recommended. This may preclude the need for further treatment because there is a significant spontaneous recovery rate from obstetric neurologic injury. If the biofeedback measures become necessary, and electrodiagnostic testing shows no neuropathy, then an EAUS could be considered looking for occult defect that might benefit from a sphincteroplasty. Should a neuropathy be present, no occult defect be identified, or the sphincteroplasty fail, then other surgical options could be considered.

ANAL SPHINCTEROPLASTY

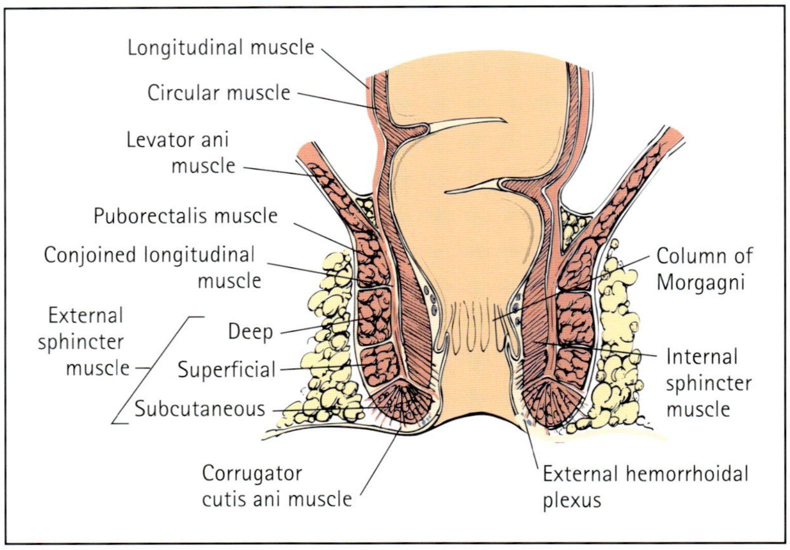

FIGURE 7-8.

Anal anatomy. An understanding of sphincter anatomy is important in accomplishing a good repair and result. The internal sphincter, an involuntary smooth muscle, has a major role of maintaining the resting sphincter tone. It is a continuation of the inner muscular layer of the rectum, which is thickened, and resides in the inner upper two-thirds of the anal canal. A problem with this portion of the sphincter can lead to problems with fine tuning of bowel control.

The voluntary sphincter mechanism consists of the medial most portion of the levator contribution, the puborectalis muscle, which is a sling wrapped posterior and lateral on the rectum and inserted bilaterally on the pubis. The distal two-thirds of the anal canal is the circumferential external sphincter, which extends about 1.5 cm distal to the lower extent of the internal sphincter. The external anal sphincter is innervated by the pudendal nerve from below. The puborectalis is innervated most likely by the direct bundles of the pelvic plexus from above. The internal anal sphincter is innervated by sacral parasympathetics and visceral (prevertebral) sympathetics. The external sphincter and puborectalis are responsible for the voluntary contraction squeeze pressure that closes the anus. Minor defects may be asymptomatic. Major defects in this mechanism may lead to significant symptoms of incontinence, but not necessarily. It is critical to repair both the voluntary and involuntary sphincter mechanism to its full length to obtain optimal results. The repair has to be such that from the baseline tonic state it would allow both relaxation with opening of the canal and contraction with tight closing. The result needs to be as close to normal anatomy as possible, otherwise patulence or stenosis can occur.

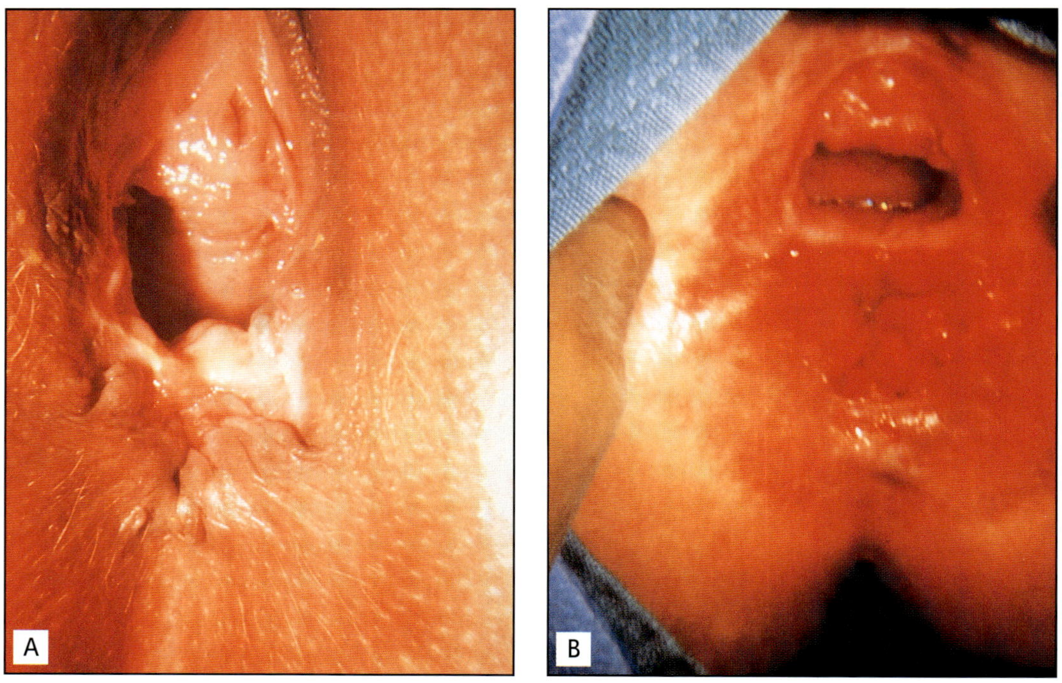

FIGURE 7-9.

Childbirth trauma. **A**, This major, easily identified sphincter defect was caused by trauma from childbirth. There is complete absence of the perineal body and anterior sphincter with major patulence of the anal canal. **B**, This is another example of a major sphincter defect from childbirth injury. There is retraction of both the internal and external sphincter musculature to about the 3 and 9 o'clock positions with anterior being 12 o'clock.

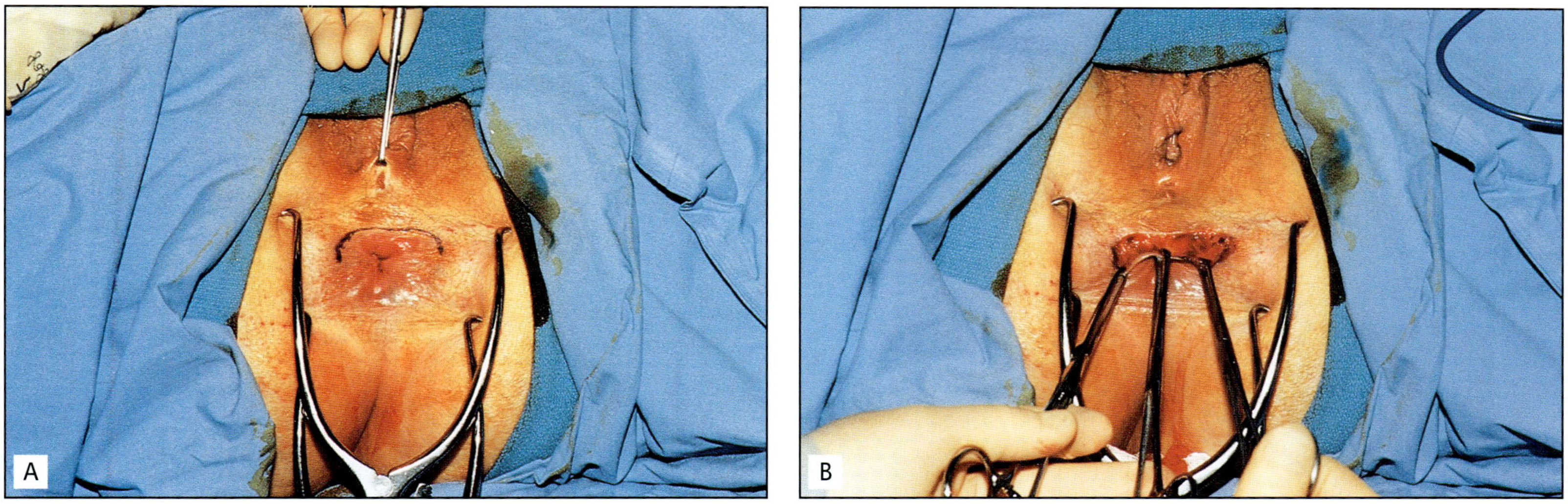

FIGURE 7-10.

Technique. This series of figures gives a detailed description and visualization of the location of the incision, technique of exposure, technique of instrument placement, and the steps to ensure adequate dissection of the sphincter. **A**, One will notice that the initial incision is a SAD incision (concentric curved) with an inverted Y closure as the sphincter ends are brought together and the anal canal closed. This illustration shows a lithotomy position with a Betadine preparation. The defect in this patient is a minor defect that was easily identified on physical examination. **B**, The skin incision is performed with a no. 15 blade and clamps are placed on the skin flap as the perianal skin is dissected up into the anal canal. The internal sphincter is beginning to be exposed and a space developed to bring the sphincters together. Gelpi retractors are used for exposure.

In a case with significant loss of perineal length, a SAD incision is made anterior to the anus combined with a smile incision posterior to the vagina with the incisions meeting in the middle. This allows for better exposure, wide dissection, and a greater area in the midline to reconstruct the perineum (not shown).

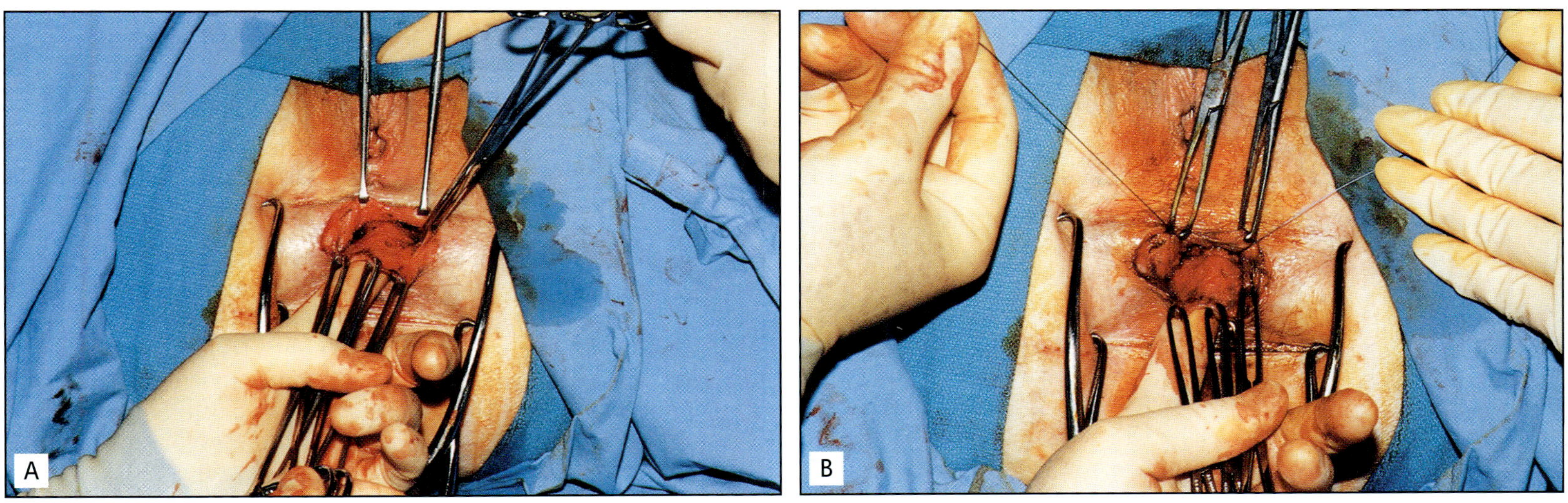

FIGURE 7-11.

Internal sphincter. **A**,With a gloved hand in the anal canal holding the inferior skin flap, retractor clamps are placed on the midline perineal scar tissue and a portion of the retracted external sphincter. The dissection is extended superiorly at least to the same level as the puborectalis, which is superior and lateral. This depth of dissection is important so that a satisfactory length on the internal sphincter repair will be accomplished. Next, the right lateral clamp is placed on the sphincter in the 2 o'clock position and retracted anteriorly while the anal canal digit is palpating the location of the internal sphincter during this retraction. As the clamp is gently and repeatedly tugged, the location of the internal sphincter is identified. **B**, This exposure allows for the complete identification of the internal sphincter superiorly to lead to a satisfactory length to the internal sphincter repair. This illustration shows the first suture being placed in the internal sphincter at the superior extent of the anal canal at the level of the puborectalis. Sutures with 2-0 Vicryl^{R} are placed and ideally the assistant would tie so that the surgeon could leave the anal canal digit in place, therefore avoiding the need to continually change gloves to tie knots. After each layer of dissection and closure is done, the wound is irrigated with saline or Betadine.

(Continued on next page)

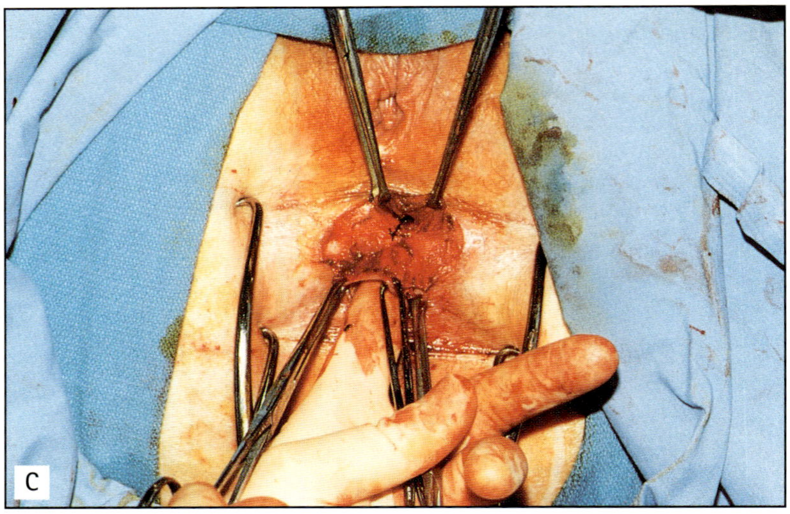

FIGURE 7-11. *(Continued)*
C, These interrupted sutures are continued to the same inferior position as the posterior internal sphincter, which can be palpated with the anal canal digit.

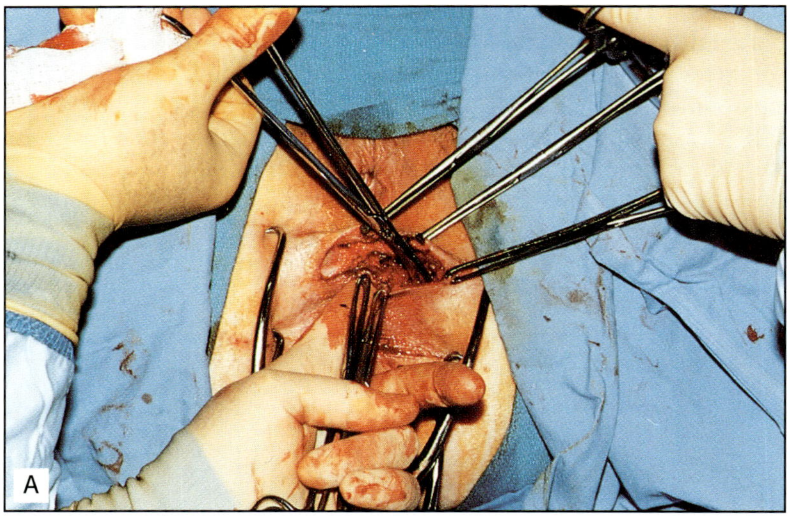

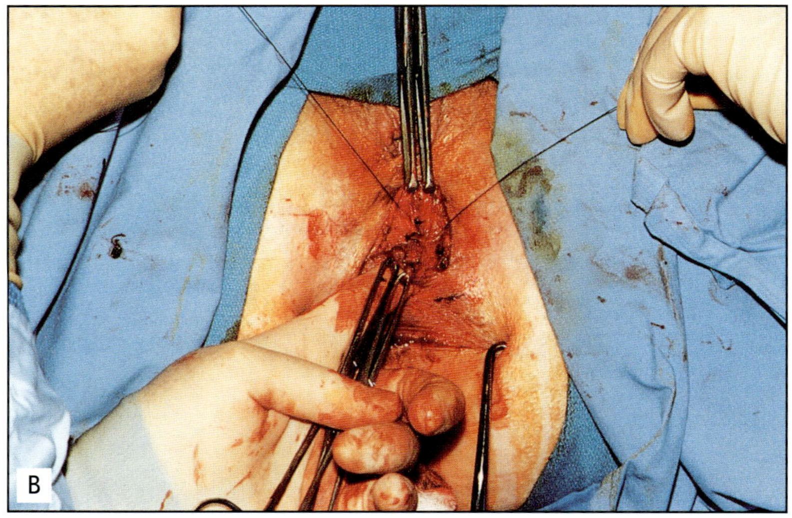

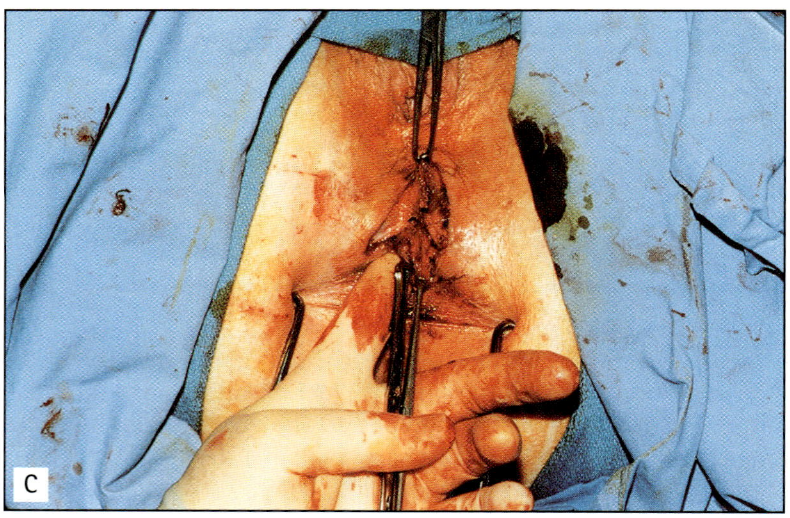

FIGURE 7-12.
External sphincter. **A**, The external sphincter is then elevated from the scar tissue and the perianal skin laterally and posteriorly bilaterally. This is only done at the skin level, as illustrated, and not dissected lateral to the sphincter in the ischial rectal space. Limiting the lateral dissection will help to avoid injury to the anal branch of the pudendal nerve. The sphincter only needs to be dissected so that it can be brought to the midline without excessive tension. Sharp dissection is necessary to allow freeing of this muscle and to avoid skin dimpling. **B**, Using clamps for exposure and retracting the external sphincter superiorly, apical superior sutures are placed in the external sphincter with the goal of providing a satisfactory length to the external sphincter. The first suture is placed in the external sphincter near the level of the puborectalis, which can be felt posteriorly and laterally. Sutures of 2-0 Vicryl^{R} are used for each layer, except for the skin where 3-0 or 4-0 Vicryl^{R} sutures are used. It should be noted that the scar tissue is not excised at any time during the sphincter dissection. In fact, it is used to anchor and secure the sutures. **C**, The repair is then continued externally so that the external sphincter is repaired to a level about a 1.0 to 1.5 cm distal to the lower extent of the internal sphincter. The external sphincter should be repaired to the same level as the palpable external sphincter posteriorly. Some degree of imbrication occurs at this distal point. The sphincter should be snug, but the examining index finger should be able to be inserted fairly easily.

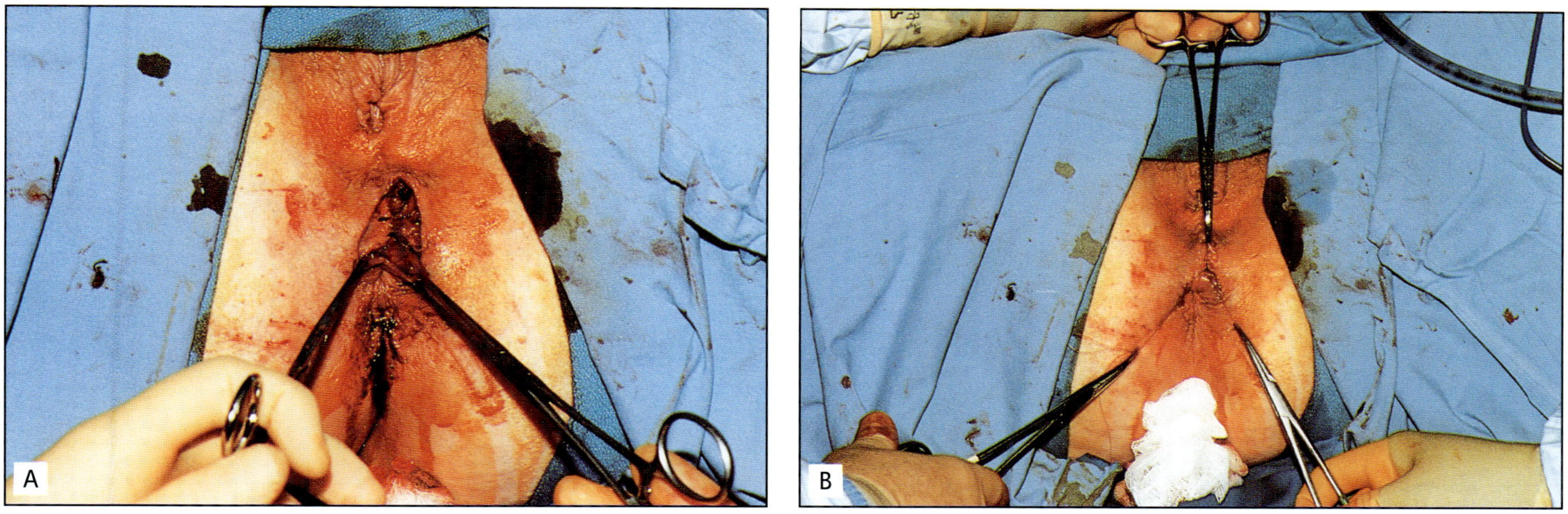

FIGURE 7-13.

Perineal body. **A**, Sutures are also placed in the perineal body and, at this point, it can be seen that the perineal body is lengthened, especially in cases where there are major sphincter injuries. The wound is then irrigated and closed. Some surgeons do a sphincterotomy at the 5 o'clock position to decrease tension on the suture line and prevent stenosis [16]. **B**, This closure has an inverted Y appearance. It is helpful to try not to trim off any skin if possible to help decrease the risk of anal stenosis. The clamps are on the tails of the knots on the Y limb. This patient had an excellent result.

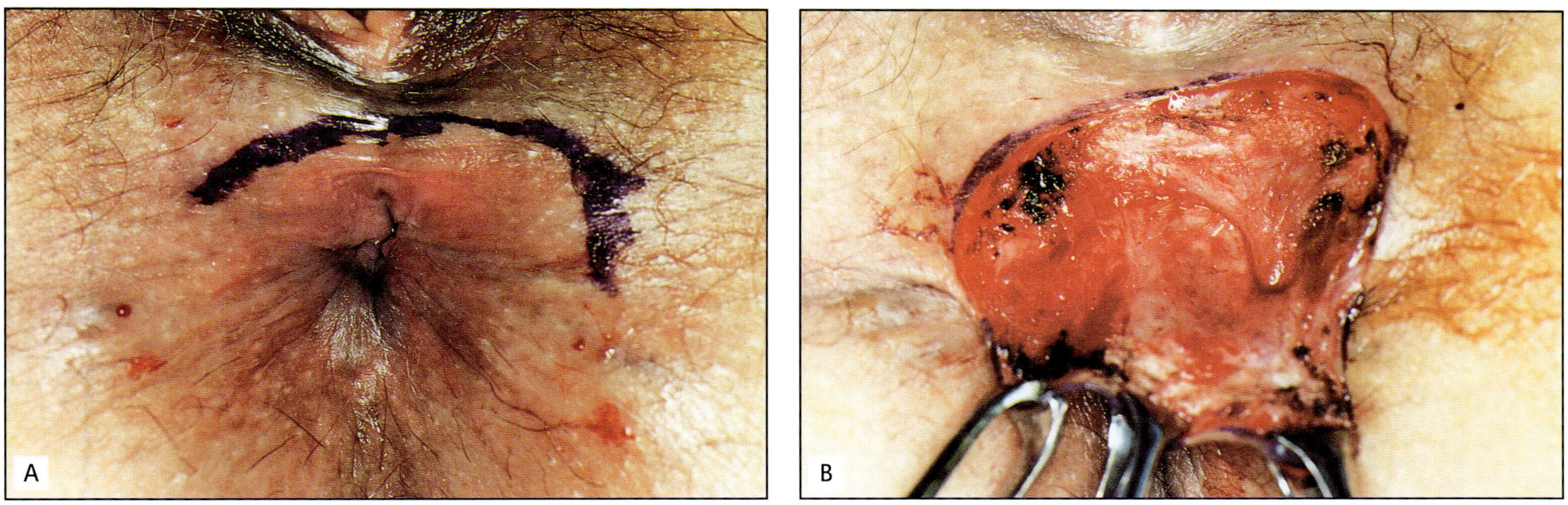

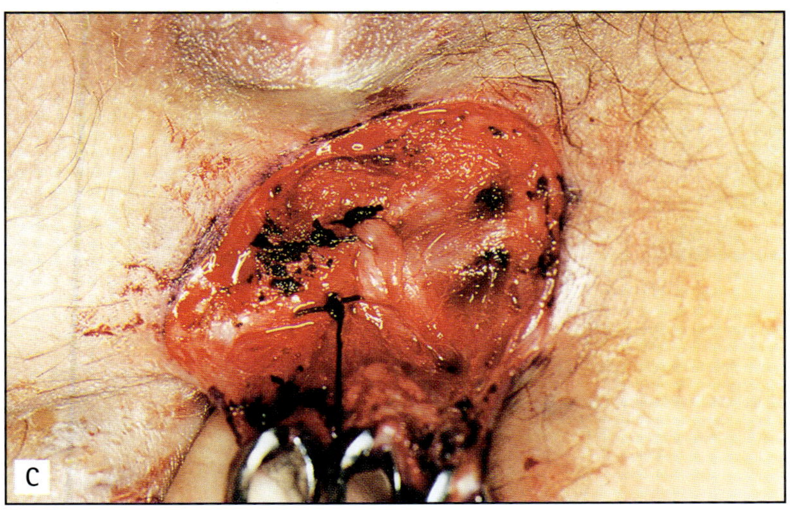

FIGURE 7-14.

Minor sphincter defect. **A**, A closer view of an obvious minor sphincter defect on physical examination is seen, again with a SAD incision from the 10 o'clock to 3 o'clock position. The incision is extended just past the edge of the palpable retracted external sphincter. Again, anterior is up. **B**, The anoderm is elevated off of the scar tissue superiorly to the level of the puborectalis, which could be palpated posteriorly. Care is taken to avoid a hole in this flap because this may result in an abscess or fistula. The scar is left intact and used to secure the suture material. **C**, The interrupted sutures are placed in the internal sphincter. The finger in the anal canal is used to identify the internal sphincter so that it can be repaired to the appropriate proximal and distal extent.

(*Continued on next page*)

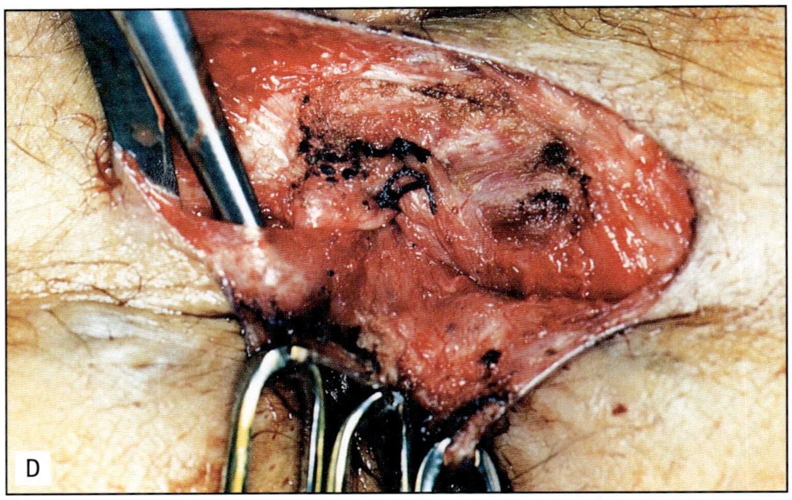

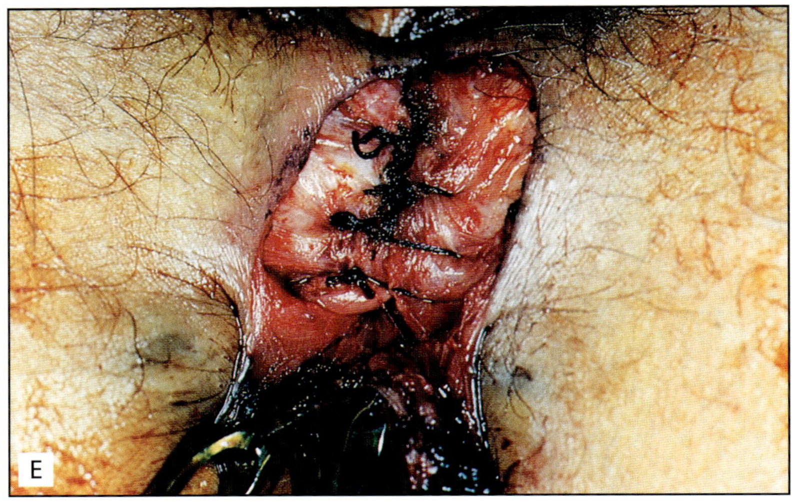

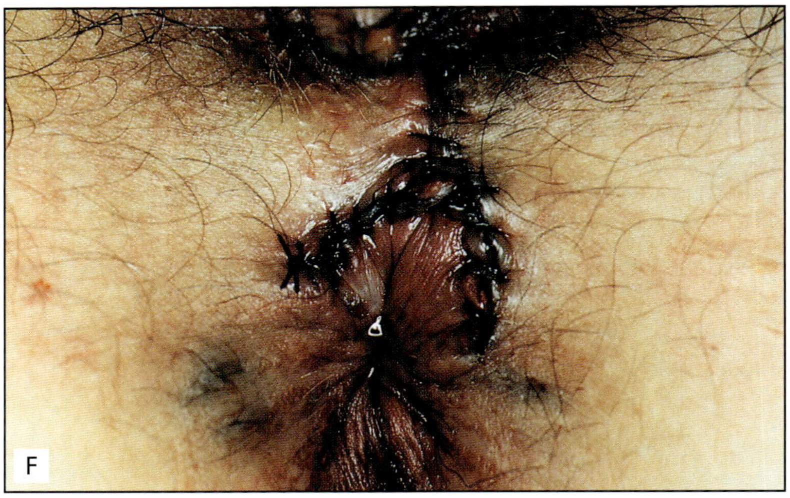

FIGURE 7-14. *(Continued)*
D, The external sphincter is then freed from the scar in the skin using sharp dissection with Metzenbaum's scissors. **E**, Interrupted sutures are used to close this external sphincter and imbricate it to the appropriate tension as previously mentioned. **F**, A Y closure can be accomplished with a running Vicryl^{R} suture.

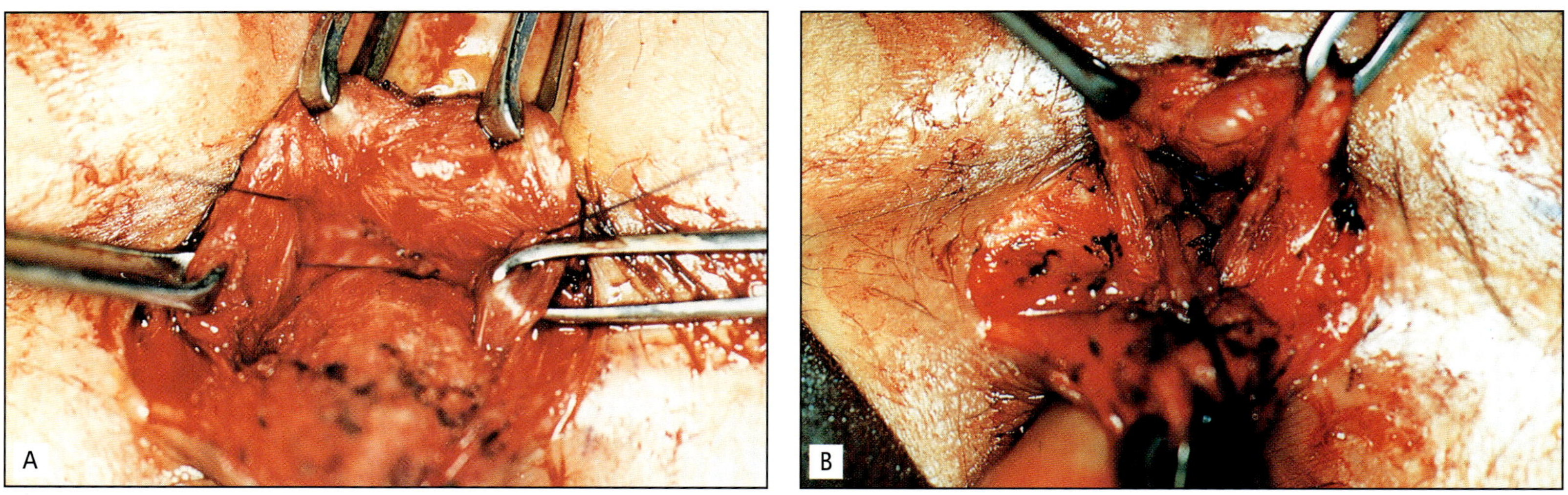

FIGURE 7-15.
Depth of dissection of anal flap. **A**, These photographs illustrate the significant depth of dissection of the anal flap. Clamps are placed laterally on the most inferior internal sphincter. The first interrupted suture is being placed in the proximal internal sphincter. Anterior clamps are placed on the skin and perineal scar for exposure. **B**, The internal sphincter repair leaves a small cavity to allow closure of the external sphincter and perineal body. This is done with interrupted sutures.

(Continued on next page)

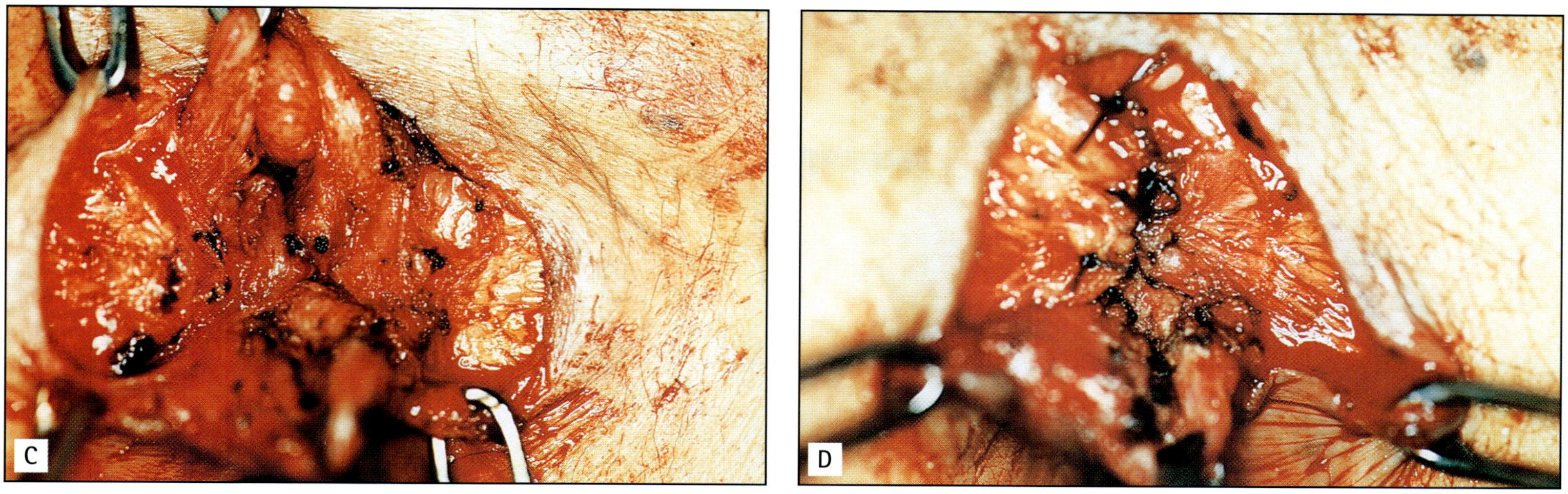

FIGURE 7–15. *(Continued)*
C, The skin flaps are then dissected giving better exposure to the external sphincter. **D**, Finally, this is closed with some degree of imbrication in the midline. The anal canal finger should be fairly easily insertable with slight resistance as an indication of the tension of the repair.

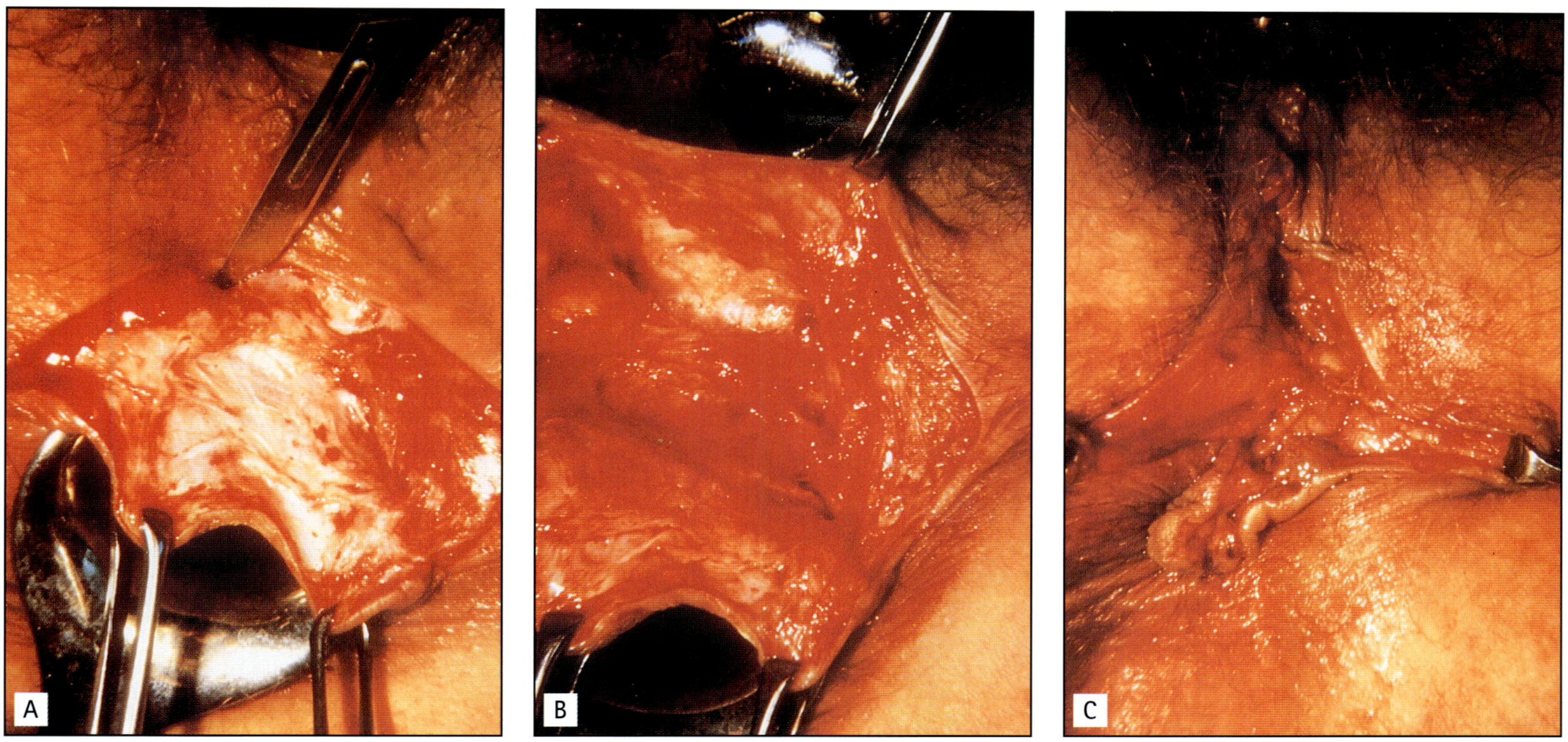

FIGURE 7–16.
Dissection in major sphincter defect. **A**, This next case illustrates the amount of dissection necessary in the repair of a patient with a major sphincter defect. A large incision is necessary with major anoderm elevation superiorly and laterally to identify the internal and external sphincter. **B**, Once these flaps are elevated in all directions, exposing the muscles, there is a large midline space giving room to bring these muscles into the midline. Again, the scar tissue is left intact to allow secure suture placement. **C**, Multiple layers of sutures are placed in the internal and external sphincter, as well as the perineal muscles, to reconstruct the perineum. What was once a SAD-shaped incision is now a vertical incision in the midline radiating between the anus and the vagina. Excessive skin may be trimmed if necessary.

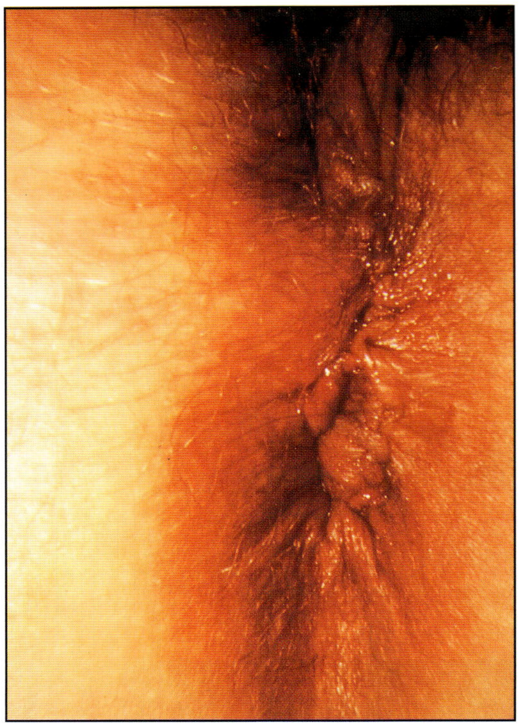

FIGURE 7-17.

Mobilization. In this case, so much mobilization was necessary that a linear skin closure was accomplished. Ideally, a good repair should be performed at the time of the initial sphincter damage using excellent lighting and sphincter exposure and identification of the same anatomic elements as discussed in this chapter. However, delayed sphincter repairs lead to good to excellent resolution of symptoms in the range of 60% to 90% of cases. Complications are uncommon but include infection, fistula, and stenosis. This can generally be performed on an outpatient basis and the postoperative care would include the use of a high-fiber diet, fiber supplements, plenty of fluids, laxatives until the first bowel movement occurs, and sitz baths. Some surgeons try to delay bowel movements in their patients with constipating agents, such as codeine. I have not found that necessary and am concerned about the risk of impaction and resultant damage to the repair.

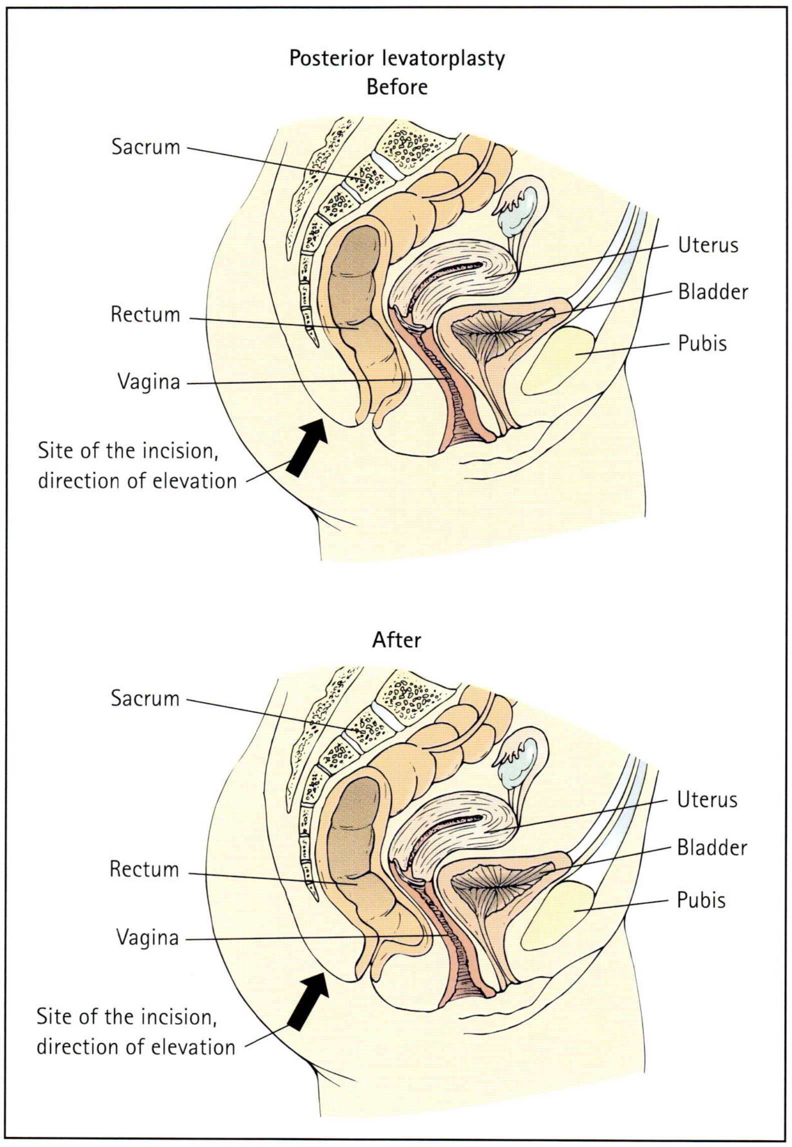

FIGURE 7-18.

Posterior levatorplasty. For idiopathic/neurogenic incontinence, various levatorplasties have been performed when nonoperative measures have been unsuccessful and when the sphincter is intact but insufficient in controlling stool. The posterior anal levatorplasty plication of the iliococcygeus, pubococcygeus, puborectalis, and external sphincter through an intrasphincteric approach has had modest initial success, but marginal long-term success. Theoretically, these procedures result in an elevation of the pelvic floor resulting in a decrease in the anorectal angle, which was thought to be a significant factor in continence. This has subsequently been disproved. Because there is not agreement on beneficial results, the anterior levatorplasty was added to plicate the puborectalis and external sphincter. The success rate of this "total pelvic floor" procedure has been modest, 33% improvement [9], and any success may be due to a lengthening of the sphincter. These procedures have limited use for the treatment of fecal incontinence. *Arrow* indicates the site of the incision, direction of elevation.

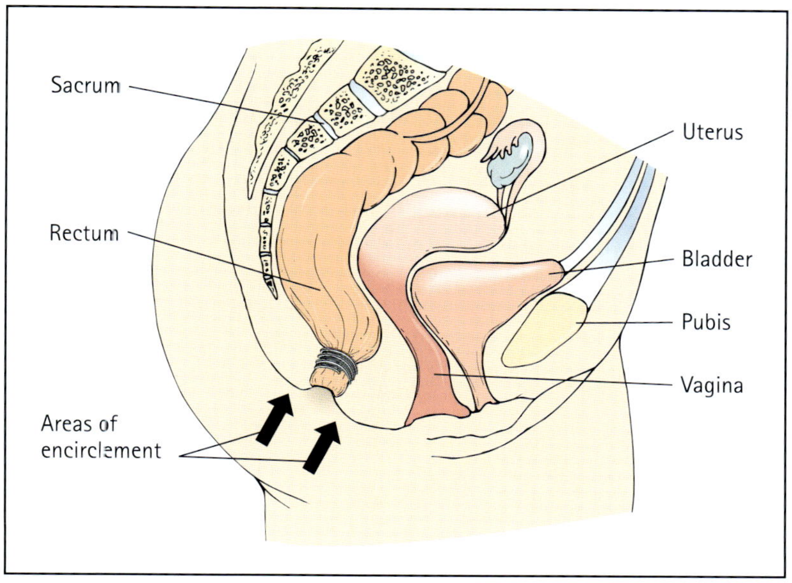

FIGURE 7-19.

Foreign material encirclement. The first of the encirclement procedures to be mentioned is encirclement of permanent foreign material (i.e., silk, wire, Silastic) about the anal sphincter (if present) or anal canal. This can be placed at various depths about the canal through two skin incisions below the levators. It has the problems of erosion, infection, obstructive-noncompliance, or laxity. This may be considered in someone with a poor health risk. It is for these reasons, autologous tissue is being used for patients in reasonable health who can tolerate the more involved procedures. *Arrow* indicates the area of encirclement.

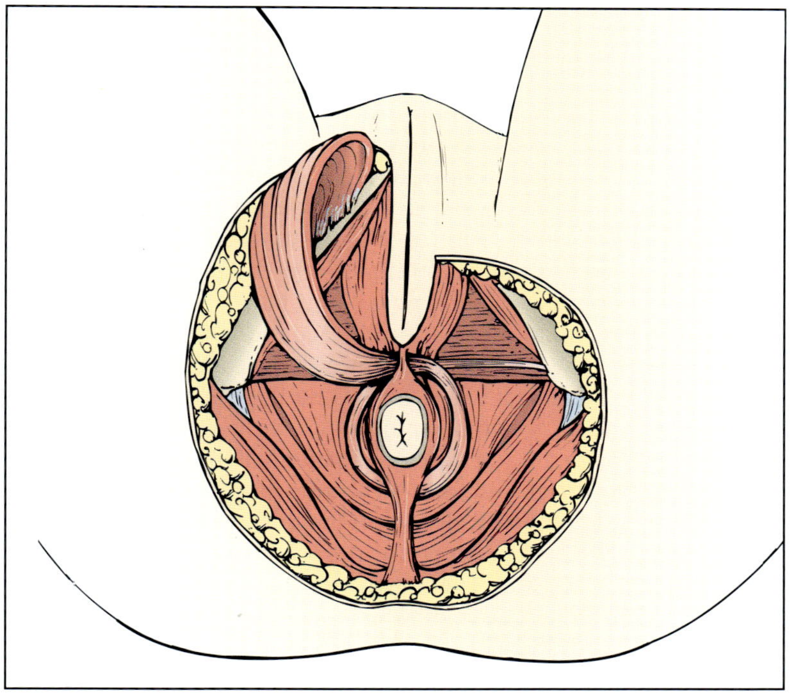

FIGURE 7-20.

Gracilis transposition. Muscle transposition with a wrap of either the gracilis or gluteus around the anus is attractive because it is autologous, unlike the foreign inert adynamic encirclements mentioned. The gracilis is dissected from the medial thigh and wrapped around the anus. It is then sutured to the contralateral ischium, preserving the nerve and vessels from the upper third of the muscle body. This procedure has been performed in one to three stages with or without a diverting stoma.

Relaxation of the neosphincter occurs with adduction of the thigh to allow for a bowel movement. More recently, attempts have been made to apply steady electrical stimulation to the innervating nerve or muscle to increase the baseline resting tone. A magnet is then passed over the battery pack to turn off the stimulus to allow the wrap to relax and a bowel movement to occur. The initiation of the stimulus is usually delayed for several weeks after surgery. As one might anticipate, there have been multiple technical complications along with the usual anticipated potential problems with any surgery. The continence rates with this procedure have been as high as 78%. However, a complication rate of 70% has been reported [10]. Some authors contend that this procedure should be done only in a research setting [11].

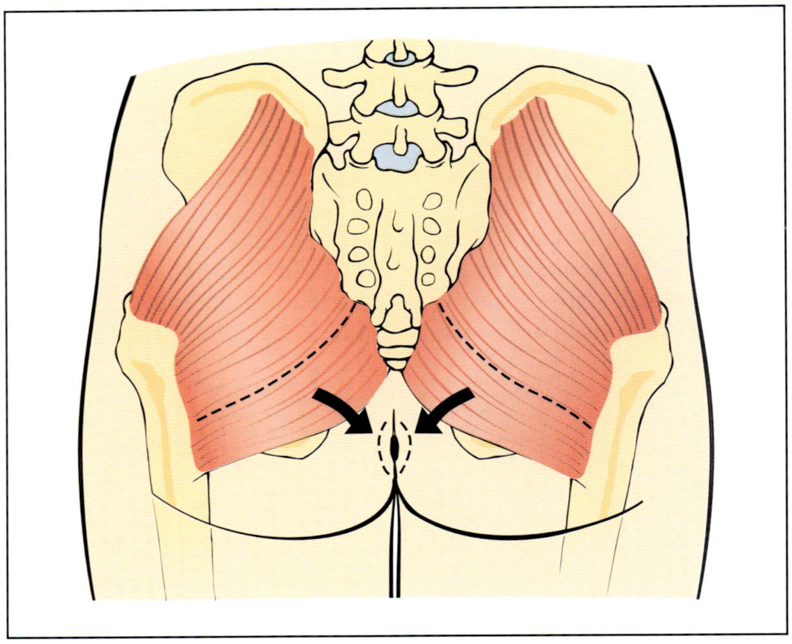

FIGURE 7-21.

Gluteus transposition. Bilateral inferior gluteal muscles have been used to create a neosphincter. They are transposed off of the sacrum, preserving the nerve supply. They are then manipulated to encircle the anus by either splitting the gluteal ends or wrapping one side anterior and one side posterior anchoring each to the contralateral muscle. Theoretically, this is a dynamic wrap with a muscle that retains the ability to contract and relax. The results of this technique are also reasonable (53% satisfactory continence) but imperfections have led investigators to consider electrical stimulation or pudendal nerve transplantation to this muscle and its nerve [12,13].

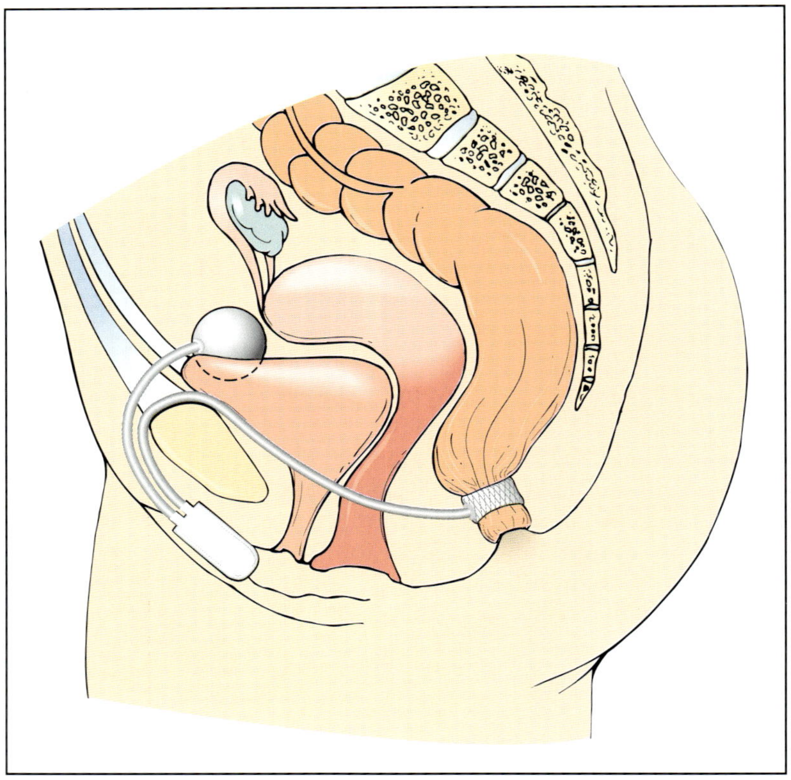

FIGURE 7-22.

Artificial sphincter. The use of the artificial sphincter has similar indications as the muscle transpositions and can be used when those muscles are not available. It does not bear the same risks involved with muscle harvest such as a defunctionalizing injury to the nerves. The device has three parts: an inflatable cuff placed around the anus, the control pump implanted in the scrotum or labia, and the pressure-regulating balloon placed in the abdomen. Deflation of the cuff allows for fecal evacuation. The artificial sphincter carries the risks of mechanical failure and infection. Despite this, the artificial sphincter has had reasonable success: 75% success and 33% complication rates, similar to the muscle transpositions with greater ease of placement [14]. Another experimental artificial sphincter technique is being engineered to be placed transabdominally, deep into the pelvis, along the rectum, just above the levators. Theoretically, it works by kinking/folding the bowel under low pressure. The drawbacks to this technique would be significant including the risks of major abdominal surgery [15].

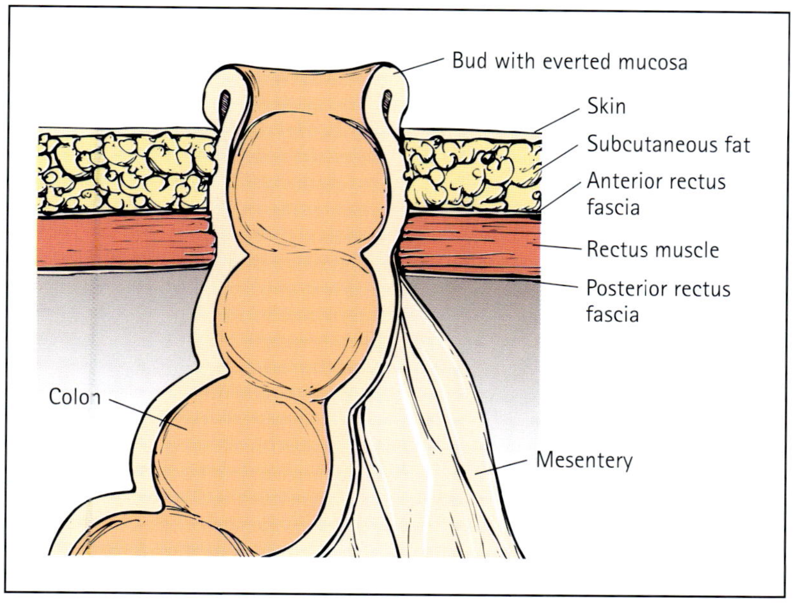

FIGURE 7-23.

Colostomy. When the other appropriate medical and surgical measures are unsuccessful in managing fecal incontinence, colostomy placement, usually at the level of the left colon, is a good option. Although it is a major operation, it is a very familiar technique to colon and rectal surgeons and is successful in controlling anal incontinence. A laparoscopic approach may decrease operative morbidity. Colostomy placement can be difficult in obese patients or in those with a history of multiple previous abdominal operations. It is important to make sure that there is an adequate length to allow an everted bud external to the skin. This ensures a better fit of the ostomy collection device and thus prevents leakage and skin excoriation. The most common long-term complication is a peristomal hernia. This is usually repairable but may require a repeat laparotomy. It is important that the physician and the enterostomal therapist work together to provide education, appropriate equipment and emotional and technical support. This will help the patient to accept the stoma and pursue a normal life-style with few, if any, limitations.

REFERENCES

1. Rieger NA, Wattchow DA, Sarre RG, *et al.*: Prospective trial of pelvic floor retraining in patients with fecal incontinence. *Dis Colon Rectum* 1997, 40:821–826.
2. Pescatori M, Pavesio R, Anastasio G, Daini S: Transanal electrostimulation for fecal incontinence: clinical, psychologic, and manometric prospective study. *Dis Colon Rectum* 1991, 34:540–545.
3. Mortensen N, Humphreys MS: The anal continence plug: a disposable device for patients with anorectal incontinence. *Lancet* 1991, 338:295.
4. Matzel KE, Stadelmaier U, Hohenfellner M: Electrical stimulation of sacral spinal nerves for treatment of fecal incontinence. *Lancet* 1995, 346:1124–1127.
5. Engel AF, Kamm MA, Sultan AH, *et al.*: Anterior and sphincter repair in patients with obstetric trauma. *Br J Surg* 1994, 81:1231–1234.
6. Jensen LL, Lowry AC. Biofeedback improves functional outcome after sphincteroplasty. *Dis Colon Rectum* 1997, 40:197–200
7. Ternent CA, Shashidharan M, Blatchford GJ, *et al.*: *Dis Colon Rectum* 1997, 40:462–467.
8. Sentovich SM, Wong WD, Blatchford GJ: Accuracy and reliability of transanal ultrasound for anterior and sphincter injury. *Dis Colon Rectum* 1998, 41:1000–1004.
9. VanTets WF, Kuijpers JHC. Pelvic floor procedures produce no consistent changes in anatomy or physiology. *Dis Colon Rectum* 1998, 41:365–369.
10. Geerdes BP, Heineman E, Konsten J, Soeters PB, *et al.*: Dynamic graciloplasty. *Dis Colon Rectum* 1996, 39:8, 912–917
11. Wexner SD, Gonzalez-Pardon A, Rius J, *et al.*: Stimulated gracilis neosphincter operation. *Dis Colon Rectum* 1996, Sept 39:9, 957–964.
12. Devesa JM, Fernandez Madrid JM, Rodriguez Gallego B, *et al.*: Bilateral gluteoplasty for fecal incontinence. *Dis Colon Rectum* 1997, 40:957–964.
13. Christiansen J, Ronholt Hansen C, Rasmussen O: Bilateral gluteus maximus transposition for anal incontinence. *Br. J Surg* 1995, 82:883–888.
14. Wong WD, Jensen LL, Bartolo DC, Rothenberger DA: Artificial anal sphincter. *Dis Colon Rectum* 1996, 39:1345–51.
15. Hajivassiliou CA, Carter KB, Finlay IG: Assessment of a novel implantable artificial anal sphincter. *Dis Colon Rectum* 1997, 40:711–717.
16. Tancer ML, Lasser D, Rosenblum N: Rectovaginal fistula or perineal and anal sphincter disruption, or both, after vaginal delivery. *Surgery, Gynecology and Obstetrics* 1990, 171:43-46.

Nonsurgical Management of Prolapse

CHAPTER 8

Stephen B. Young

A pessary is a device worn in the vagina to support the uterus, remedy a malposition, or prevent conception; it is also considered a vaginal suppository [1]. In this chapter we confine our discussion to the contemporary use of flexible silicone devices used to nonsurgically treat pelvic organ prolapse. Our goal is to guide the practitioner as to which pessary to chose and how to use it in the conservative treatment of each woman's pelvic floor problem.

Pessaries are excellent devices to prepare for, postpone, or prevent surgical intervention. Many postmenopausal women with exteriorized prolapse present with atrophic, dry, thin, cracked, and frequently ulcerated vaginal skin outside the vulva. To prepare for optimal surgical intervention, a minimum of 2 months of topical intravaginal estrogen cream should be applied. A pessary will keep the exteriorized bulge in situ allowing for improvement in the local environment by relieving vascular kinking, air-drying, and decreasing friction from contact with clothing. The now replaced vagina can maintain prolonged contact with the estrogen cream, which is inserted each night. This will allow thickening, increased vascularity, and perhaps even improvement in the dissection planes to permit optimized surgical technique. Other patients with prolapse want to wait a period of months before surgery. The schoolteacher, the "snowbird," and the caregiver of a sick husband may need to postpone definitive correction to a more appropriate time. Many older women have multiple significant medical conditions that render them poor candidates for lengthy definitive reconstructive pelvic surgery. They may be managed effectively with long-term pessary use.

The history of pessaries dates back to the Greek and Roman eras and is rich and fascinating in the varieties of organic and inorganic materials used for replacement of vaginal contents. Famous medical names through ancient and medieval times are associated with the development of pessaries. Hippocrates and later Soranus and Diocles used half of a pomegranate sometimes soaked in vinegar. Near the end of the Roman Era emollient, astringent, and aperient drug-soaked pledgets tied to string were used. In the Middle Ages, around 1050 AD, Trotula, the first recorded female gynecologist, made a ball pessary of linen strips, which she held in place with a T-binder. In 1559, Caspar Stromayr used a tightly rolled sponge, bound with string, dipped in wax and covered with oil or butter. The great physician Ambrose Pare invented an oval pessary of hammered brass and waxed cork as well as pear-shaped and ring pessaries. The anatomist William Harvey used pessaries. The first operative gynecology textbook by Hendrik Van Roonhuyse in 1663 described a cork with a hole dipped in wax [2]. When complications from pessary use, including discharge and viscous perforation, were discovered, the field evolved. In 1783, Jean Juville invented a soft rubber pessary that could be self-inserted.

During the past 200 years, pessaries have been used for a variety of illusory conditions including uterine inflammation, displacement, or retroversion. The invention and development of rubber vulcanization, plastics, and more recently, silicone-based materials over the past 150 years has facilitated the evolution of better materials for pessary manufacture. Most pessaries currently in use for the treatment of pelvic organ prolapse are simple, soft, flexible, inert devices made of silicone and supplied in various shapes and sizes.

In choosing a particular pessary for an individual patient's needs we try to use the least invasive device that will remain in the vagina, hold the pelvic organs in situ, cause the least number of local symptoms, and require the gentlest and most infrequent change. A properly sized and positioned pessary will sit obliquely behind the symphysis and will just barely appear, if at all, on lithotomy Valsalva with the labia separated. A device that is too small will fall out with any activity. A device that is too large may not sit properly intravaginally behind the symphysis and will cause discomfort and pressure. It may also interfere with micturition and defecation.

When possible, we instruct the patient in self-removal, cleaning, and reinsertion. This allows her to change her own pessary in the privacy of her home, taking it out at night and reinserting in the morning so that the vagina can be free of the foreign body while she is at rest. This markedly decreases pessary-related vaginitis and local erosions, by far the most frequent complications of pessary use. It also makes her more independent, requiring far fewer visits to have the pessary changed.

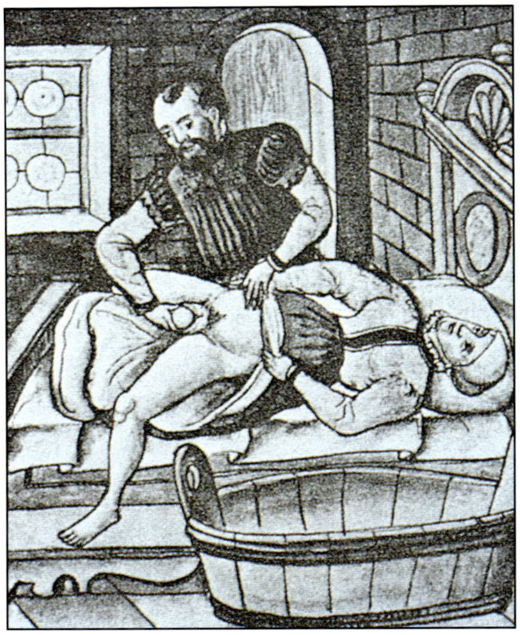

FIGURE 8–1.
Woodcut of Caspar Stromayr inserting a wax ball pessary circa 1559. (*From* Miller DS [2], with permission.)

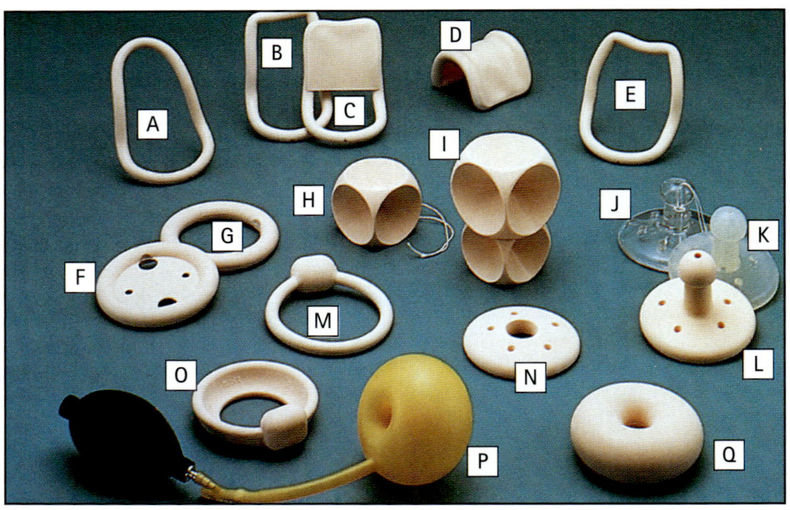

FIGURE 8–2 .
Milex pessaries. The Milex Company distributes a wide selection of largely silicone-flexible pessaries. **Bold** indicates the pessaries most frequently used and detailed in this chapter.
A. Smith (silicone, folding)
B. Hodge without support (silicone, folding)
C. Hodge with support (silicone, folding)
D. **Gehrung with support (silicone, folding)**
E. Risser (silicone, folding)
F. **Ring with support (silicone, folding)**
G. **Ring without support (silicone, folding)**
H. **Cube (silicone, flexible)**
I. Tandem-Cube (silicone, flexible)
J. Rigid Gellhorn (acrylic, multiple drain)
K.95% Rigid Gellhorn (silicone, multiple drain)
L. **Flexible Gellhorn (silicone, multiple drain)**
M. Ring incontinence (silicone)
N. Shaatz (silicone, folding)
O. Incontinence dish (silicone, folding)
P. Inflato Ball (latex)
Q.**Donut (silicone)**
In decreasing order of choice and increasing order of invasiveness we use the ring, donut, Gehrung, Gellhorn, and cube pessaries in the conservative treatment of pelvic organ prolapse. (*From* Milex Products, Inc., Chicago, IL)

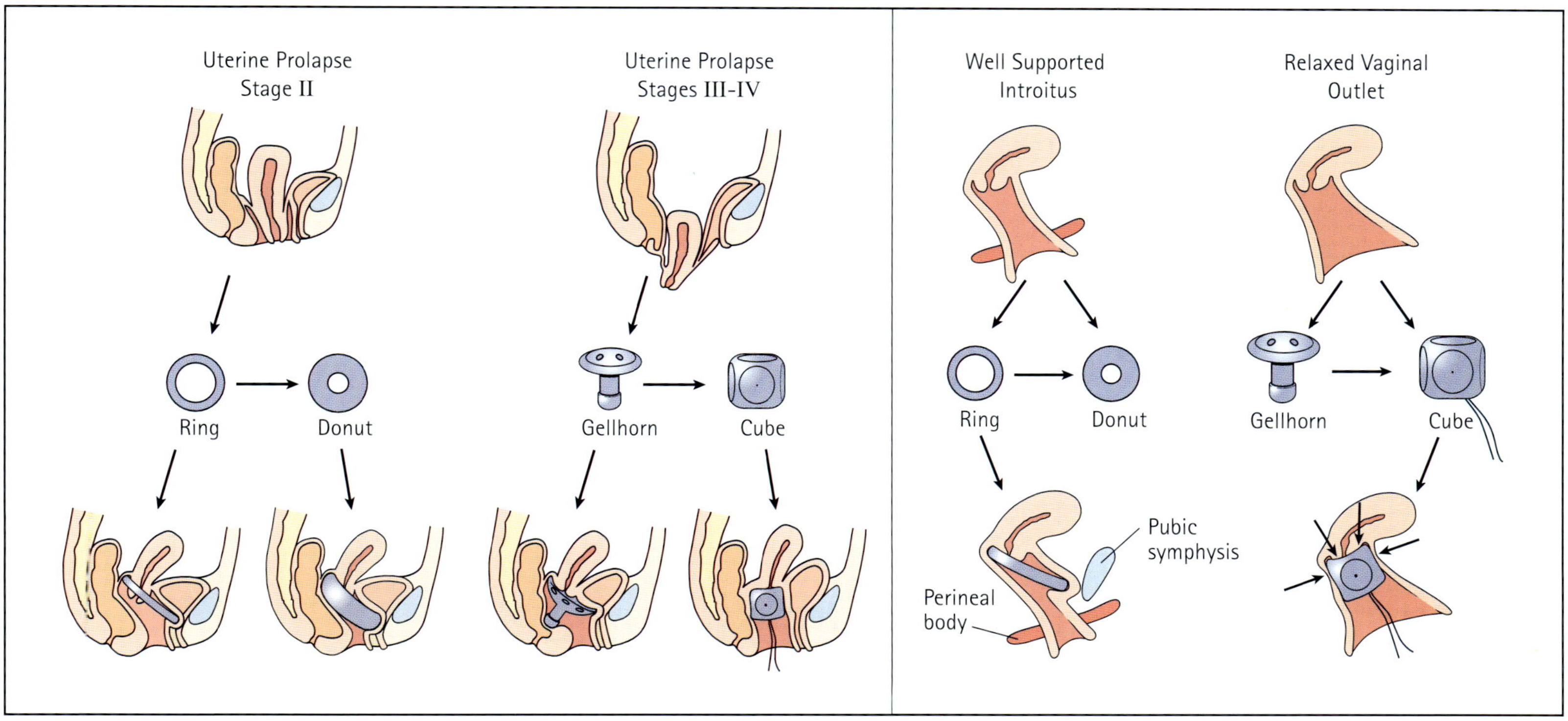

FIGURE 8-3.

The two determinants of pessary choice. The two factors determining pessary choice are the degree of pelvic organ prolapse (*left*) and the integrity of the pelvic outlet (*right*). Lesser degrees of pelvic organ prolapse are usually managed quite adequately with the less invasive, gentler ring or donut pessary. More severe or exteriorized lesions, however, may require the Gellhorn or cube device. An intact pelvic outlet consists of a cylindrical, nonfunneled vagina with a well-supported introitus, admitting only two to three fingerbreadths and a thick, long, intact muscular perineum. Many older women with stages III and IV pelvic organ prolapse, however, have a funneled vagina with a gaping relaxed vaginal outlet and a markedly deficient perineum. Although all pessaries sit obliquely in the vagina behind the pubic symphysis, the ring, donut, and Gehrung types are merely space-occupying objects and rely on a well-supported intact introitus/perineum to stay in the vagina. They will fall out of a funneled vagina with a gaping introitus and deficient perineum with any significant increase in intra-abdominal pressure, such as defecation. The Gellhorn and cube types, on the other hand, will usually hold up even massive exteriorized lesions with a gaping introitus because they stay in by a different mechanism. The single large dish of the Gellhorn and the multiple cups of the cube pessaries become attached to the vaginal walls by a partial suction effect. This keeps both prolapse and pessary in situ through full activities of daily living.

INSERTION

- Empty bladder and bowels
- Gently replace prolapse if massive and exteriorized, use Trendelenburg and steady gentle pressure
- Lubricate pessary:estrogen cream/Metrogel
- Make device as small as possible
- Widest diameter in A/P direction
- Insert during patient exhalation
- After placement intravaginally, have patient valsalva and assess fit
- Fit largest device that can be worn comfortably

FIGURE 8-4.

General pessary insertion.

TEST PESSARY FIT

- 15 minutes in the exam room: walking, sitting, attempting to void
- If no discomfort or significant pressure, try at home
- Extrusion with activity: larger or different pessary
- Significant pressure or discomfort: smaller or different pessary
- Instruct patient to report: discomfort, inability to void or defecate

FIGURE 8-5.

Testing the fit and comfort.

PESSARY CARE

- Topical creams
  - Estrogen cream (Metronidazole gel, Trimosan)
- Self insertion or removal
- Follow-up
  - Time varies with pessary type
  - Remove and wash device, inspect vagina
    - Mild vaginitis: irrigate, betadine painting
    - Severe vaginitis, erosion, or ulceration: discontinue temporarily

FIGURE 8-6.

Pessary care.

COMPLICATIONS

- Vaginal odor or discharge (dilute vinegar or betadine douch may relieve)
- Severe anaerobic vaginitis
- Urinary or fecal retention, pressure
- Urinary tract infections
- Ulcerations, erosion
- Entrapped, embedded pessary
- Recto or vesicovaginal fistula
- Cytological atypias, ? vaginal or cervial cancers

FIGURE 8-7.
Complications of pessary use.

SELECTION OF INDIVIDUAL PESSARIES

RING PESSARY WITH AND WITHOUT SUPPORT MEMBRANE

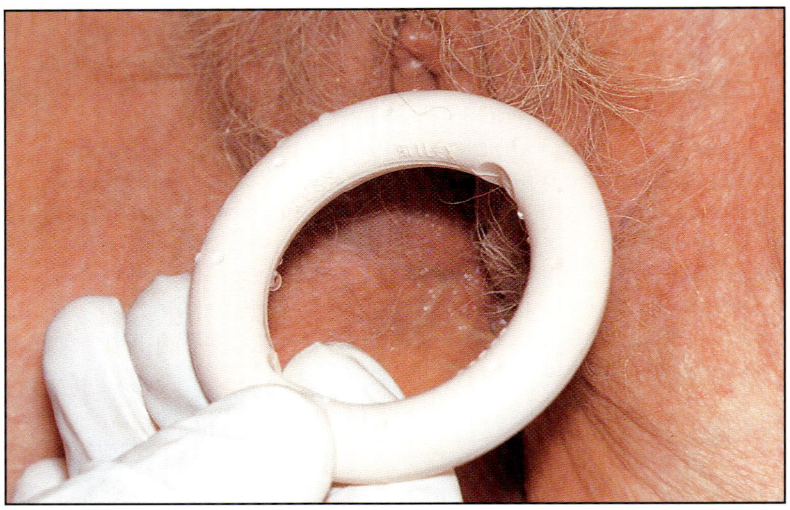

FIGURE 8-8.
Ring pessary. The ring pessary is available with or without a supportive membrane for mild to moderate prolapse. The flaccid funneled outlet equals extrusion membrane if the cervix or vagina comes through the ring. It is the least invasive and rarely causes heavy discharge. It requires infrequent visits, allows easy self-insertion and removal, and permits coitus. This ring is used in a very healthy, independent, 80-year-old, multipara woman who suffered from symptomatic stage II uterovaginal prolapse. She had a strong desire to avoid pelvic surgery if possible and also a well-supported perineum and intact introitus. We were able to prevent surgery with a folding ring pessary, which is cleaned and reinserted every 4 to 6 months.

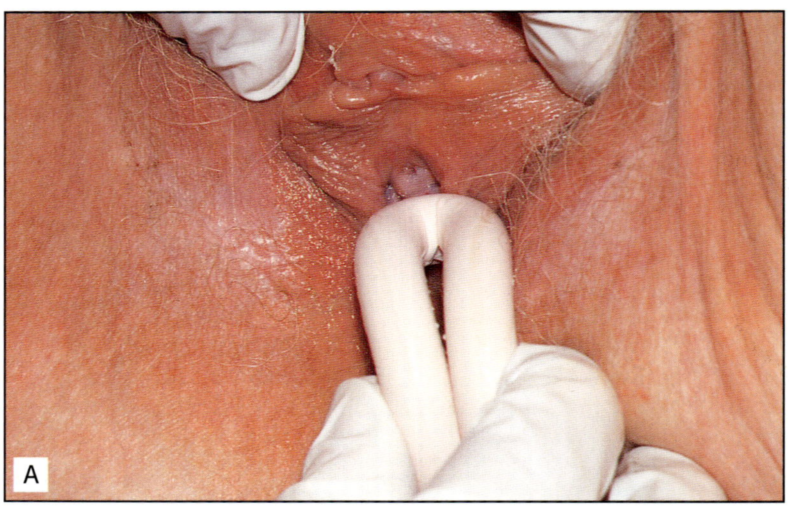

FIGURE 8-9.
Insertion. **A**, The ring is grasped with the index finger and thumb where it says "press" and will fold in half on its notches.

(*Continued on next page*)

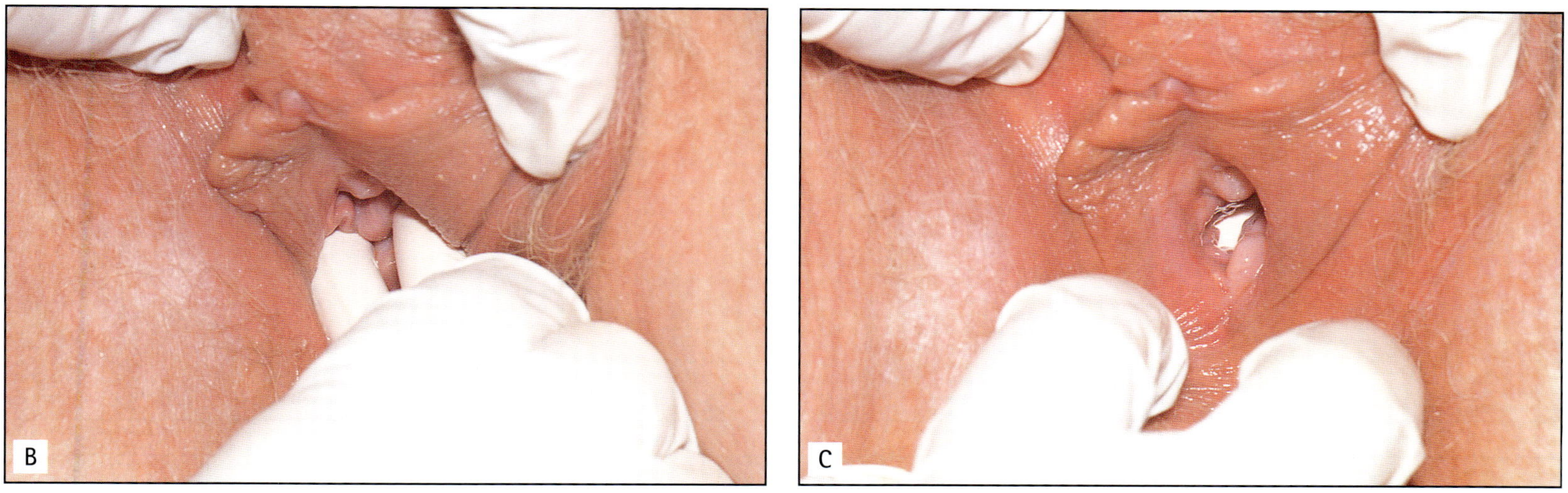

FIGURE 8-9. *(Continued)*

B, This semicircle is inserted over the perineum, through the introitus with the convexity upward while the contralateral hand holds the labia apart. **C**, Once the lubricated pessary has slipped into the vagina, it is released. It will open up into its semirigid circular form and assume an oblique axis with its anteriorly inclined distal rim just cephalad to the pubic symphysis and its posteriorly inclined proximal rim just behind the cervix. Rotate the notch 90° so that it will not flex on its own and be spontaneously extruded. This demonstrates a well-positioned pessary.

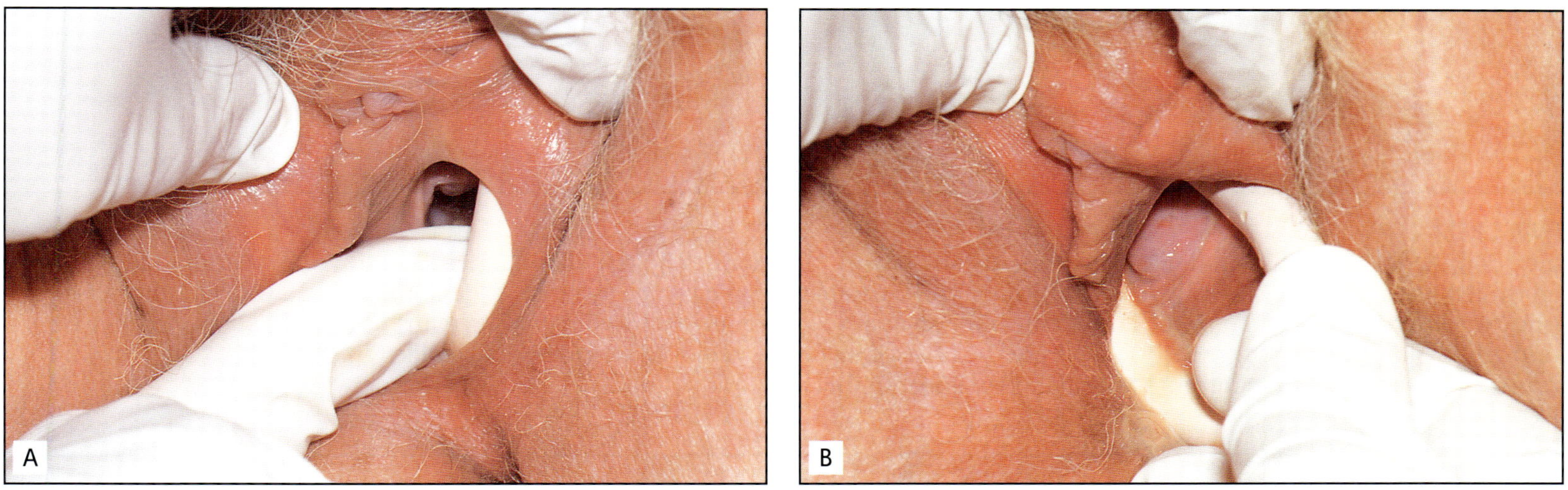

FIGURE 8-10.

Removal. **A**, To remove , insert an index finger inside the ring and find the notch located along the inner surface. **B**, Gently pull down and out while turning and the ring will fold, decreasing its diameter for gentle removal.

Donut Pessary

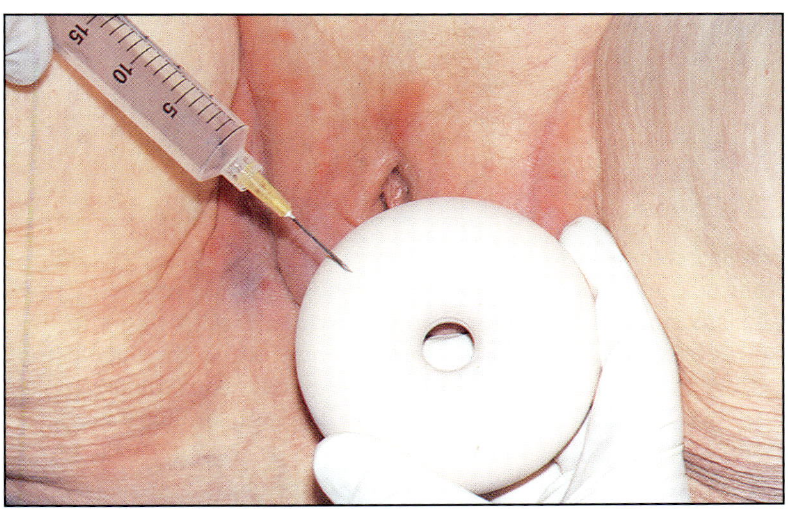

FIGURE 8-11.

Donut pessary. If the ring fails, the donut pessary is the next choice. It requires outlet integrity and occludes the upper vagina to support prolapse. It requires monthly changes in the beginning, then generally changes every 1 to 3 months are sufficient. After approximating the most appropriate size, the air is removed via a 21-gauge needle and 20-cc syringe. With the plunger out, the pessary is compressed and after maximizing deflation, the needle is removed.

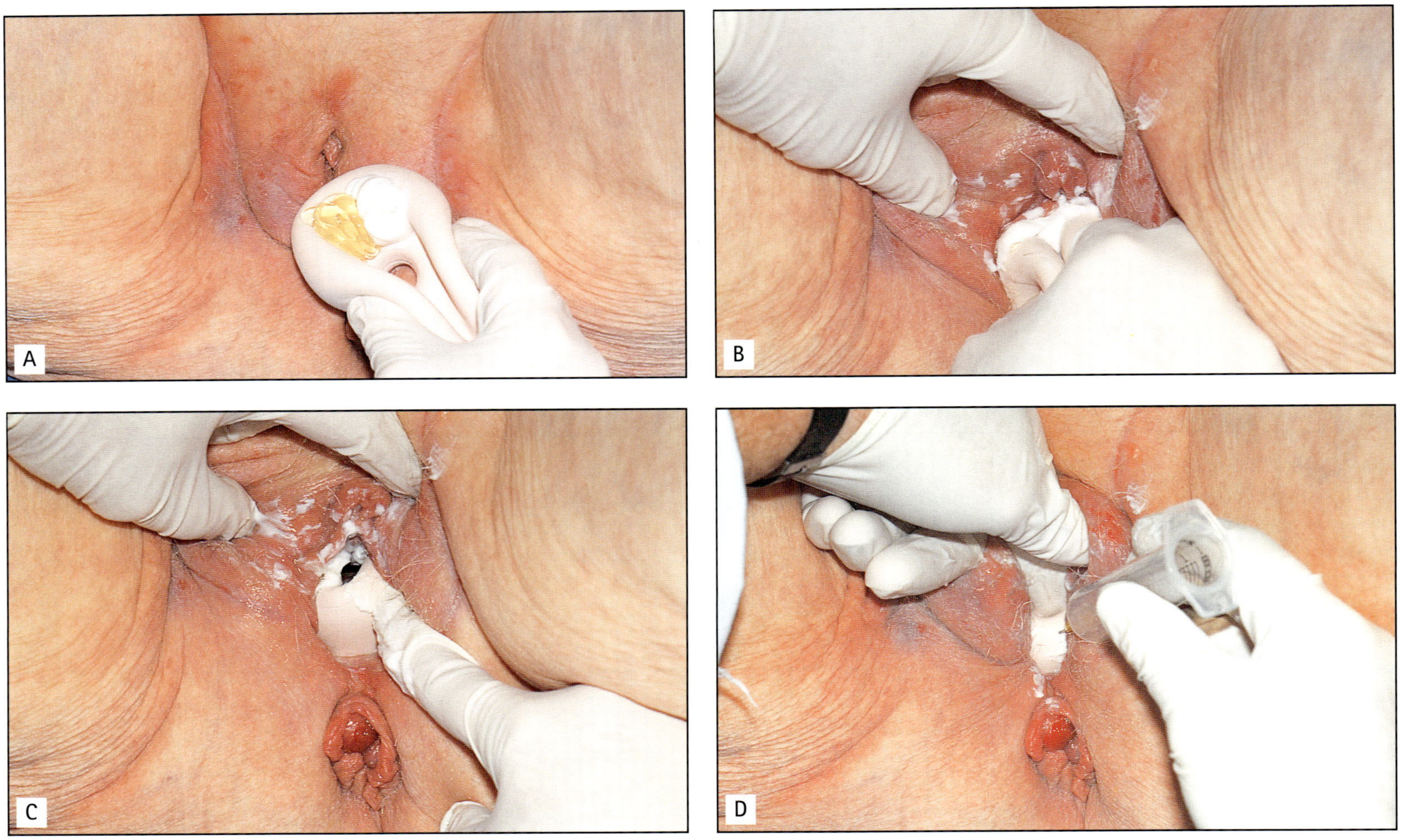

FIGURE 8-12.

Insertion. **A**, The deflated donut occupies less space. **B**, When lubricated, the donut is very easily inserted through the separated labia. **C**, Once the widest part of the donut enters the vagina through the introitus, it tends to slip away from the physician's grasp. **D**, It is held near the introitus with an index finger in the donut's hole so that the needle and syringe without plunger can again be inserted through the silicone wall and the pessary reinflated by equilibrating with room atmosphere. The needle is removed and the pessary slides apically.

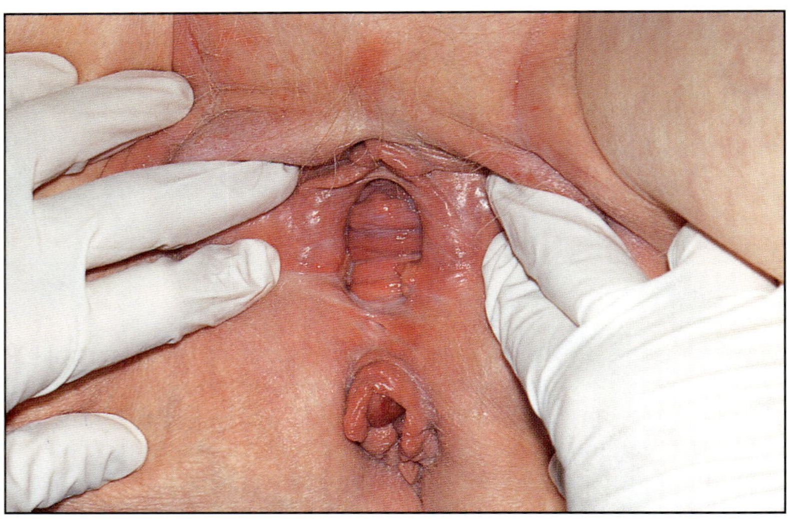

FIGURE 8-13.

Correct position. A properly positioned donut pessary in a 91-year-old woman with massive stage IV uterovaginal prolapse. This patient has been completely asymptomatic through 9 years of treatment with a donut pessary. She visits every 6 weeks for pessary cleaning and in between uses occasional povidone-iodine douches and metronidazole gel applications for her sometimes copious vaginitis.

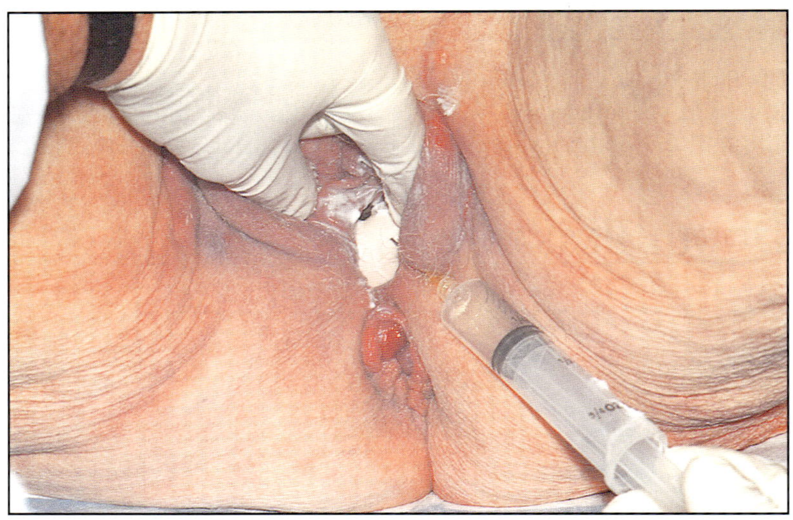

FIGURE 8-14.

Removal. Atraumatic removal is facilitated by first removing the air. The intravaginal donut is grasped with an index finger in the donut hole and brought down near the introitus. The needle and syringe, now with plunger in, are used to draw out the 30 to 60 cc of air. This now deflated donut can be gently and easily removed with simple traction.

Gehrung Pessary

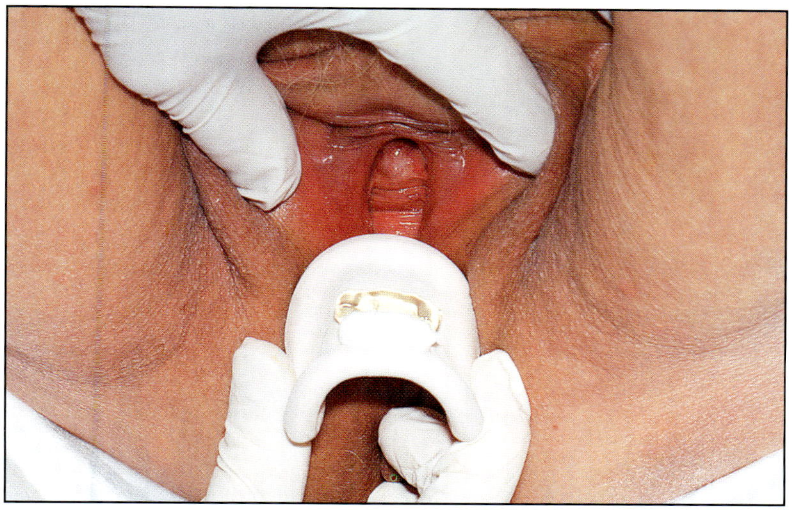

FIGURE 8-15.

Gehrung pessary. This type is specifically designed for cystocele but may also be used for rectocele. It sits as a double arch under the anterior wall with its legs directed posteriorly. Its use requires monthly follow-up visits initially, then every 2 to 3 months. The Gehrung pessary with estrogen cream and metronidazole gel is positioned outside the introitus as it will sit intravaginally to treat cystocele. Its two arches will act as a bridge to support the anterior wall. This 68-year-old morbidly obese woman with a symptomatic stage III isolated cystocele and severe anxiety regarding surgery has been successfully treated with a Gehrung pessary.

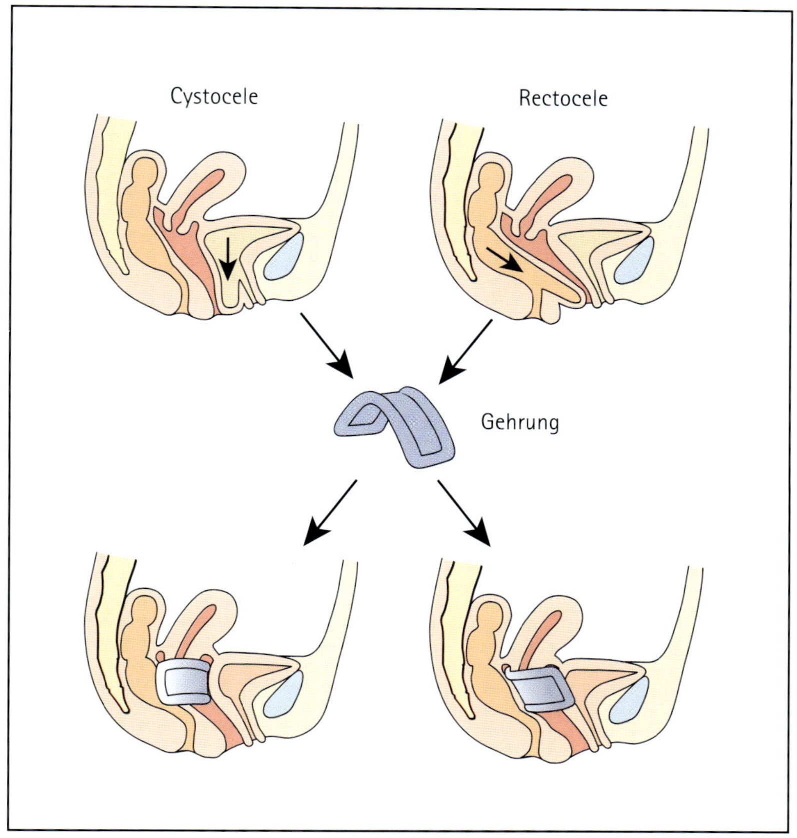

FIGURE 8-16.

Position schematic. The Gehrung pessary with its semirigid double arches sits perpendicular to the long axis of the vagina and is designed specifically as a bridge to support isolated anterior (cystocele) or posterior (rectocele) defects.

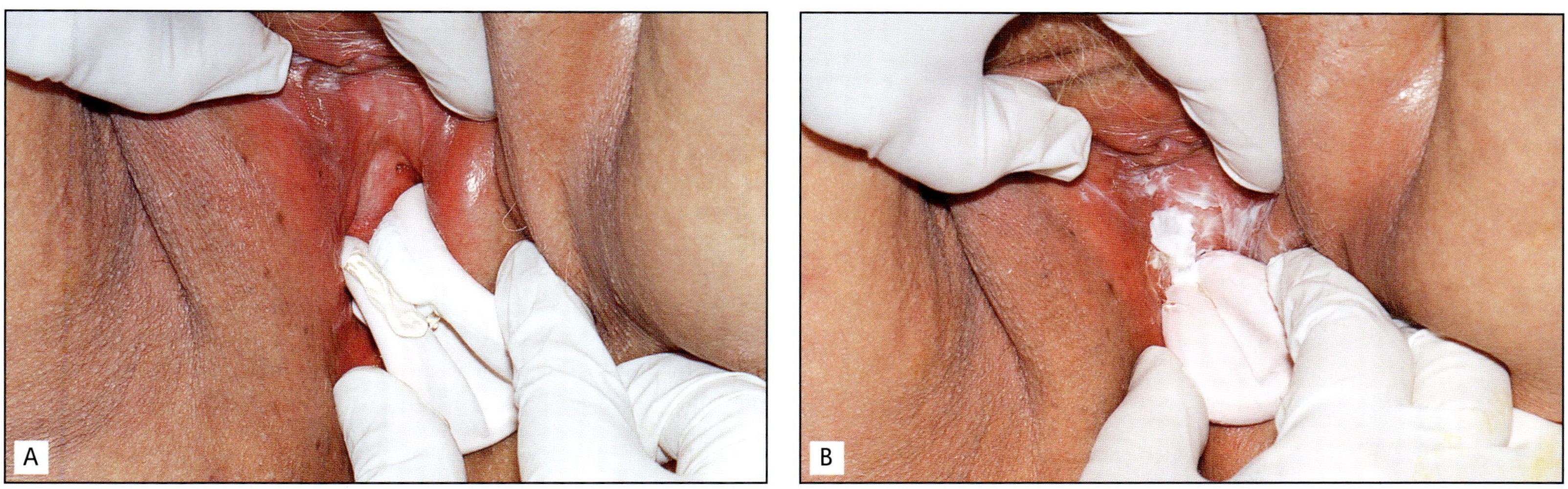

FIGURE 8-17.

Insertion and position. **A**, The two arches are pushed together to decrease its overall size. As such, its insertion is similar to that of a folded ring pessary. **B**, It is slipped into the vagina, convexity upward over the posterior forchette. It is then rotated 90° so that the more distal arch sits transversely behind the symphysis and the more proximal arch sits transversely under the anterior vaginal apex.

(Continued on next page)

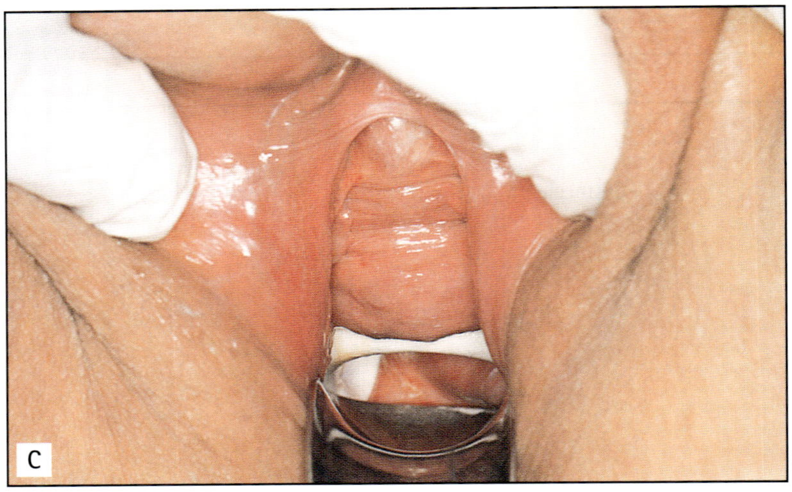

FIGURE 8-17. *(Continued)*
C, This shows a properly positioned Gehrung pessary supporting a cystocele as visualized with Sim's speculum retracting posteriorly.

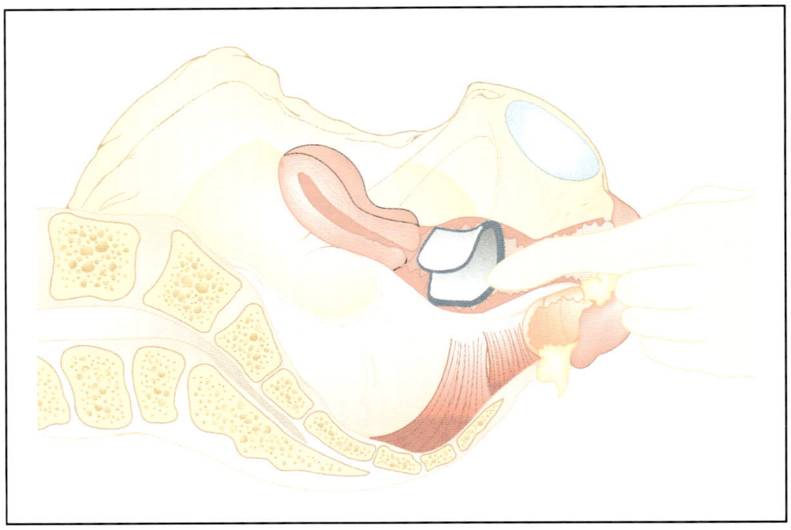

FIGURE 8-18.
Removal. To remove the pessary, insert the index finger and gently turn the pessary as you pull its presenting part down toward, through, and out of the introitus. It will compress as it is twisted.

GELLHORN PESSARY

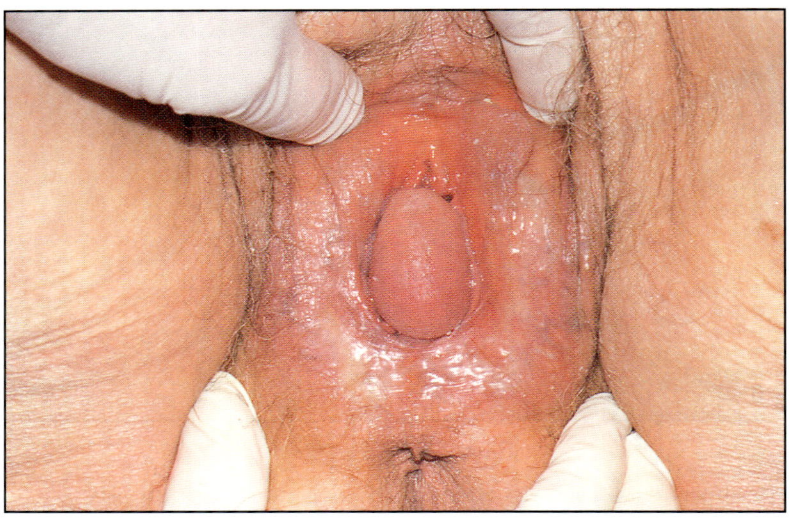

FIGURE 8-19.
Gellhorn pessary. A Gellhorn pessary is an effective device, especially for stages III and IV prolapse. It is strong and supportive because of its size, structure, and partial suction effect. It is successful in those with less outlet support, but its insertion and removal can be difficult. Careful attention to details will minimize patient discomfort. Cleanings are necessary every 2 weeks, initially, and then every 1 to 2 months. This 92-year-old patient has stage III vaginal vault prolapse and has been unable to hold a ring or donut pessary. The bulge is very bothersome to her and definitive reconstructive surgery is not an option.

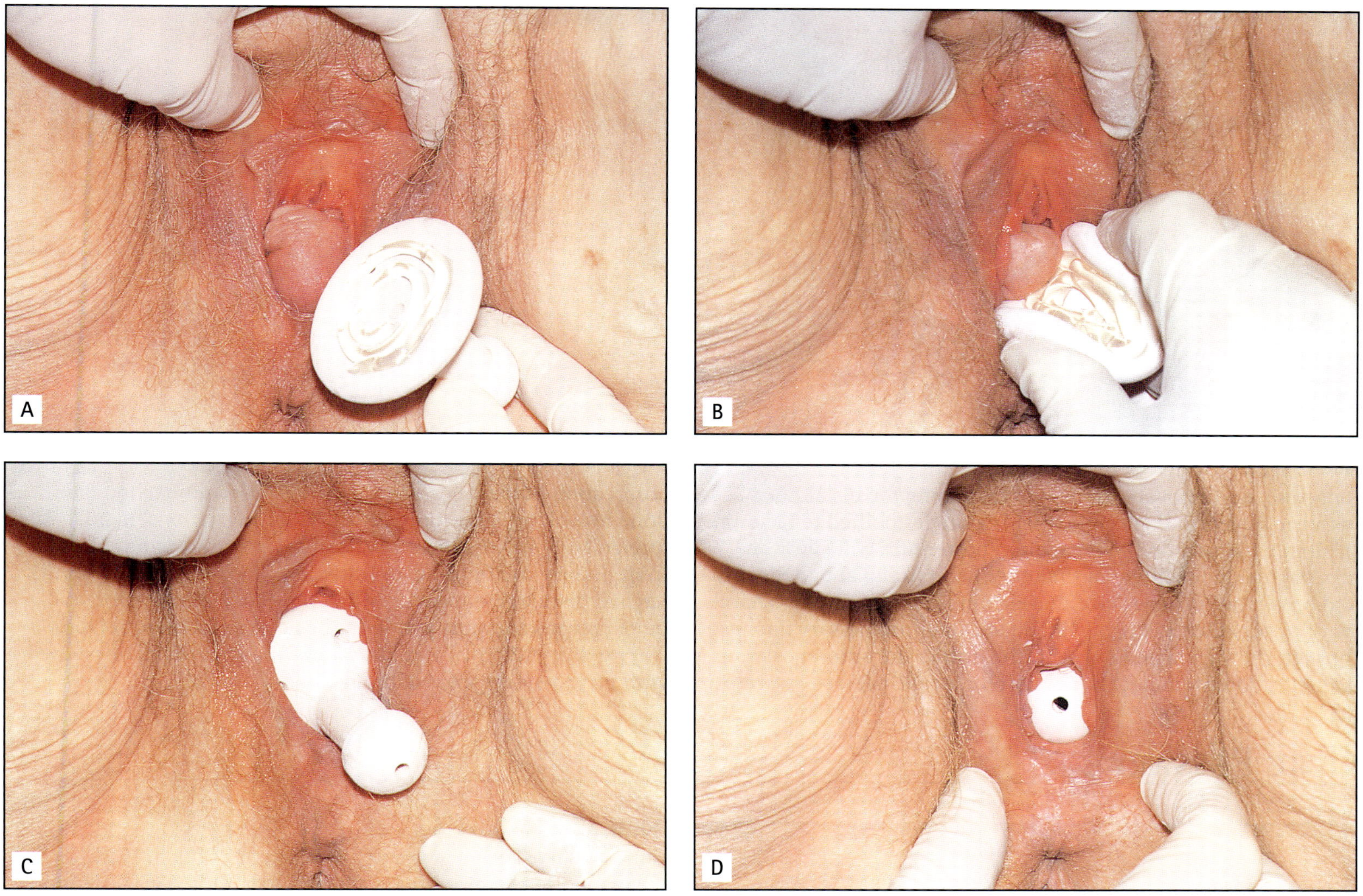

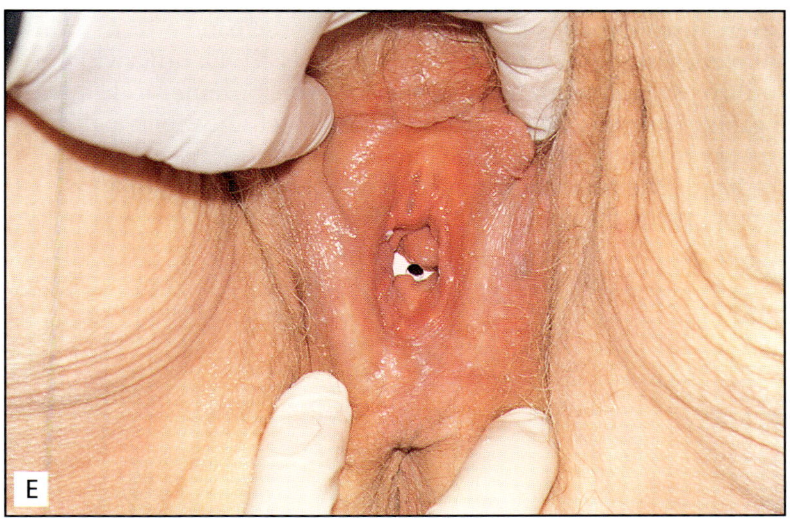

FIGURE 8-20.

Insertion and position. **A**, Metronidazole gel is copiously applied with Gellhorn and cube pessaries to counteract anaerobic growth in the hypoxic environment above the Gellhorn dish or cube cup. Small Gellhorns like the one pictured ($2\,{}^{1}/_{4}''$) can be inserted directly with the dish parallel to the anteroposterior diameter of the introitus, inserting the side of the dish first. **B**, Alternatively, and particularly with larger Gellhorns, the dish can be pinched or folded to compress its size and inserted obliquely through the vulva held open with the contralateral hand. **C,** Once the dish is in the vagina, it will spontaneously and easily turn into the proper axis. It should sit obliquely with the dish positioned under the vaginal apex and the horn pointing toward the perineum. **D**, After giving the patient a chance to relax, the pessary is pushed up into the vaginal apex. **E**, A properly positioned Gellhorn pessary has its presenting horn pointing down toward the perineum and just barely visible with the vulva held apart and the patient performing a Valsalva maneuver.

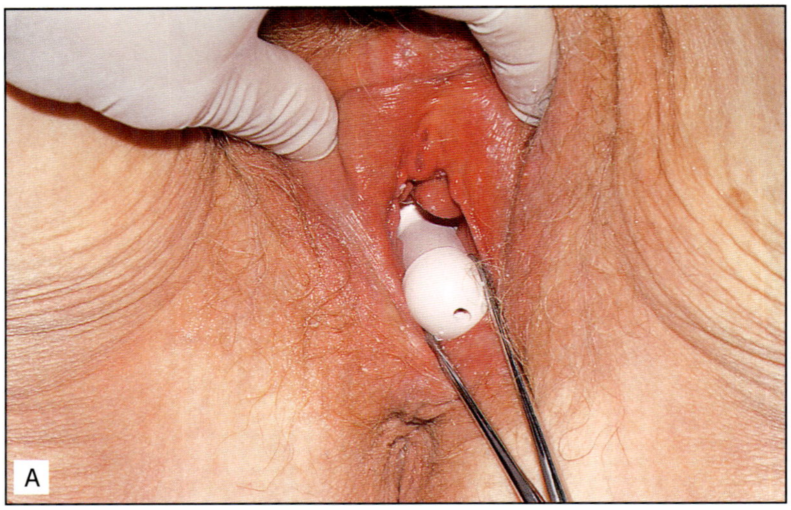

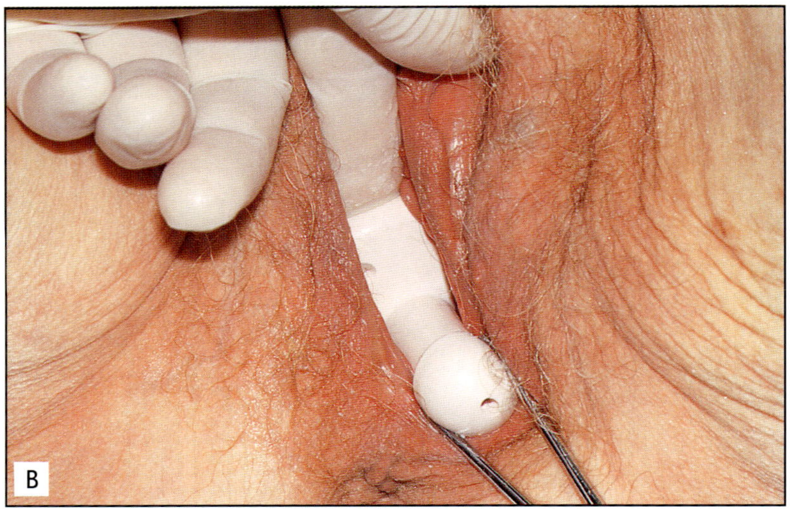

FIGURE 8-21.
Removal. **A**, Removal is facilitated by finding the distal horn with the fingers and grasping it with a single-toothed tenaculum. **B**, Gentle traction on the tenaculum posteriorly will allow an intravaginal index finger of the other hand to slip above the dish and break the suction. Once the suction is broken, the two hands working together will gently guide the Gellhorn pessary down through the vagina and out with the dish in the anteroposterior diameter. After removing a Gellhorn or a cube pessary, a careful observation of the vaginal walls, using a speculum, should be done to look for lacerations, erosions, or ulcerations. Significant foreign body-related lesions warrant a temporary moratorium from pessary use until topical estrogen-mediated healing occurs. Vaginal discharge can occur with any pessary and is sometimes quite copious and purulent with the cube and Gellhorn types. After pessary removal and inspection, the vagina can be painted with procto-swabs soaked in povidone-iodine.

Cube Pessary

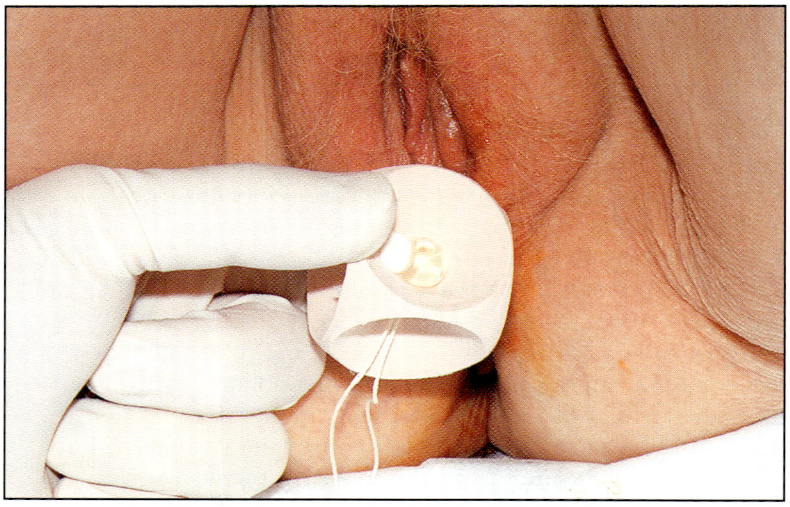

FIGURE 8-22.
Cube pessary. The cube pessary is the choice of last resort, used when all others fail. It has six suction cups and is self-positioning and very soft. It creates an hypoxic environment and may cause severe discharge. It is removed nightly by the patient or requires frequent visits, every 2 to 4 weeks. A 78-year-old, otherwise healthy woman, with massive vaginal eversion/enterocele and a gaping introitus was unable to undergo definitive pelvic reconstructive surgery because she had to care for her terminally ill husband. She received complete temporary relief of prolapse symptoms with a cube pessary, allowing her to postpone surgery.

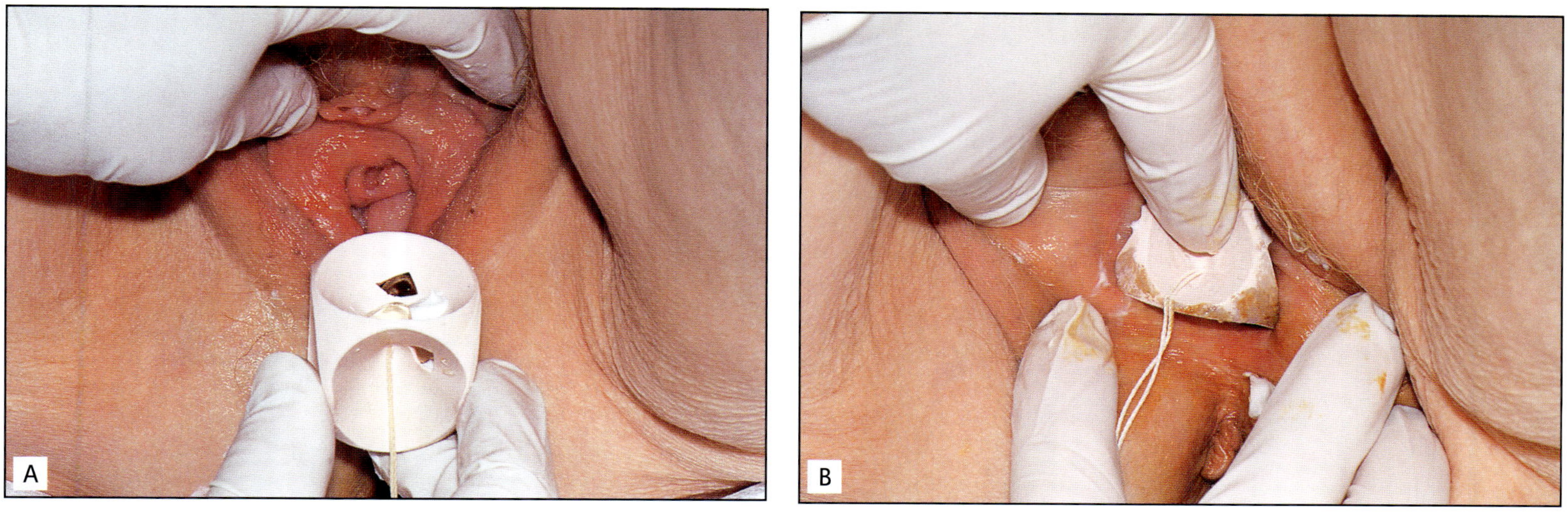

FIGURE 8-23.

Insertion. **A**, Holes may be cut between cups allowing air to get at an otherwise hypoxic environment. Metronidazole gel and estrogen cream are used together. **B**, The very soft cube is easily compressed and atraumatically inserted into the vagina. The device is moved from the distal vagina up into the apex with steady digital pressure in a cephalad direction.

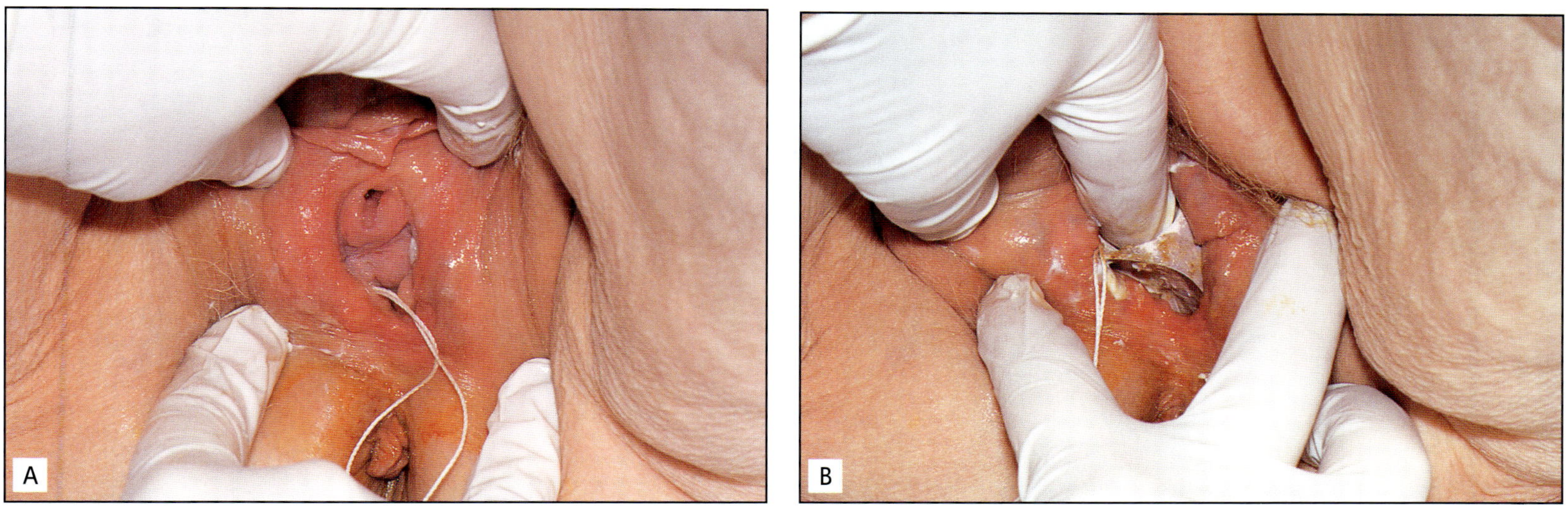

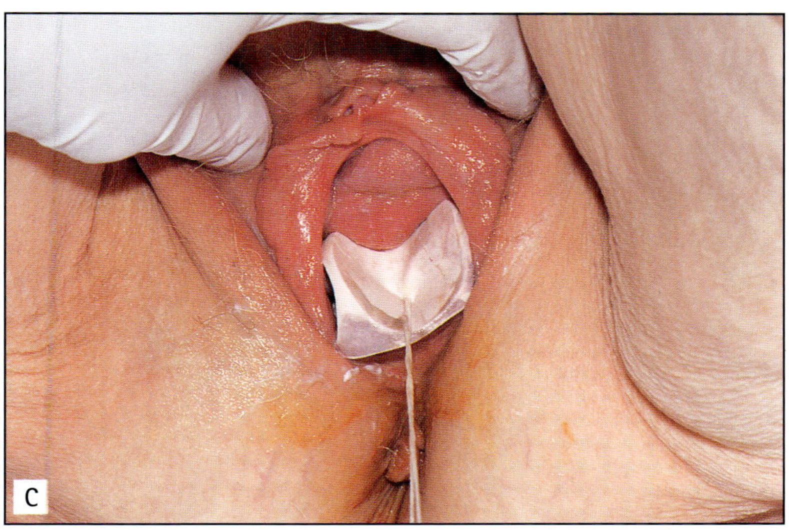

FIGURE 8-24.

Removal. **A**, The labia are separated and the cube string identified and grasped. **B**, With gentle traction on the string, use the contralateral index finger high in the apex to break the suction-cup effect. Then grasp that edge and gently pull down while maintaining traction on the string. **C**, Continued gentle traction on the string will easily complete removal of the cube.

GUIDE TO COMMONLY USED PESSARIES

Pessary	Mechanics	Requires Vaginal Outlet Integrity	Coitus Possible with Pessary In situ	Self-removal and Insertion	Vaginitis	Follow-up (if patient is not self-removing)	Tips/comments
Ring with or without membrane	Fits obliquely behind pubic symphysis	✓	✓	Easiest	None to mild	Initially 3 mo then q 3-6 mo	Least invasive Use ring with membrane for procidentia which may prolapse through open ring
Donut	Occludes upper vagina by filling the space to support prolapse	✓		No	Moderate	Initially 3 mo then q 1-3 mo	Removing the air from the donut with a syringe will markedly facilitate insertion and removal.
Gehrung	Sits as a double arch under the anterior wall, legs directed posteriorly	✓	✓	Yes	Mild	Initially 1 mo then q 2-3 mo	Designed especially for cystoceles (may also be used for rectoceles)
Gellhorn	Shallow cup is directed anteriorly and obliquely holding up the prolapse while the horn is directed toward the posterior forchette			No	Moderate to severe	Initially 2 wks then q 1-2 mo	Removal is not always easy and may be aided by the use of single-tooth tenaculum traction on the horn while the contralateral index finger breaks the suction on the cup to gently ease it out.
Cube	Size fills vagina and suction cups adhere to vaginal walls			Yes	Severe	Initially 2 wks then 2-4 wks	It will remain intravaginal, relieving significant external protrusions, despite a gaping introitus and deficient perineum when all others are extruded. Cutting holes to decrease the hypoxic environment and to facilitate egress of vaginal discharge is helpful.
Inflato	Occludes upper vagina by filling space to support prolapse			Yes – specifically designed for self-care	None to mild	prn	

FIGURE 8-25.

Guide to commonly used pessaries. Pessaries are extremely useful devices to prepare for, postpone, or prevent pelvic reconstructive surgery. With minimal experience any obstetrician-gynecologist can become comfortable in the use of pessaries. Many patients with prolapse, hesitant to initially undergo surgery, will become more receptive after an initial trial of conservative pessary treatment. There are almost no contraindications to pessary use other than a noncompliant patient. A neglected pessary may be trapped behind a rigid vaginal cicatrix. A severely neglected pessary, especially of the Gellhorn variety, may cause deep ulceration and even, on rare occasion, cause a fistula into the bladder and rectum [3]. However, with proper care an extremely valuable clinical function can be served by the lowly vaginal pessary.

REFERENCES

1. *Merriam Webster's Medical Desk Dictionary*. Springfield, MA: Merriam-Webster; 1993.
2. Miller DS: Contemporary use of the pessary. In *Gynecology and Obstetrics*, Volume 1. Edited by Sciarra JJ. Philadelphia: Lippincott; 1995:1–12.
3. Goldstein I, Wise GJ, Tancer ML: A vesicovaginal fistula and intravesical foreign body. *Am J Obstet Gynecol* 1990, 163:589–591.

Surgical Management of Pelvic Organ Prolapse

CHAPTER 9

Douglass S. Hale

Surgery for pelvic organ prolapse is one of the most commonly performed gynecologic procedures in the United States. It is estimated that a woman living in the United States has an 11.1% lifetime chance of undergoing a single surgery for pelvic organ prolapse or urinary incontinence [1]. As the aging population grows, the number of women suffering from these problems will only increase [2]. When treating these problems the philosophy to address the pelvic floor as a whole and not fragment it into separate, unrelated compartments has been realized [3]. Rarely do defects in one area of the pelvic floor exist alone. More often, multiple defects are present. In a study of 100 consecutive patients referred for radiographic evaluation of pelvic organ prolapse, 95% were found to have defects in all three vaginal vault compartments [4]. Failure to identify all defects may stem from oversight by the practitioner or ineffective evaluative techniques. In either case, incomplete repair at the time of prolapse surgery risks an unsatisfactory result and potential need for secondary repair. The goal of the surgeon should be relief of the patient's symptoms balanced with restoration of normal anatomy and function.

Realization of the symbiotic relationship between the neuromuscular system and the connective tissue support system is leading to a change in prolapse procedures. Incomplete understanding of normal versus abnormal, parous versus nulliparous, and symptomatic versus asymptomatic contributes to the confusing state of evaluation and management of prolapse. Sorely lacking are scientific studies that are standardized in regard to evaluation, management, and follow-up. Our knowledge is largely drawn from case series and expert opinions, among the weakest types of scientific evidence. To date only one prospective randomized study has compared surgical techniques for pelvic organ prolapse. This study found that abdominal reconstructive procedures had twice the success rate when compared to vaginal procedures for pelvic organ prolapse [5]. This does not mean that vaginal surgery should be abandoned; however, it does question the majority of current management techniques. Despite little change since their inception over a century ago, anterior and posterior colporrhaphies remain among the most commonly performed procedures for gynecologic prolapse. Attention to paravaginal support, apical vaginal support, and perineal body support combined with preservation of the neuromuscular integrity of the pelvic floor and organs is emerging at the forefront of surgery for pelvic organ prolapse.

ANATOMY OF SUPPORT

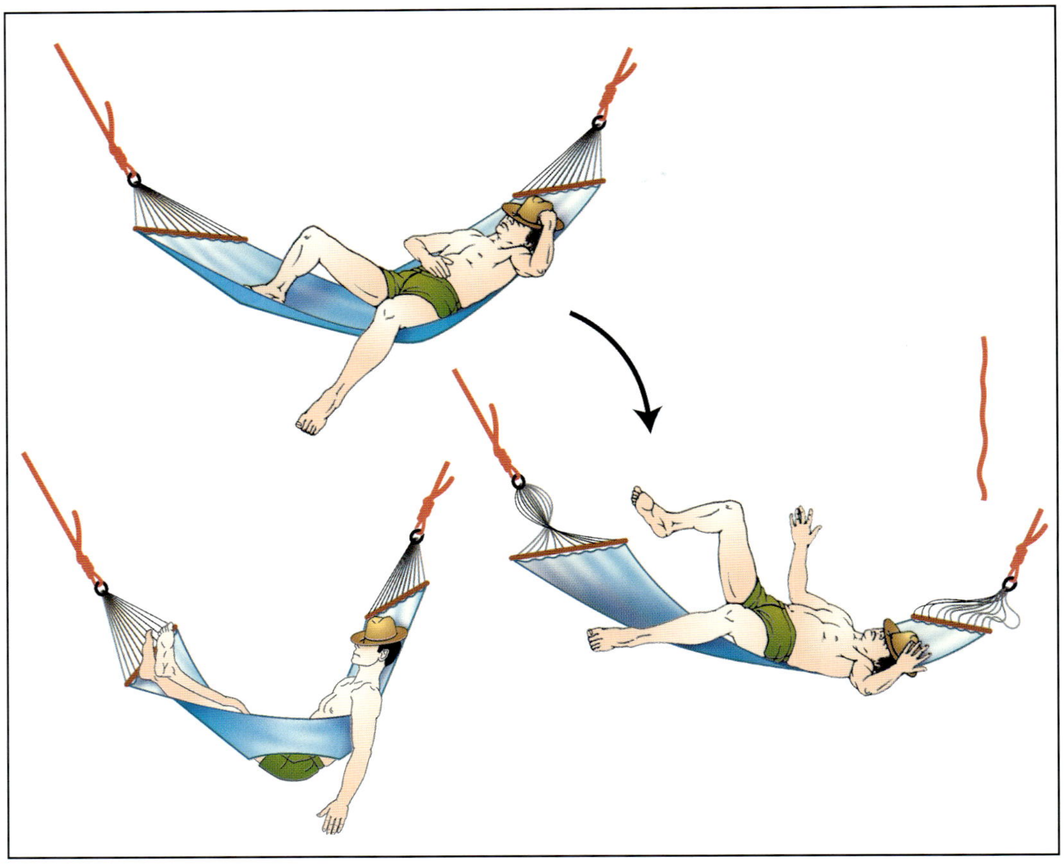

FIGURE 9–1.

Vaginal support [6] and defects in the shell. The vaginal vault should be thought of as an epithelial-lined tube surrounded by a musculofascial connective tissue shell. In the past, a layer separate from the vaginal muscularis has been described. However, the pubovesicocervical fascia, which is often described grossly, has not been a layer that can be demonstrated histologically [7]. The vaginal muscularis envelops the epithelial tube and blends with a vast endopelvic connective tissue network. This blending of tissue creates a "shell" around the vagina, which is supported at different levels. True ligamentous support of the vaginal vault and uterus does not exist. These connective tissue structures along with the levator ani provide an active platform of support [6]. (See Chapter 1)

When organs are prolapsed, the defect lies not in the organ but in the musculofascial shell or the endopelvic connective tissue supports. These defects lead to loss of organ support. An analogy between a hammock and this shell can be made. The rope support of the hammock can be cut and the person in the hammock will fall. This defect may be at the ends of the hammock, analogous to any of the three levels of endopelvic support, or the defect may be in the body of the hammock itself, analogous to defects in the surrounding musculofascial shell of the vagina. The problem is not with the person, but in the supporting hammock structure. Likewise, with a cystocele, enterocele, or rectocele the major problem originates with a defect in the enveloping or supporting musculofascial connective tissue. These defects can lead to displacement of the overlying organ.

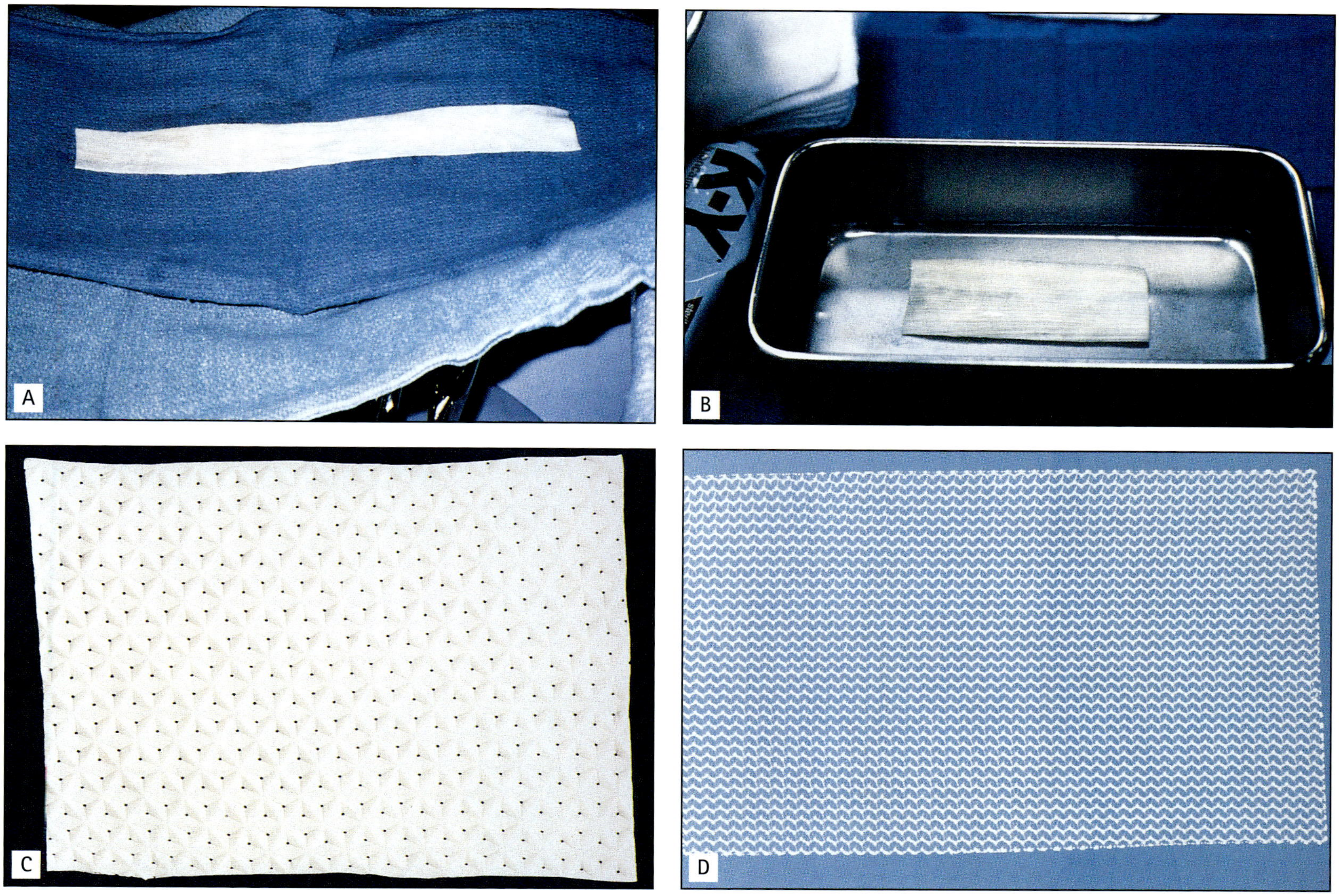

FIGURE 9–2.

Examples of graft material (**A** and **B**, donor fascia lata; **C**, Gore-tex mesh; **D**, prolene mesh). Many times defects in the supporting tissues can be recognized and repaired. However, at times this tissue is of such poor quality that its use in the repair is unacceptable. In these instances, substitution of this tissue with an autograft, allograft, or synthetic material is required. The ideal support material that eliminates erosion, infection, and foreign body reaction is still awaiting development. Autografts of rectus fascia or fascia lata have been reported [7a, 7b]. Often the sizes needed for pelvic reconstructive procedures makes the use of autografts impractical. Allografts of fascia lata, rectus fascia, dura mater, patellar tendon, and Achilles tendon are available. The most commonly used is donor fascia lata, but long-term studies in gynecology are lacking. Tissue preparation techniques (radiation, dehydration, lyophilization) differ among tissue banks and this may affect tissue performance. Synthetics include polyethylene terephthalate (Mersilene), polypropylene (Marlex, Prolene, Atrium), polytetrafluoroethylene (Teflon), and expanded polytetrafluoroethylene (Gore-tex). Erosions are the major problem, occurring in 9% to 11% of cases [8]. Until definitive answers are found, the limitations and risks of each material need to be discussed with patients before selecting them for use.

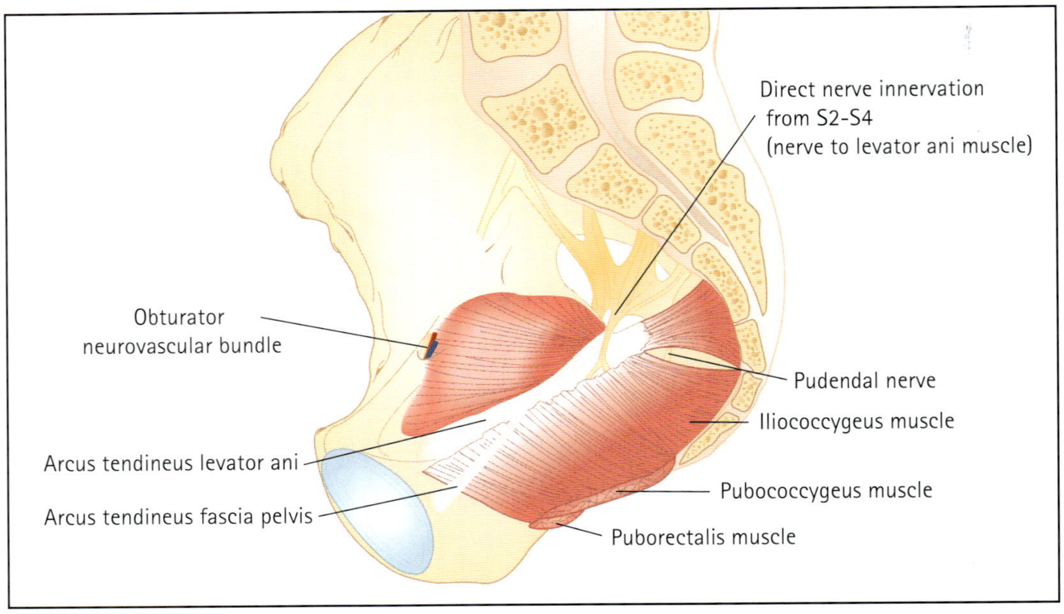

FIGURE 9-3.
Levator ani showing innervation. The musculature of the pelvic diaphragm requires intact innervation to provide an active platform that aids the connective tissue in supporting the pelvic organs. For proper support of pelvic organs both the muscular floor (pelvic diaphragm) and the musculofascial ligamentous network must be intact. Often after reconstructive efforts, little or no attention is paid to the rehabilitation of the levator ani. This misses the opportunity to address a major contributing factor to pelvic organ prolapse. Persistent weakness in the levator ani places a greater stress on the surgical repair, whereas a strong levator ani can augment the surgical repair.

ANTERIOR WALL DEFECTS

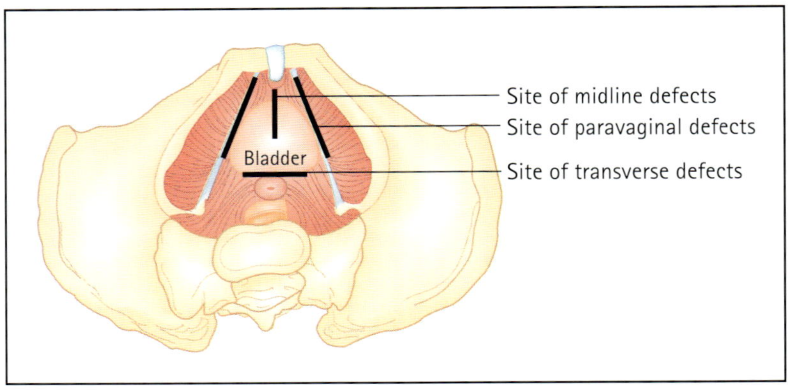

FIGURE 9-4.
Sites of defects in the anterior vaginal wall. Defects in the anterior vaginal wall can result in cystocele, urethrocele, or anterior enterocele. Pictured are the most common sites for defects in the anterior vaginal wall [9]. Paravaginal cystoceles are reported to be the most common, although no large epidemiologic study exists to confirm this. Other sites include the transverse and midline defects. Site-specific analysis examining the lateral sulci, apex, and midline is needed to identify these different defects. Because not all cystoceles have the same etiology, clinicians need different procedures to correct them. (*From* Richardson [9].)

Paravaginal Defect Repair—Abdominal Approach

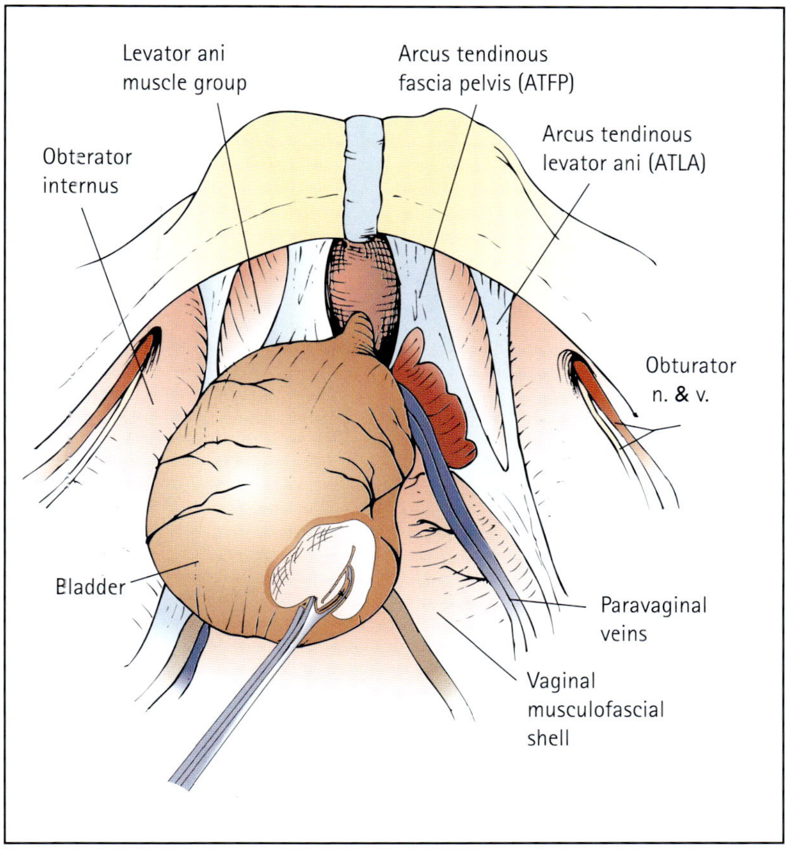

FIGURE 9-5

Space of Retzius anatomy and abdominal view of paravaginal defect. Opening the transversalis fascia at the level of the pubic symphysis enters the space of Retzius. The obturator internus muscle is located laterally with the accompanying obturator canal and obturator neurovascular bundle. The levator ani muscle is identified taking origin from the arcus tendineus levator ani (ATLA), a fascial thickening of the obturator internus muscle. The ATLA is fused posteriorly with the arcus tendineus fascia pelvis (ATFP). The ATFP begins about 1 cm superior and 1 cm lateral to the inferior margin of the pubic symphysis extending posteriorly to the ischial spine. The ATFP is the lateral support for vaginal level II. The paravaginal veins serve as a border for the lateral margin of the bladder. These vessels run in an anteroposterior direction. These are differentiated from the vessels of the bladder, which usually run in a more transverse direction.

In a paravaginal defect, the vaginal musculofascial shell has torn away from the arcus tendineus fascia pelvis (ATFP) at level II. On physical examination, the lateral vaginal sulcus is absent, and central vaginal rugation is maintained. Several variations of a paravaginal defect may exist. The ATFP may remain attached to the pelvic sidewall with the vagina torn away medially as shown. Alternatively, the ATFP may be found on the vaginal wall having torn away from the pelvic sidewall. Lastly, the ATFP may be split in two. In any of these cases, repair of the paravaginal defect is accomplished by reapproximating the vagina and the ATFP in their correct anatomic location. (*From* Richardson [9].)

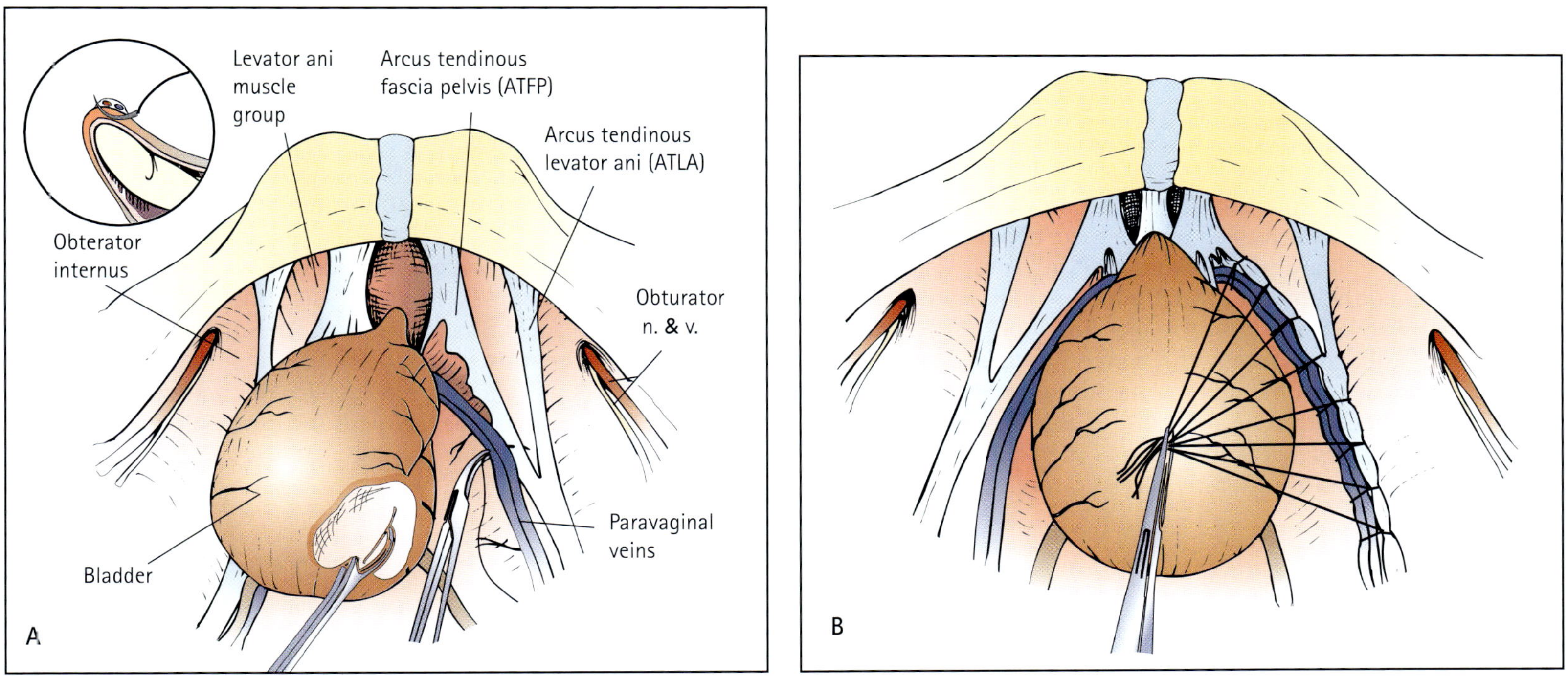

FIGURE 9-6.

Correction of paravaginal cystocele. **A**, With the operator's nondominant hand intravaginally, the extent of the defect is palpated. The bladder is gently retracted medially over the vaginal hand, exposing the glistening white musculofascial tissue of the vagina. Before suture placement, pressure should be removed temporarily from the vaginal hand to ensure a vein is not being entered. **B**, Sutures are then placed close to the bladder medially; either encircling the paravaginal veins or placed just lateral to them. A full thickness vaginal suture is used. The suture is completed by placement in the arcus tendineus fascia pelvis (ATFP) on the sidewall or in the anatomic location of the ATFP if it has torn away. Successive sutures extending from the ischial spine to the urethrovesical junction are placed. When repairing a bilateral defect, the first side should be tied down before proceeding with the second side to prevent overcorrecting of the anterior vaginal wall. As the sutures are tied, the operator should feel the lateral vaginal sulci returning and correction of the cystocele occurring. (Part A *from* Richardson [9].)

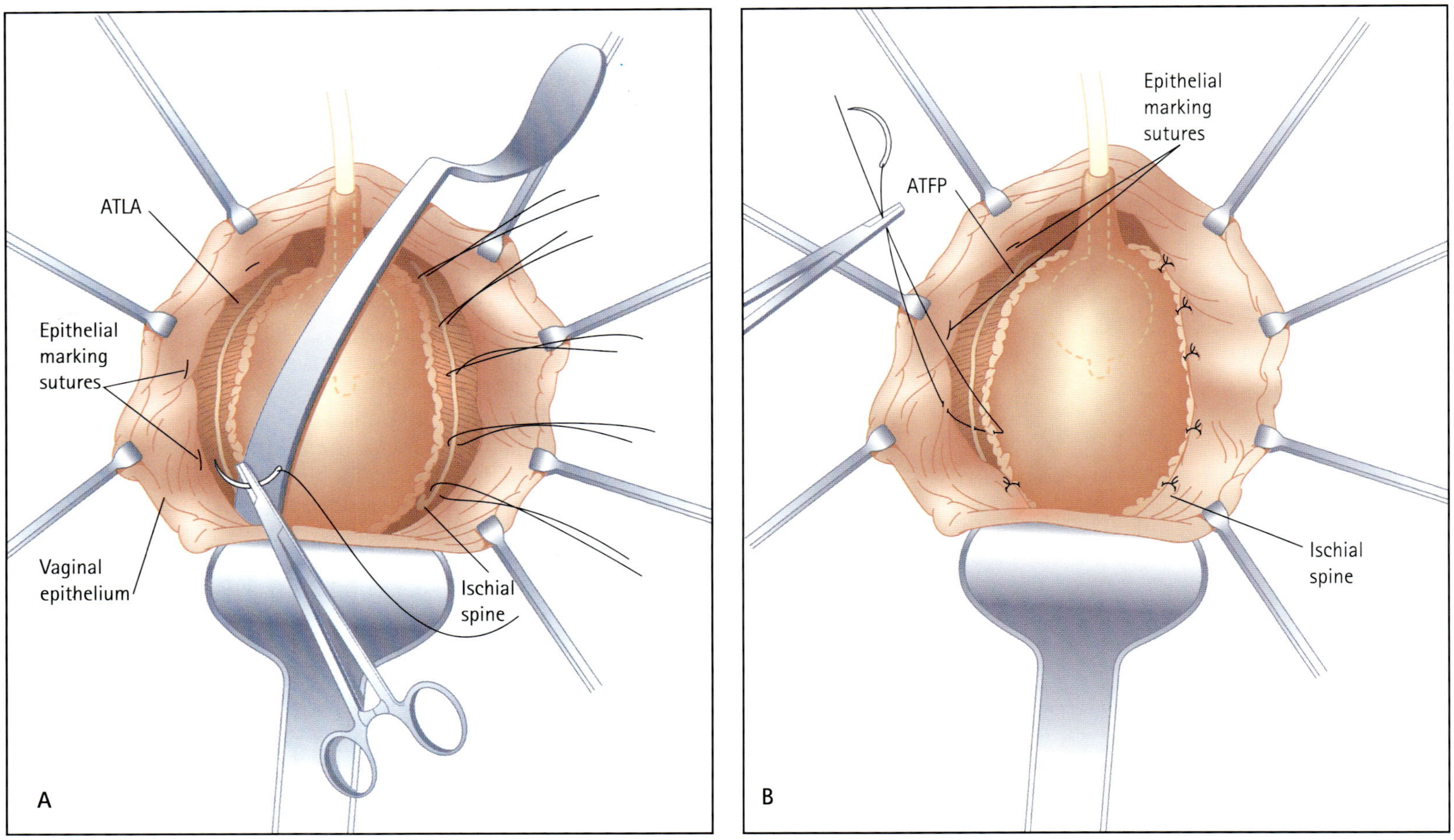

FIGURE 9-7.

Marking sutures and vaginal suture placement into ATFP. Several vaginal incisions including a midline, parasagittal, or an inverted U incision may be used to gain access to the space of Retzius. A midline incision damages the perineal nerve, which may affect urethral sphincter function [9a, 9b].The other incisions have not been studied with respect to perineal nerve damage. Before making any incision, marking sutures are placed in the vaginal epithelium to approximate final location of the vaginal wall. This will aid in suture placement once the vaginal epithelium is opened. Typically three marking sutures are used: anterior to the level of the ischial spine, midway between the spine and the symphysis, and close to the symphysis.

A, The space of Retzius is entered and the bladder is retracted medially and superiorly. Breisky-Navratil retractors along with a lighted suction irrigation device aid in visualization. The vaginal musculofascial tissue may be dissected into a separate layer or left intact on the vaginal epithelium. The ATFP is located, and sutures are placed along it extending from just anterior to the ischial spine to the insertion of the ATFP on the pubis. To prevent these sutures from becoming entangled, a device such as the McIntosh suture holder (V. Mueller, Allegiance Healthcare Corporation, Deerfield, IL) can be used. **B**, Sutures are then placed through the musculofascial connective tissue shell and the vaginal epithelium at the level of the marking sutures. Sequential tying begins with the deepest suture working toward the symphysis. The repair is completed with epithelial closure.

Anterior Vaginal Wall Graft for Multiple Defects

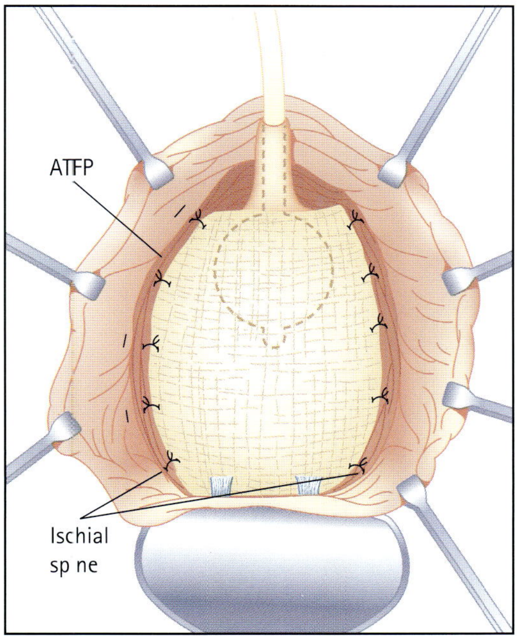

FIGURE 9–8.

Graft in anterior vaginal wall. If paravaginal defects exist with a central defect, an alternative to correcting each site individually is to use a graft. In this figure a donor fascia lata graft is used. The repair is exactly as that used for a vaginal paravaginal repair, with the exception of the intervening graft. The superior edge of the graft should be sutured to the supported vaginal apex and include the uterosacral-cardinal complex. A double-layer vaginal wall closure over the graft may help prevent graft erosion. ATFP—arcus tendineus fascia pelvis.

Anterior Colporrhaphy for Central Defects

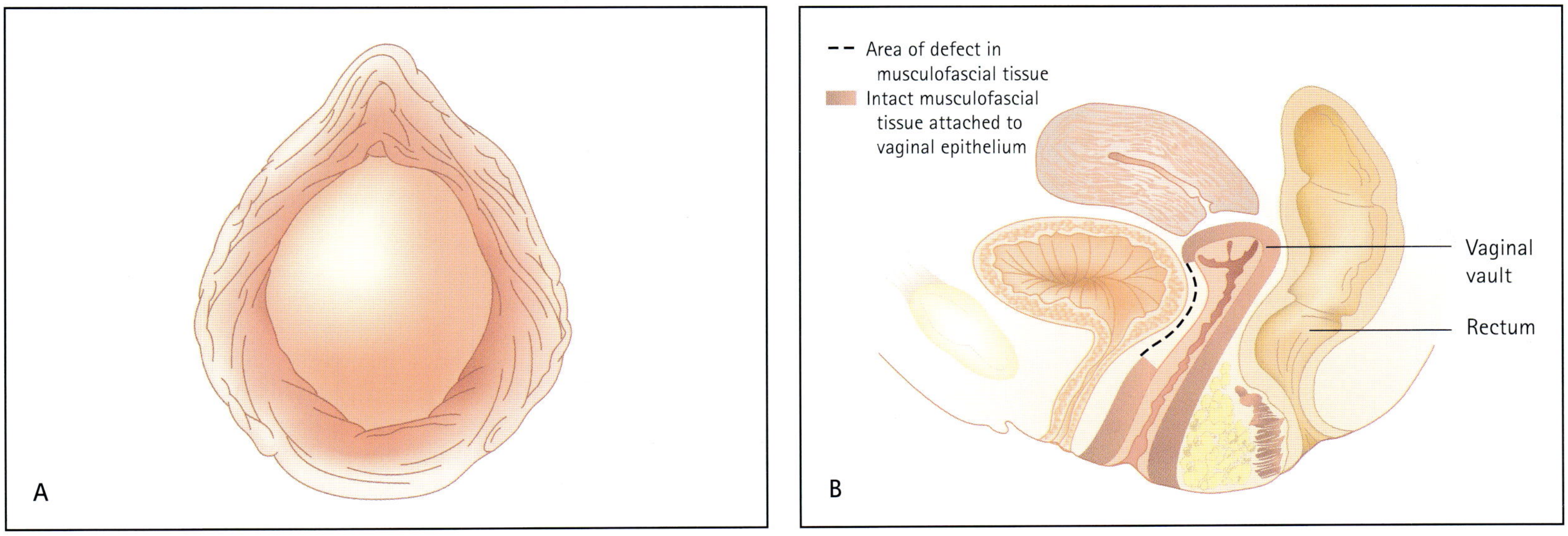

FIGURE 9–9.

Bladder "herniation" in a central defect. The anterior colporrhaphy is used for correction of a defect in the central vaginal wall. The extent of the defect can often be appreciated by looking for the presence or absence of vaginal rugae. Rugae indicate vaginal epithelial attachment to the underlying musculofascial tissue. With a central vaginal wall defect, the lateral sulci (paravaginal attachment) will be intact as will support to the vaginal cuff. **A**, The bladder can be visualized herniating through the central defect in the musculofascial tissue. This leads to bladder muscularis in direct contact with vaginal epithelium. **B**, *Dotted line*—area of defect in musculofascial tissue; *solid line*—intact musculofascial tissue attached to vascular epithelium.

In anterior colporrhaphy, repair is begun with a midline or an inverted U anterior vaginal epithelial incision. A subepithelial injection of saline or a dilute vasoconstricting solution may aid in this dissection. The extent of the defect is identified and the separated musculofascial connective tissue is reapproximated while reducing the herniating bladder. Vaginal epithelial trimming should be limited because this adds little to the support and may lead to vaginal shortening.

VAGINAL APEX

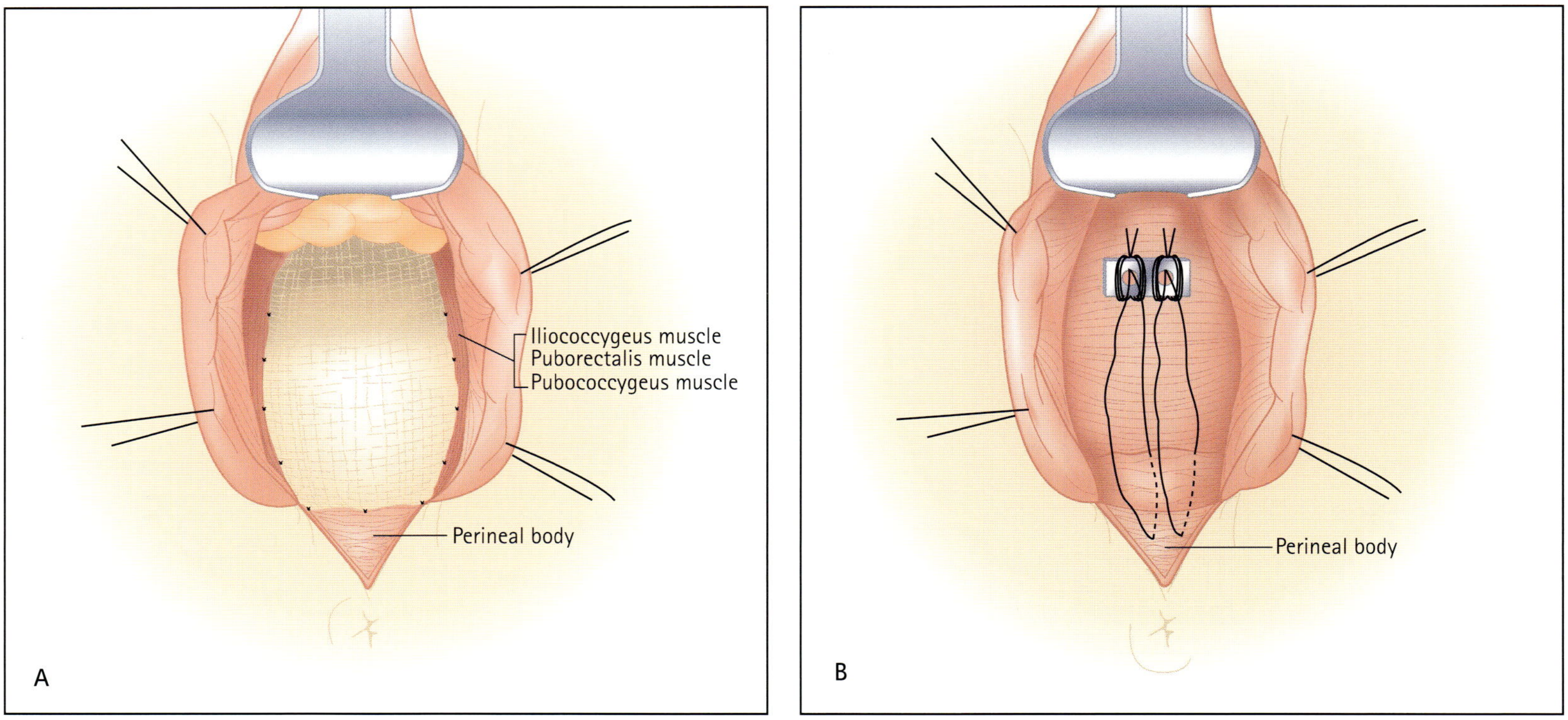

FIGURE 9–10.

Abdominal sacral colpoperineopexy [10,11] with perineal graft. Procedures for support of the vaginal apex involve restoring the continuity of level I vaginal support. Choices for apical support include use of native uterosacral-cardinal complex, a graft material substitute for the native ligaments, or an alternative support site such as the sacrospinous ligament or levator plate. Abdominal sacral colpoperineopexy allows for simultaneous correction of multiple vaginal wall defects and has evolved from the abdominal sacral colpopexy [12]. The basic premise is rebuilding the vaginal musculofascial "shell" using a graft to envelop the vagina epithelium and then recreate the vaginal levels of support. Two leaves are involved in graft placement. A posterior graft restores the continuity of the rectovaginal septum correcting descending perineum, rectocele, and enterocele. This graft extends support from the perineal body to the sacrum recreating the natural support of the rectovaginal septum, musculofascial shell, and the uterosacral ligaments. An anterior graft is placed into the vesicovaginal space from just above the level of the trigone and vaginal apex to the sacrum. Additional support may need to be added to level II with a paravaginal repair.

Graft attachment to the perineal body may be attempted vaginally or abdominally. Abdominal graft fixation to the perineal body is more difficult and may lead to inadequate fixation. An initial vaginal approach allows secure fixation to the perineal body and also simultaneous perineorrhaphy. If a perineorrhaphy is required, a diamond-shaped area of vaginal and perineal epithelium is removed from the vaginal introitus allowing an introital opening of two to three fingerbreadths. If no perineorrhaphy is required, a midline introital incision is used. A posterior midline vaginal incision is made just through the vaginal epithelium and extends to the apex or high enough to enter the cul-de-sac peritoneum. The vaginal epithelium is mobilized laterally to the level of the pubococcygeus and iliococcygeus. **A**, If the enterocele sac has been entered vaginally, graft placement can begin vaginally. The graft is secured to the perineal body as widely as possible. The lateral graft margins are sutured to the crura of the levator muscles, typically involving a width of 4 to 5 cm. The apical portion of the graft is then passed through the enterocele sac opening to be retrieved during the abdominal portion of the procedure. The graft can be fixed to a small orthopedic fracture plate to aid in orientation and location of the graft once the abdomen has been entered. **B**, Adhesions or other pathology may prevent safe entry into the cul-de-sac, in which case, the perineal body sutures can be placed and left long while attaching them to the orthopedic plate. After a vaginal approach to dissect the rectovaginal space, the orthopedic plate and sutures are placed just beneath the cul-de-sac peritoneum for later abdominal retrieval. The vaginal epithelium is closed and a perineorrhaphy is performed as necessary. The abdominal portion of the procedure is begun and appropriate exposure gained.

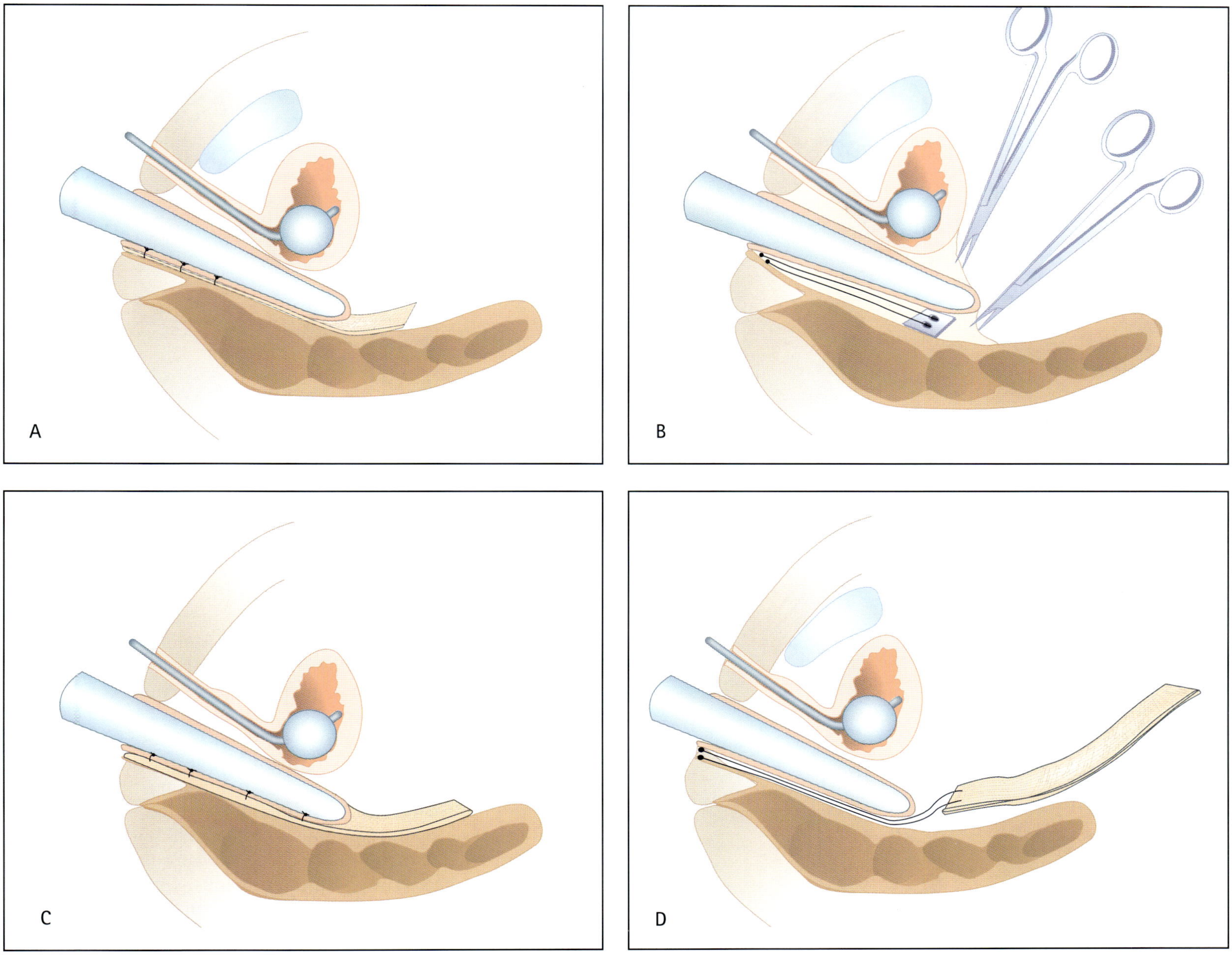

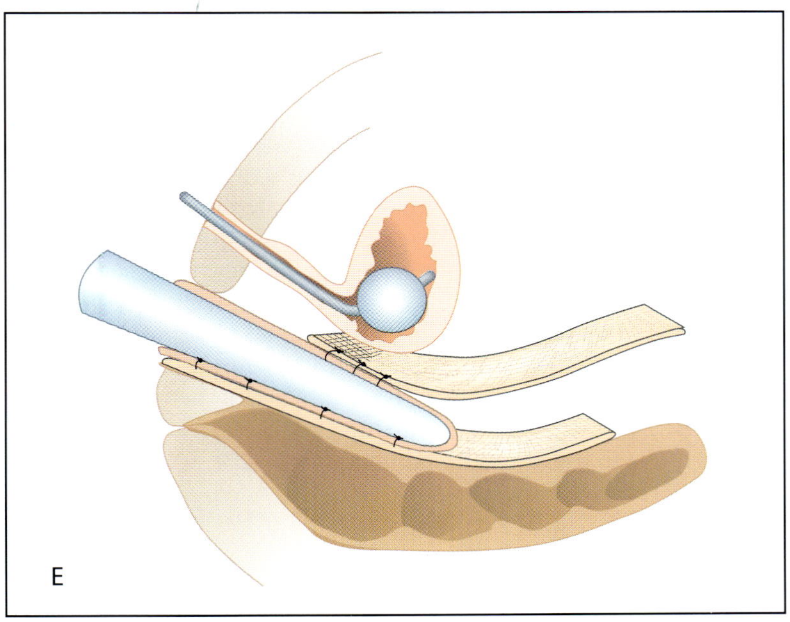

FIGURE 9-11

Graft placement. **A**, If cul-de-sac entry and distal graft placement were begun vaginally, the graft will be lying in the cul-de-sac on entering the abdomen. **B**, If the cul-de-sac could not be entered vaginally, the peritoneum overlying the orthopedic plate and sutures is incised and they are recovered. A Lucite stent placed vaginally helps dissect the vesicovaginal space, and if needed, the rectovaginal space. Dissection into the vesicovaginal space will separate the bladder from the underlying white musculofascial tissue of the vagina. This should be a bloodless dissection, and significant bleeding indicates wrong tissue planes. Laterally, this dissection extends to the bladder pillars. The vagina has now been isolated and is ready for graft placement. **C**, If the posterior graft placement had begun vaginally, it is now continued with the aid of the Lucite stent. The graft is spread as widely as possible over the posterior wall and fixed bilaterally to the vaginal apex. The graft is then sutured on each side allowing about 2 cm between rows of sutures. This typically results in a total of 8 to 10 sutures holding the posterior graft in place. **D**, If only the perineal sutures were placed vaginally, the graft is attached to these and tied down securely. The remaining posterior graft is fixed as above. **E**, The anterior graft is secured by placing gentle retraction on the bladder exposing the vesicovaginal space. With the Lucite rod serving as a guide, the graft is fixed to the anterior vaginal wall as laterally and as distally as possible. Typically, three to four rows of two sutures each are placed to secure this graft.

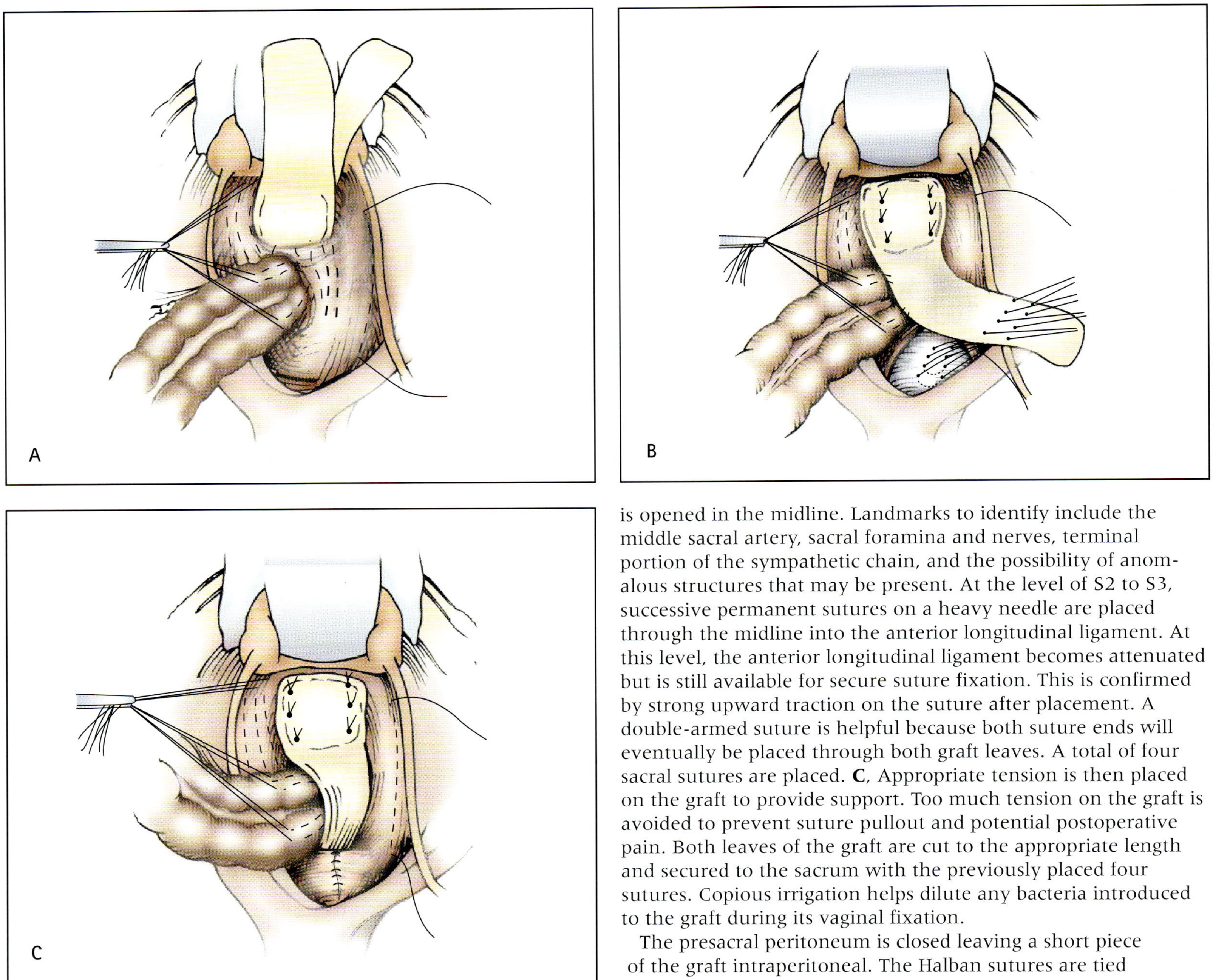

FIGURE 9-12.

Halban culdoplasty. **A**, To prevent herniation of bowel under the graft, a Halban culdoplasty is performed. This usually begins at the level of S2 to S3 on the tinea of the sigmoid colon, across the cul-de-sac, and up a portion of the posterior vaginal wall. The right-most lateral Halban suture will lie to the right of the graft and the remaining will be to the left of the graft. In general, the Halban sutures are tied down after the graft is fixed to the sacrum. This allows the cul-de-sac to be pulled up to the graft rather than the graft having to bridge over an already occluded cul-de-sac. **B**, The presacral space is now opened. The sacral promontory is located and the sigmoid colon is retracted to the left. The peritoneum overlying the S2 to S3 level of the sacrum is opened in the midline. Landmarks to identify include the middle sacral artery, sacral foramina and nerves, terminal portion of the sympathetic chain, and the possibility of anomalous structures that may be present. At the level of S2 to S3, successive permanent sutures on a heavy needle are placed through the midline into the anterior longitudinal ligament. At this level, the anterior longitudinal ligament becomes attenuated but is still available for secure suture fixation. This is confirmed by strong upward traction on the suture after placement. A double-armed suture is helpful because both suture ends will eventually be placed through both graft leaves. A total of four sacral sutures are placed. **C**, Appropriate tension is then placed on the graft to provide support. Too much tension on the graft is avoided to prevent suture pullout and potential postoperative pain. Both leaves of the graft are cut to the appropriate length and secured to the sacrum with the previously placed four sutures. Copious irrigation helps dilute any bacteria introduced to the graft during its vaginal fixation.

The presacral peritoneum is closed leaving a short piece of the graft intraperitoneal. The Halban sutures are tied down in succession completing the intra-abdominal portion of the procedure.

Uterine preservation.
In general, childbearing should be completed before a woman has major reconstructive pelvic surgery for pelvic organ prolapse. However, uterine preservation may be indicated in women desiring fertility or in those whose body self-image does not permit them to undergo a hysterectomy. Study numbers for uterine preservation with pelvic organ prolapse are small, but several techniques have been used and may be discussed with patients. Abdominal and vaginal approaches exist and are similar to the procedures described for apical support. These include use of the uterosacral ligaments [24], sacrospinous ligament [25], sacral hysteropexy [26], or grafts to the anterior abdominal wall [27].

Uterosacral Support to the Apex

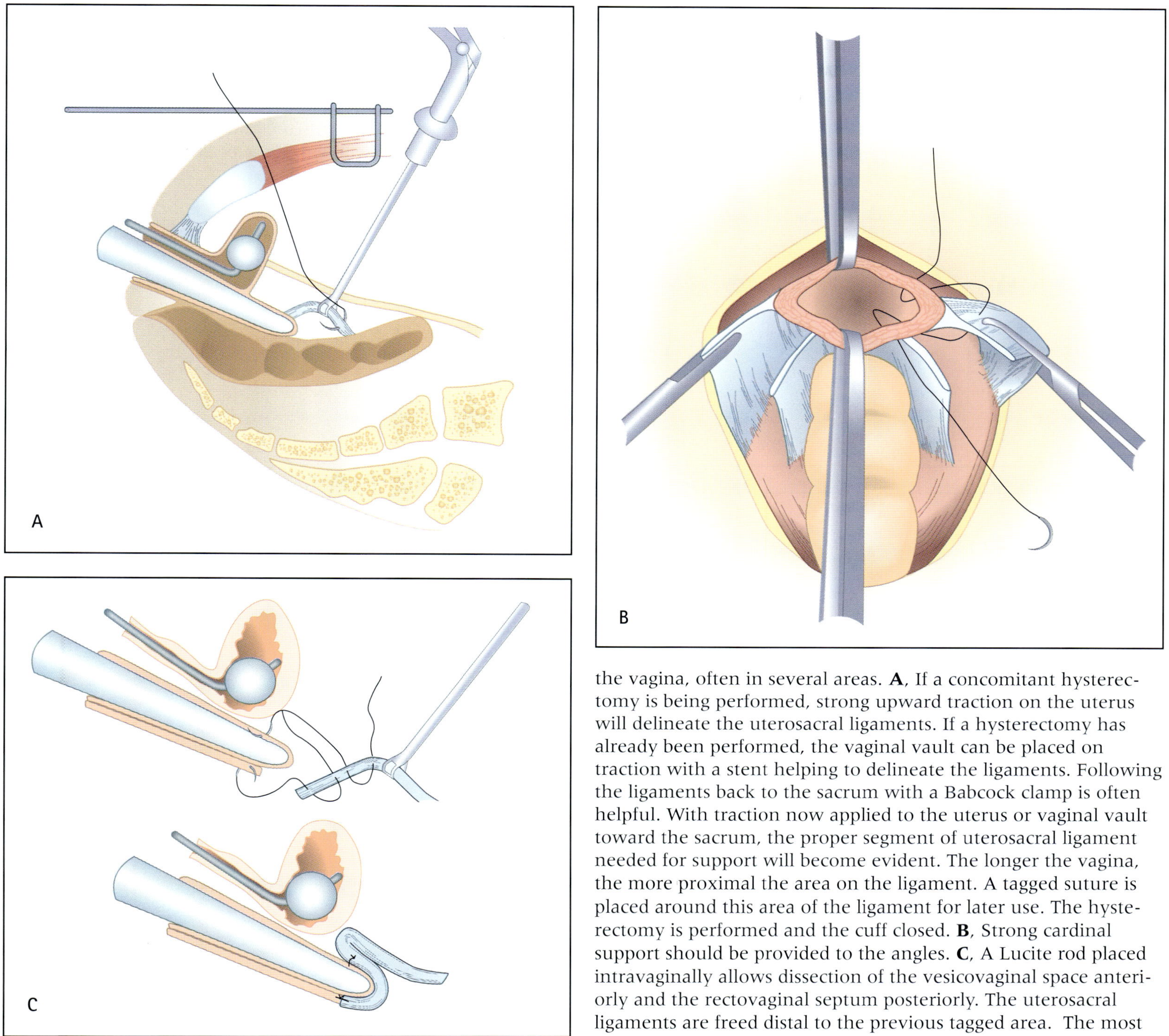

FIGURE 9-13.

Abdominal approach to uterosacral support. The native vaginal level I support is to the uterosacral-cardinal ligament complex. If identified, they can be used to reconstruct apical support abdominally, vaginally, or laparoscopically. In any of these cases, identification of ureters and surrounding vasculature is critical. A hysterectomy is performed for indicated reasons. The uterosacral ligaments are appropriately shortened and reattached to the vagina, often in several areas. **A**, If a concomitant hysterectomy is being performed, strong upward traction on the uterus will delineate the uterosacral ligaments. If a hysterectomy has already been performed, the vaginal vault can be placed on traction with a stent helping to delineate the ligaments. Following the ligaments back to the sacrum with a Babcock clamp is often helpful. With traction now applied to the uterus or vaginal vault toward the sacrum, the proper segment of uterosacral ligament needed for support will become evident. The longer the vagina, the more proximal the area on the ligament. A tagged suture is placed around this area of the ligament for later use. The hysterectomy is performed and the cuff closed. **B**, Strong cardinal support should be provided to the angles. **C**, A Lucite rod placed intravaginally allows dissection of the vesicovaginal space anteriorly and the rectovaginal septum posteriorly. The uterosacral ligaments are freed distal to the previous tagged area. The most distal uterosacral segment is attached to the rectovaginal septum and the most proximal portion of the ligament is placed to the anterior vaginal wall just inferior to the cuff. Remaining sutures are placed along the posterior vaginal wall as needed. This technique will provide support to both the anterior apex and posterior apex. The laparoscopic approach is performed exactly as above with the exception of a laparoscopic-assisted vaginal hysterectomy if indicated. The laparoscope is a means of access; its use should not change the way the basic procedure is performed.

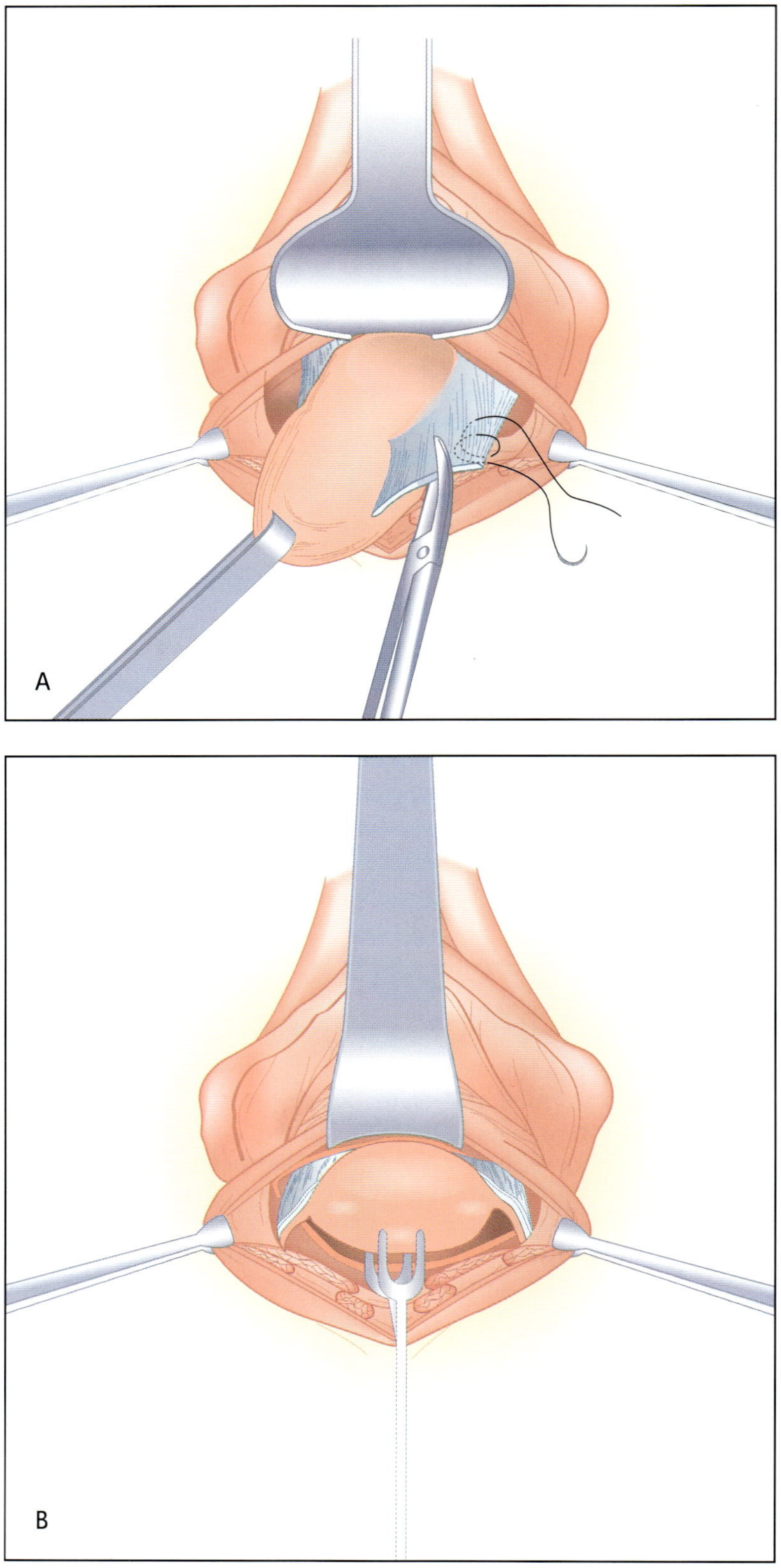

FIGURE 9-14.

Vaginal approach to uterosacral apical support. **A**, The vaginal approach involves the same identification of the uterosacral ligaments. It is made easier if a uterus is still intact to provide traction and help trace the course of the uterosacral ligaments. Some surgeons prefer the Doderlein technique to help delineate the ligaments (**B**). As in all support procedures, ureteral location is critical. Location of the ureters may be through palpation or direct visualization, or a laparoscope can be passed through the cul-de-sac vaginally to help with their localization.

(*Continued on next page*)

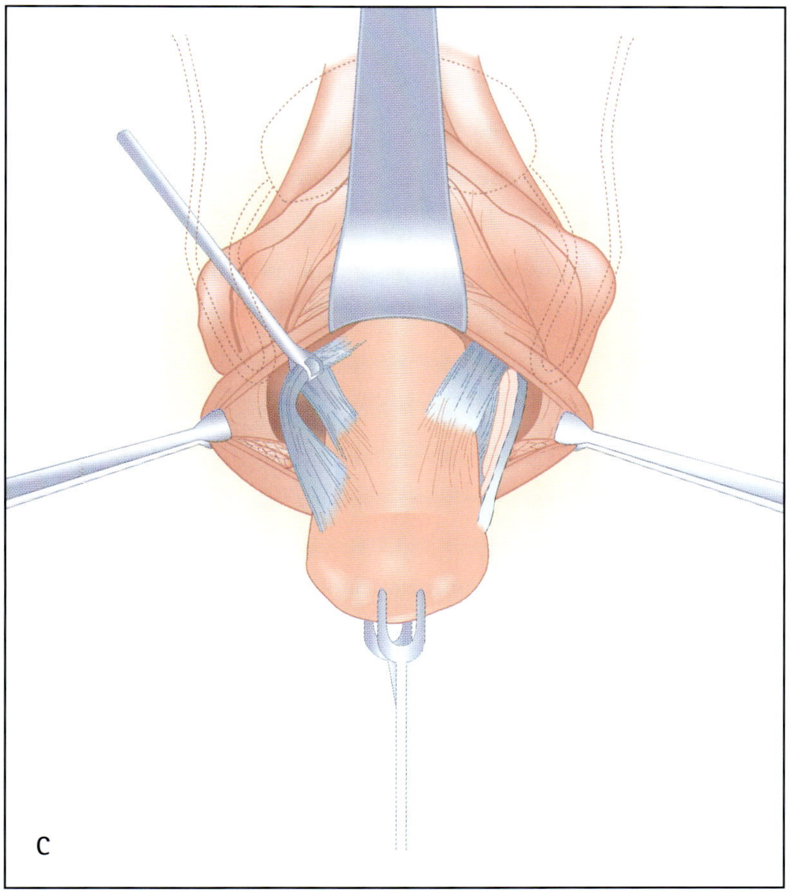

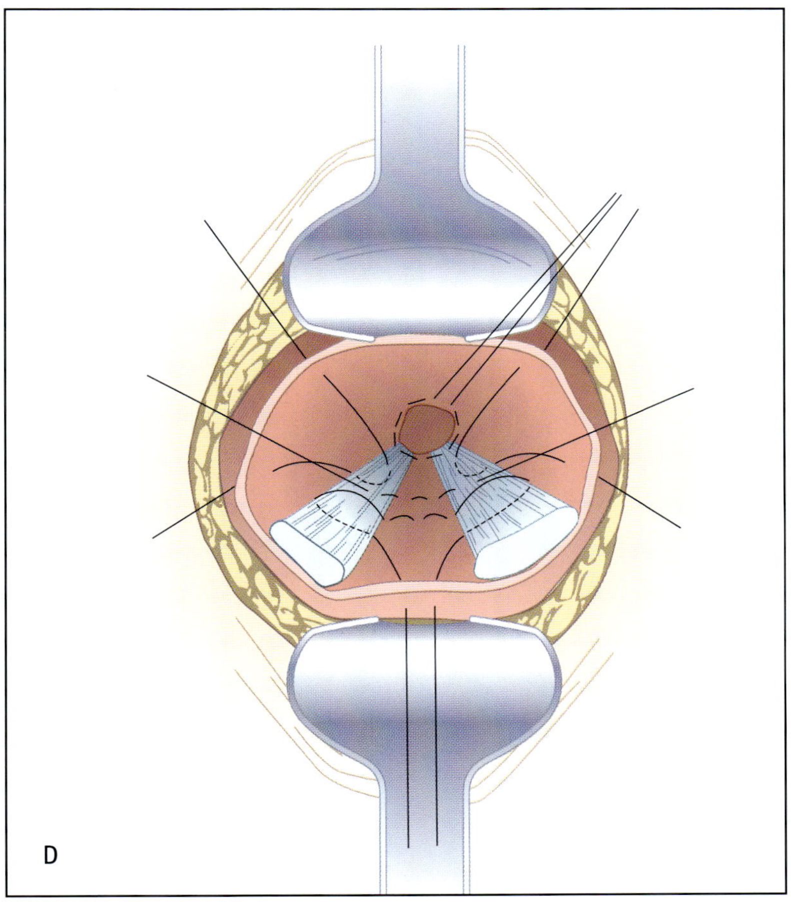

FIGURE 9-14. *(Continued)*

C, The uterosacral ligament is tagged at the level needed to support the apex and restore normal anatomic location over the levator plate. A double-armed permanent suture is used. **D**, The anterior portion of the suture is placed through the anterior vaginal muscularis and held. The posterior suture is passed through the posterior peritoneum and posterior vaginal wall muscularis. The anterior and posterior muscularis sutures are placed lateral to the midline approximately half way to the vaginal angle. The cul-de-sac is closed with an internal McCall-type culdoplasty suture. The most distal segment of the uterosacral ligament is used for an external McCall suture. If strong cardinal ligaments were identified, they are placed through the vaginal angles and lastly the cuff closed.

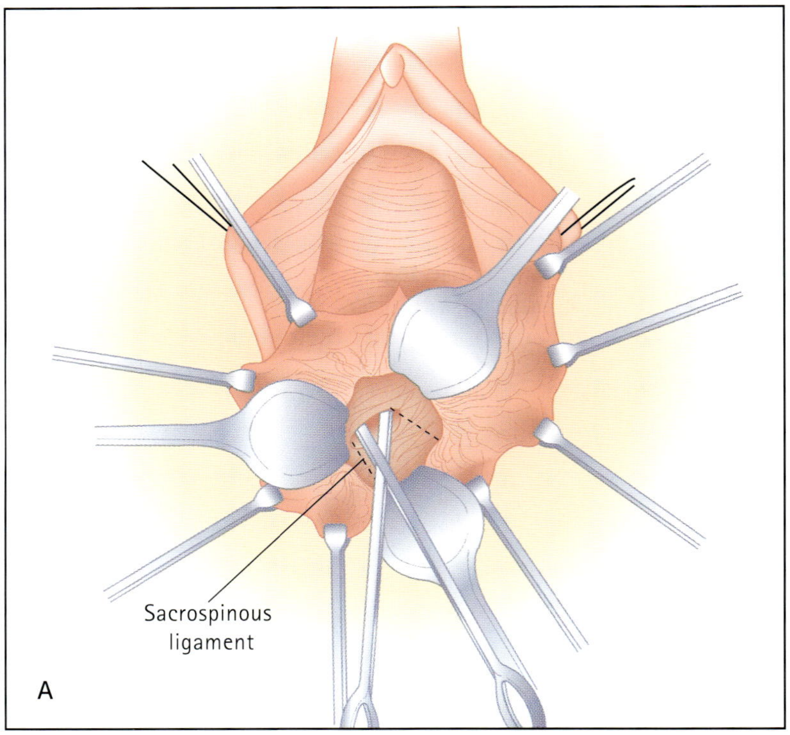

B. INSTRUMENTS FOR SACROSPINOUS VAULT SUSPENSION

Instrument	Manufacturer
Shutt punch [17]	Linvatec Corporation, Largo, FL
Laurus needle driver [18]	Laurus Medical Corporation Irvine, CA
BEI ligature carrier [19]	BEI Medical Systems, Chatsworth, CA
Endo stitch [20]	Autosuture Company, US Surgical Corporation, Norwalk, CT
Miya hook [21]	BEI Medical Systems, Chatsworth, CA

FIGURE 9-15.

Sacrospinous ligament fixation. This has been the most popular vaginal approach for correction of apical prolapse since its introduction into the United States in 1971 [13]. Various modifications using surrounding fascial points of attachment have also been described. Difficulties with supporting the anterior apical wall are seen with this technique. The sacrospinous ligament can be approached through a midline vertical incision or a midline apical incision [14,15]. Some authors propose bilateral sacrospinous vault suspension, although the utility of this has not been proven. In addition, the bilateral technique depends on adequate vaginal length and depth. Marking sutures placed on the epithelium at the anticipated site of attachment are recommended. The vaginal epithelium is separated from the underlying musculofascial tissue and the dissection taken to the level of the ischial spine. The rectal pillars, which separate the vagina from the sacrospinous ligament, are perforated with an atraumatic clamp gaining access to the sacrospinous-coccygeus ligament complex. **A**, The ligament complex is visualized using Briesky retractors to retract the bladder superiorly and the rectum medially. Under direct visualization, a permanent suture is placed about 3-4 cm medial to the ischial spine. Generally at least two sutures are placed. Numerous devices are now available for this suture placement (**B**). The surgeon must be aware of surrounding anatomic structures including the superiorly located inferior gluteal vessels and nerve. The lumbosacral plexus lies on the piriformis muscle just above the ligament complex. Just deep to the ligament complex are the pudendal vessels and nerve, sciatic nerve, and accompanying nerves of the lumbosacral plexus. Nerves running in the sacrospinous-coccygeus ligament complex may result in postoperative pain [16].

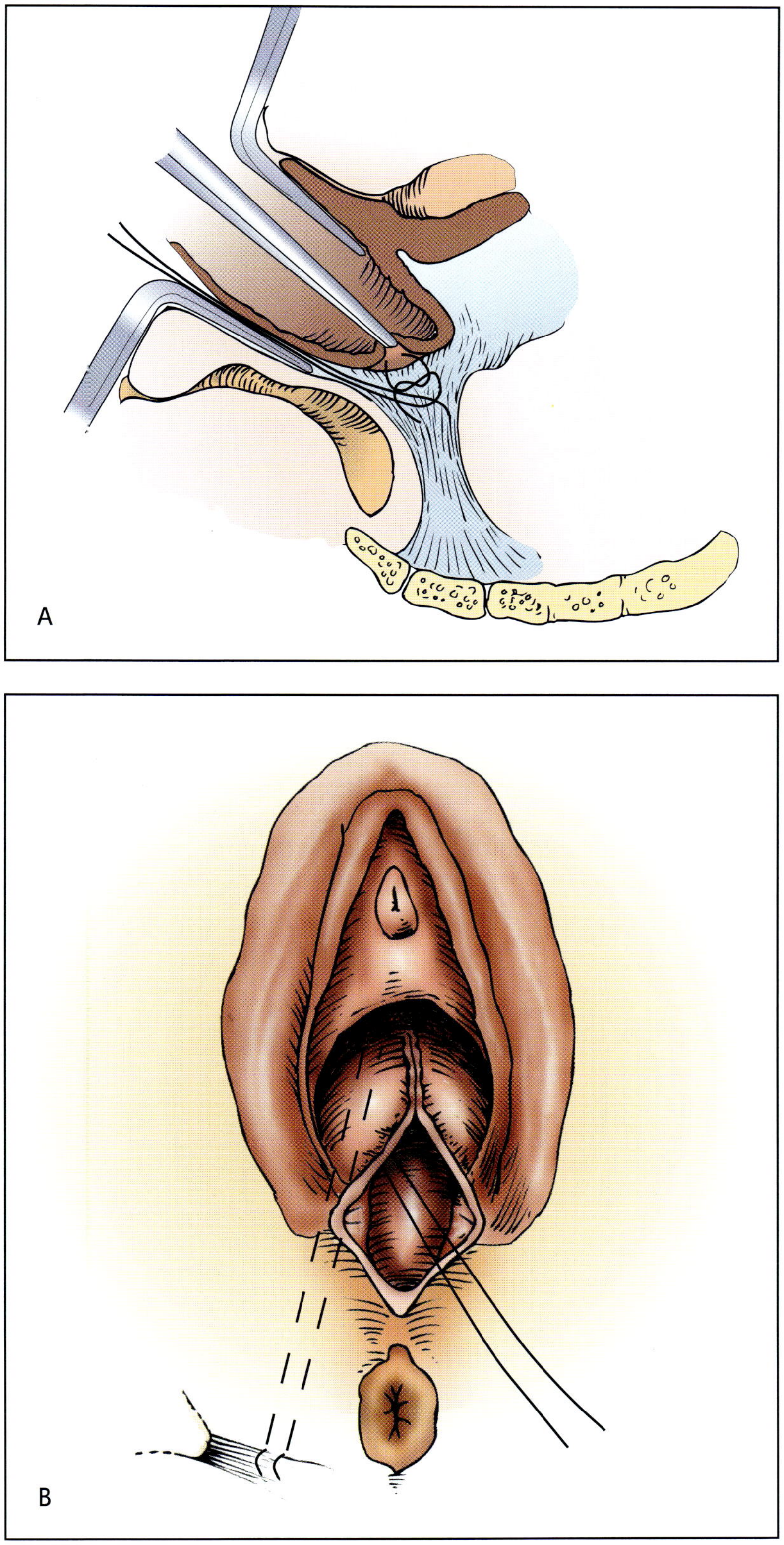

FIGURE 9-16.

Pulley stitching. **A**, After securing the sutures to the ligament complex, a pulley stitch is placed at the site of the vaginal marking suture. **B**, Before tying these down securely, the vaginal apex is partially closed to prevent difficulty reaching the apex once the pulley stitches are tied down. Suture bridging is avoided as the pulley stitches are secured bringing the vagina in direct apposition to the sacrospinous-coccygeus ligament complex. Pulley stitches are also used in iliococcygeus vault suspension, which uses iliococcygeus fascia or the levator plate as points of vaginal fixation [22,23]. The approach is similar to that of the sacrospinous vault suspension with a midline posterior vaginal wall incision. The epitheliun is separated from the rectovaginal septum and the dissection extended laterally and superiorly to the levator muscles. Lateral to the rectum and anterior to the ischial spine is the location of the iliococcygeus fascia. Sutures are anchored in this fascia as the rectum is retracted medially Pulley stitches are used for fixation and secured after partial closure of the midline incision.

OBLITERATIVE PROCEDURE

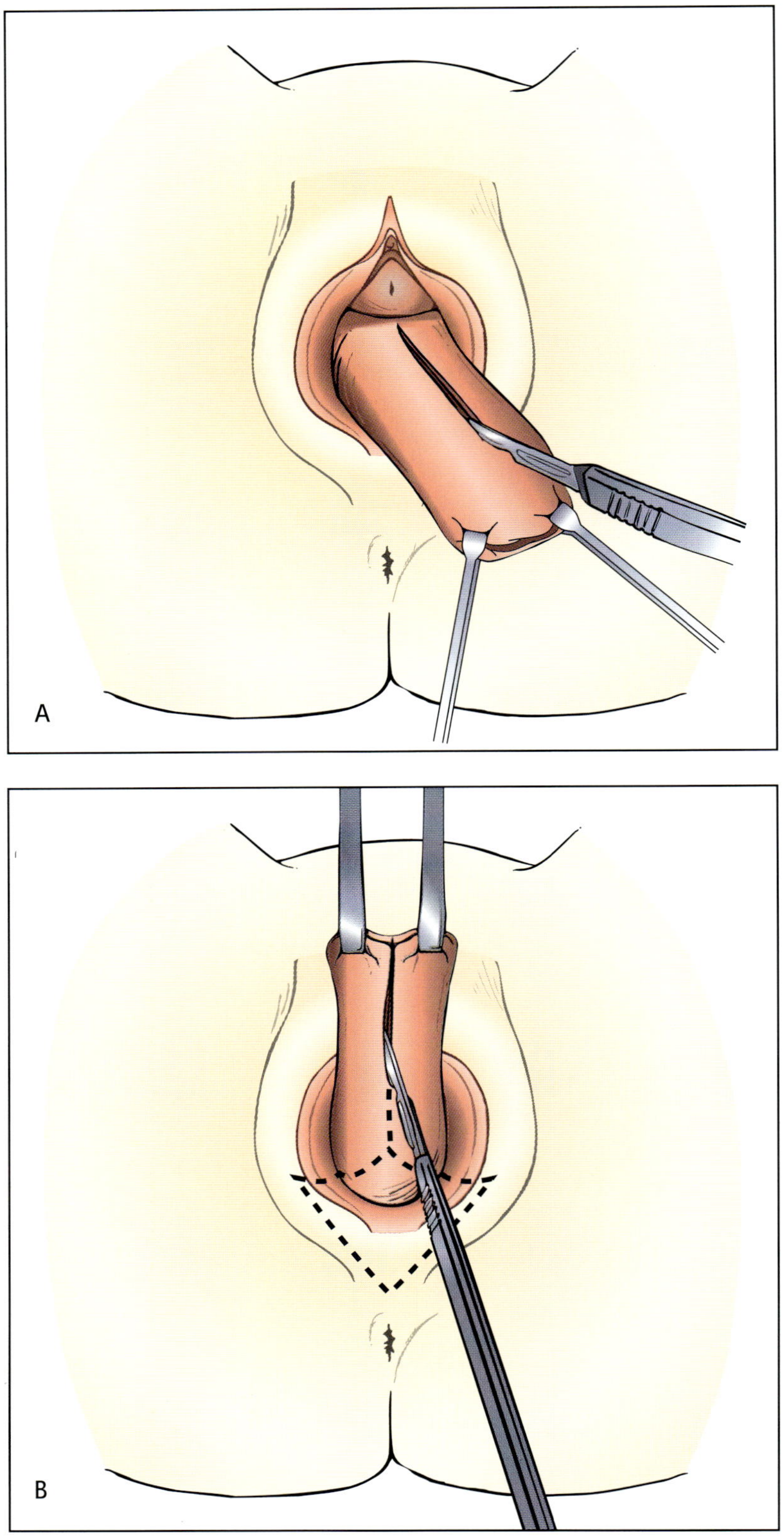

FIGURE 9-17.

Obliterative surgery is reserved for the patient who no longer desires sexual intercourse or in whom body self-image is not an issue. A LeFort colpocleisis may be used if the uterus is still present. An alternative approach uses a vaginal hysterectomy, if a uterus is still present, combined with a complete colpocleisis [28] and levator plication. **A**, After performing a vaginal hysterectomy, the vaginal epithelium is undermined with a subepithelial solution of saline. Kocher clamps placed at the vaginal angles help maintain orientation as the dissection proceeds. Either a circumferential epithelial incision just inside the hymen can be made or a standard midline anterior and posterior incision is used. **B**, A wide perineorrhaphy is made by removing a large diamond shaped-area of perineum and distal vaginal epithelium.

C–E, Using sharp and blunt dissection, the vaginal epithelium is dissected away from the underlying musculofascial tissue. The bladder, enterocele, and rectocele are all freed from the vaginal epithelium. The operator's nondominant hand is placed immediately on the vaginal epithelium and an assistant places countertraction on the prolapsing organs. Metzenbaum scissors are used to sharply divide the vaginal epithelium. The epithelium is removed leaving behind the prolapsing structures.

(*Continued on next page*)

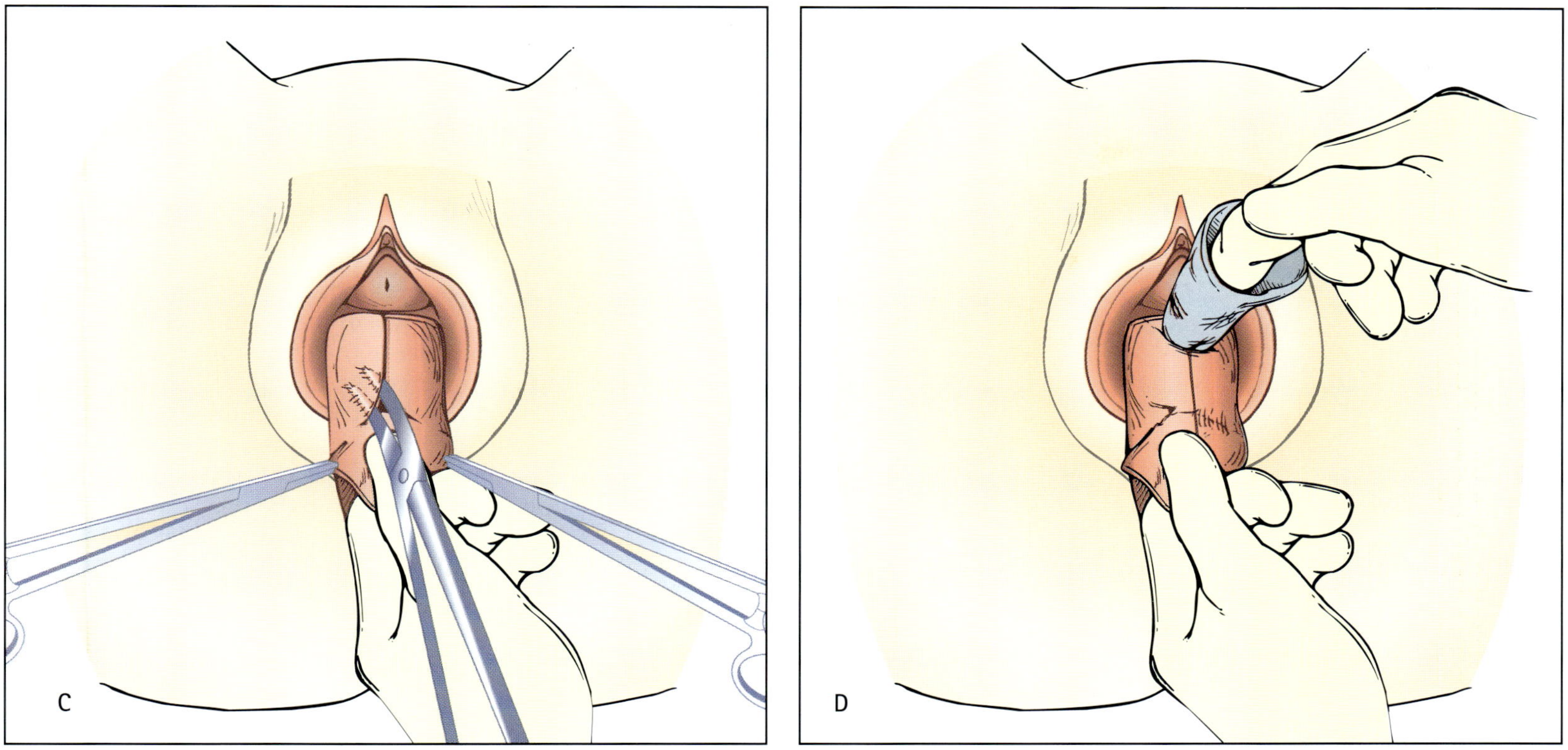

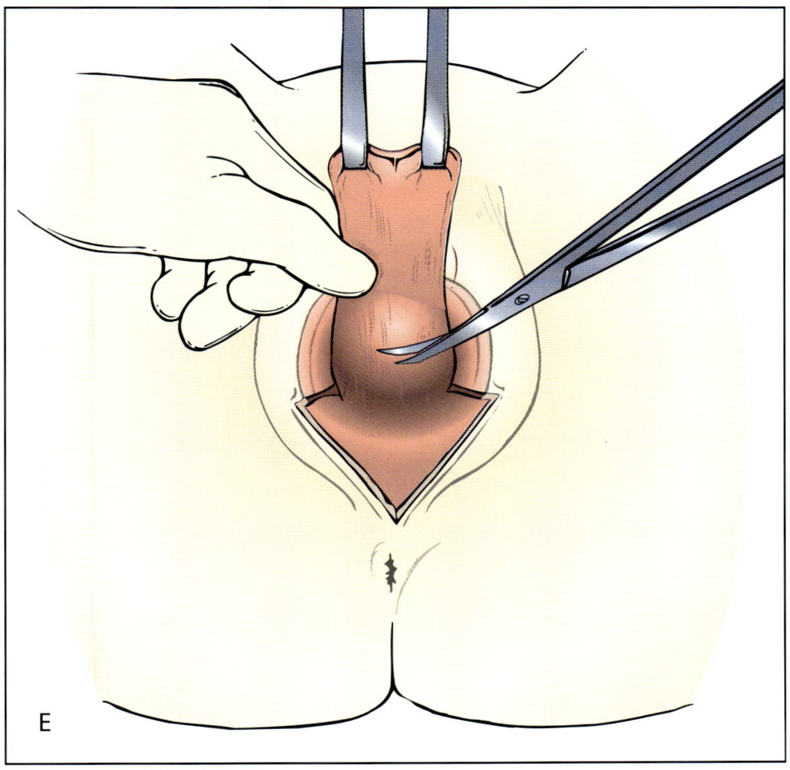

FIGURE 9-17. *(Continued)*

C–E, Using sharp and blunt dissection, the vaginal epithelium is dissected away from the underlying musculofascial tissue. The bladder, enterocele, and rectocele are all freed from the vaginal epithelium. The operator's nondominant hand is placed immediately on the vaginal epithelium and an assistant places countertraction on the prolapsing organs. Metzenbaum scissors are used to sharply divide the vaginal epithelium. The epithelium is removed leaving behind the prolapsing structures.

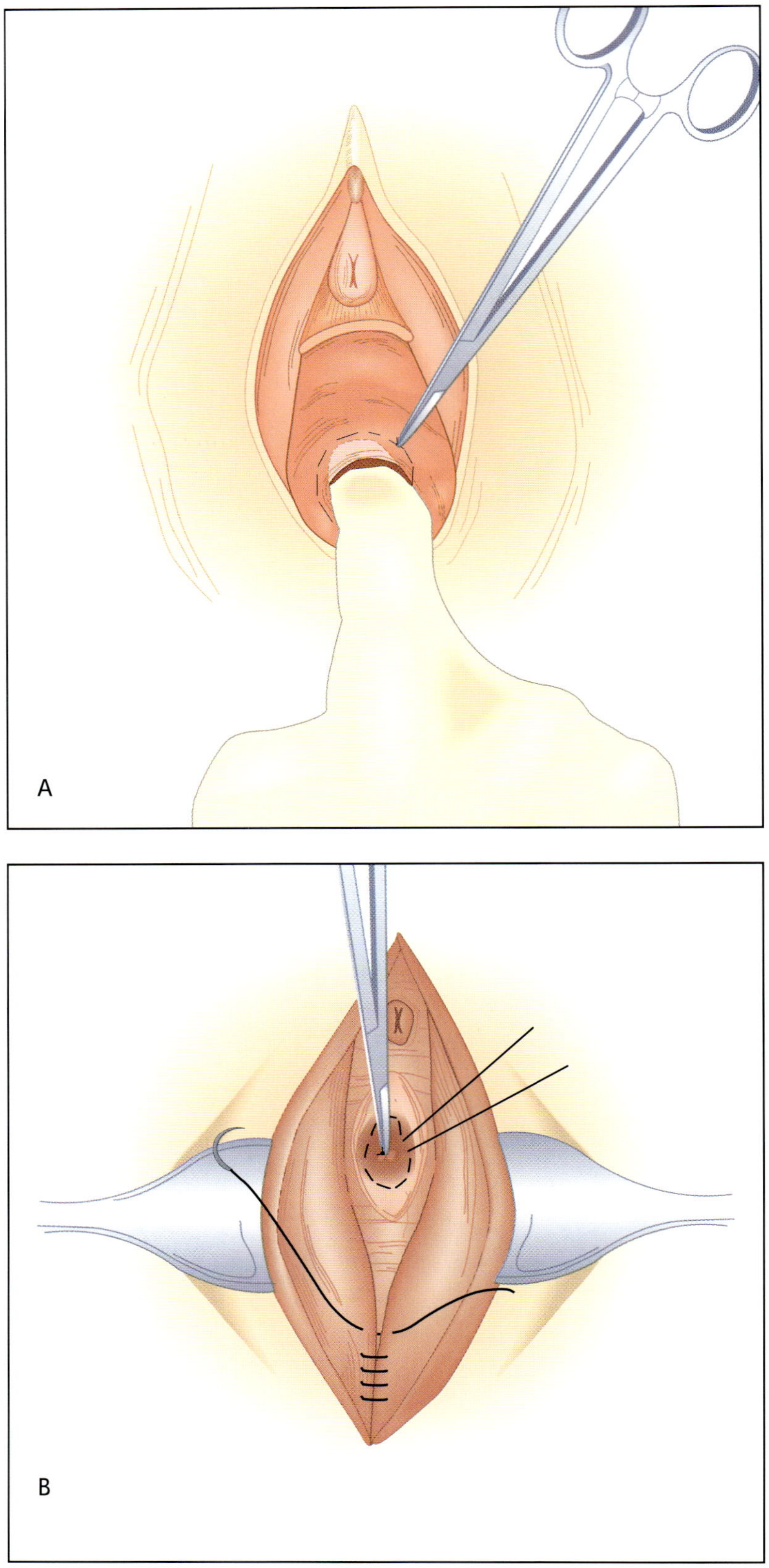

FIGURE 9-18.

Suturing. **A**, The leading edge of the prolapse is identified and pursestring sutures placed around it. As the suture is tied down and the tissue reduced, a hemostat is placed on the knot and the suture cut. The next pursestring suture is then placed with the tagged suture serving as the center. The hemostat helps reduce the tissue as the next suture is tied. This is carried on until the prolapsing tissue is above the level of the levator plate. **B**, The levator muscles are palpated and approximated using a 0 or #1 permanent or delayed absorbable suture. They should be closed from above the rectum to the level of the urethrovesical junction (UVJ). The ureters must be clear of the levator muscles and the operator should place a finger rectally to help with suture placement. A Kelly-type plication at the UVJ helps prevent downward traction on the UVJ from the levator plication. A tight perineorrhaphy is performed so that at most one fingerbreadth can be placed below the urethra. At completion the typical vaginal vault will be reduced to 3 cm in length and only one finger should fit below the urethra to the posterior fourchette.

POSTERIOR VAGINAL WALL

REPAIR OF DEFECTS

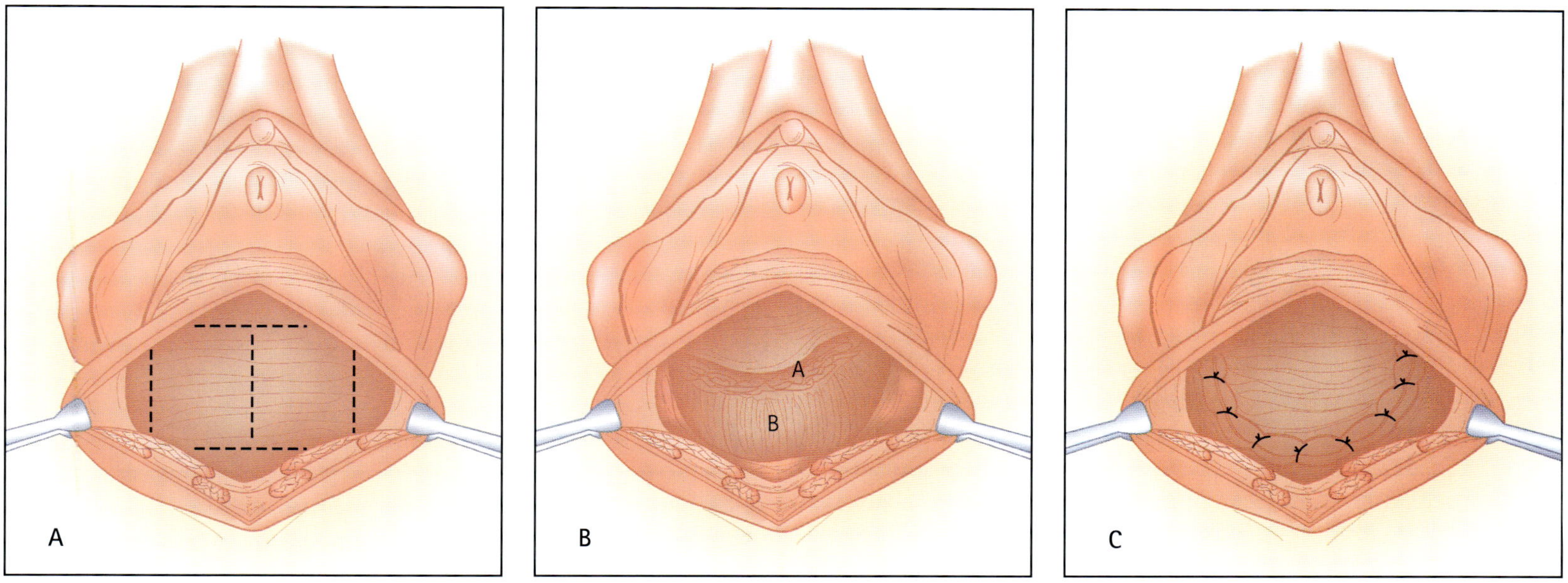

FIGURE 9-19.

Sites and types of rectovaginal septal defects. Defects in the posterior vaginal wall may be enterocele, rectocele, or sigmoidocele. Ancillary imaging such a dynamic cystoproctogram may be helpful in differentiating these entities. Symptoms vary widely in patients with posterior wall defects, a fact that underscores the importance of discussing patient and physician expectations of surgery. Successful correction of the bulging does not always equate to relief of the patient's symptoms. Rectoceles have several methods described for their correction although no one technique has proven superior. They include a defect repair, graft replacement, traditional posterior colporrhaphy, rectal wall imbrication, and transanal repair. **A**, The defect approach to rectocele repair [29] involves identifying the defect in the musculofascial tissue or the rectovaginal septum and correcting it. It avoids the mass closure technique of the posterior colporrhaphy. The support tissue may be torn at the perineal body, lateral sidewall, or apex. The concept is the same as that for defects involved in the anterior wall. **B**, The dissection is begun in the posterior midline and carried out laterally. The dissection should be kept as thin as possible below the vaginal epithelium. A finger placed rectally will aid in this dissection and help delineate the margins of the defect. *A* is the torn rectovaginal septum; *B* is the rectal muscularis. **C**, Once identified, the defect is repaired with interrupted sutures and the epithelium closed.

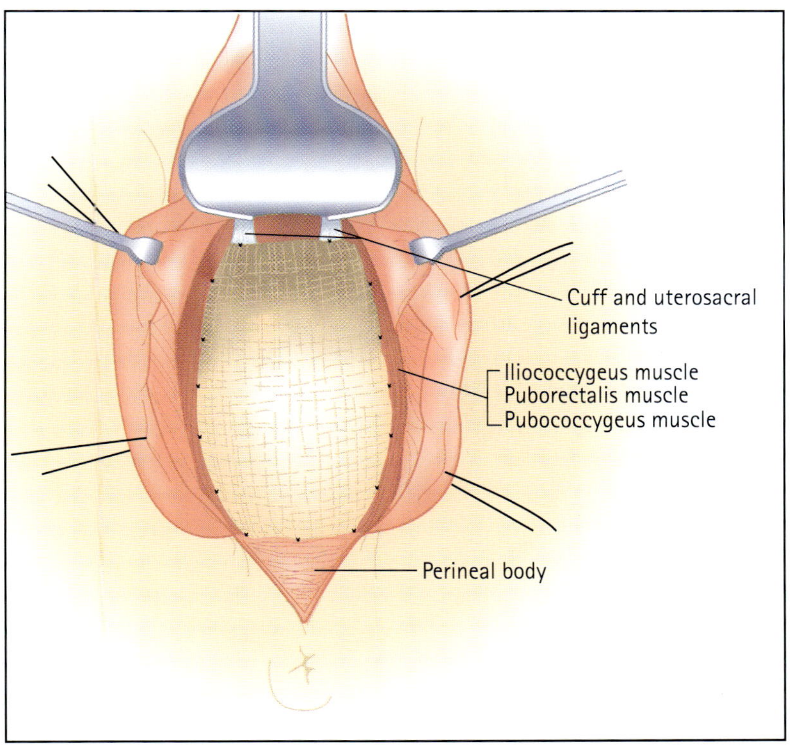

FIGURE 9-20.

Graft replacement of rectovaginal septum. When the rectovaginal septum is inadequate for repair, a graft can be substituted. Studies indicate the rectovaginal septum does not reach the vaginal apex and may in fact be only 2 to 3 cm in length [30]. This makes the native septum too short to reach the vaginal apex or if used will result in a markedly foreshortened vagina. In these cases a graft can be used. The dissection is begun in the posterior midline and widened laterally to the level of the levator muscles. Vaginal apical support is also identified. The graft is measured and sutured to the perineal body, vaginal apex, and laterally to the levator muscles. This recreates a full-length rectovaginal septum. At times, a voluminous rectum may require some imbrication before laying the graft.

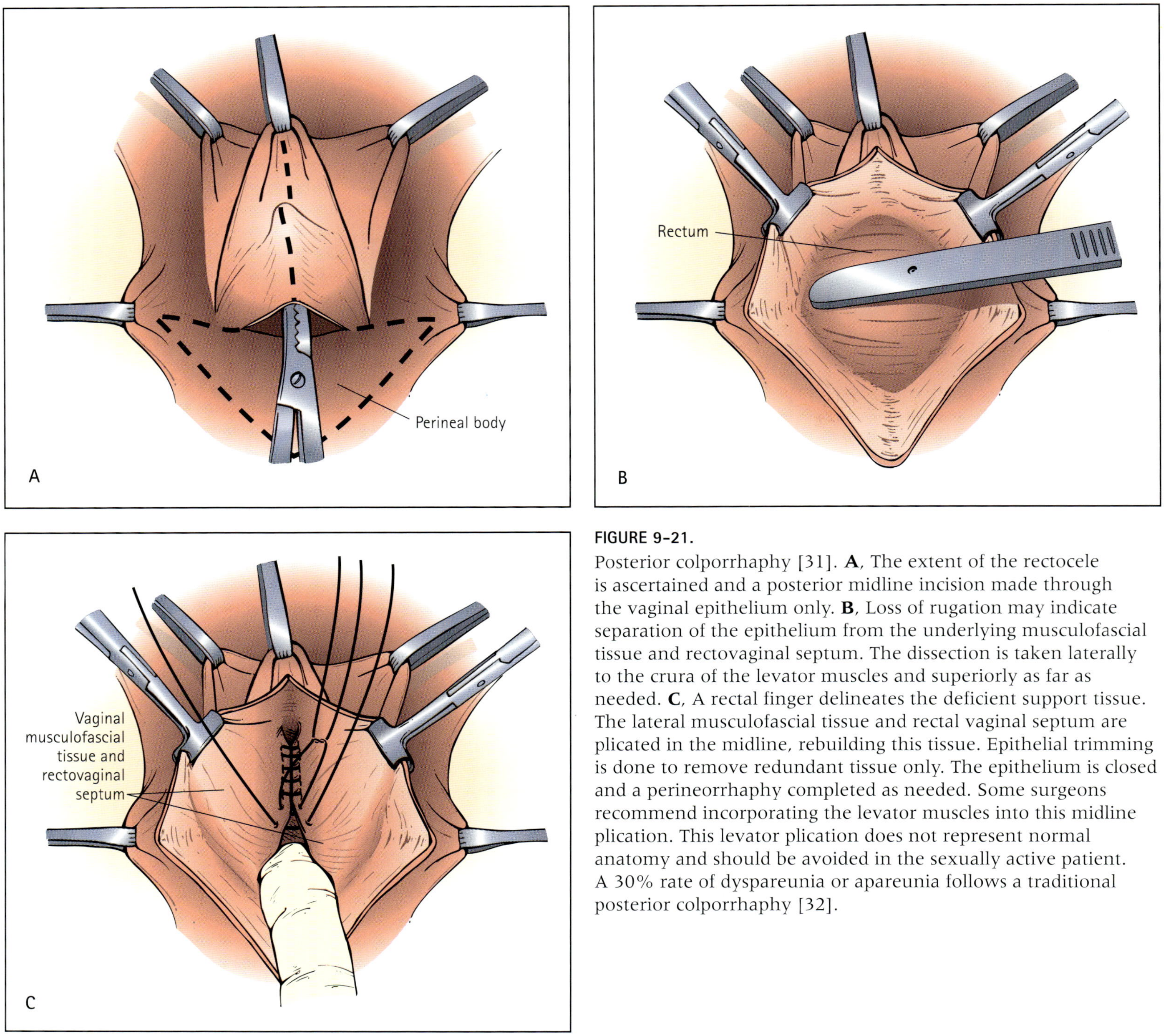

FIGURE 9-21.

Posterior colporrhaphy [31]. **A**, The extent of the rectocele is ascertained and a posterior midline incision made through the vaginal epithelium only. **B**, Loss of rugation may indicate separation of the epithelium from the underlying musculofascial tissue and rectovaginal septum. The dissection is taken laterally to the crura of the levator muscles and superiorly as far as needed. **C**, A rectal finger delineates the deficient support tissue. The lateral musculofascial tissue and rectal vaginal septum are plicated in the midline, rebuilding this tissue. Epithelial trimming is done to remove redundant tissue only. The epithelium is closed and a perineorrhaphy completed as needed. Some surgeons recommend incorporating the levator muscles into this midline plication. This levator plication does not represent normal anatomy and should be avoided in the sexually active patient. A 30% rate of dyspareunia or apareunia follows a traditional posterior colporrhaphy [32].

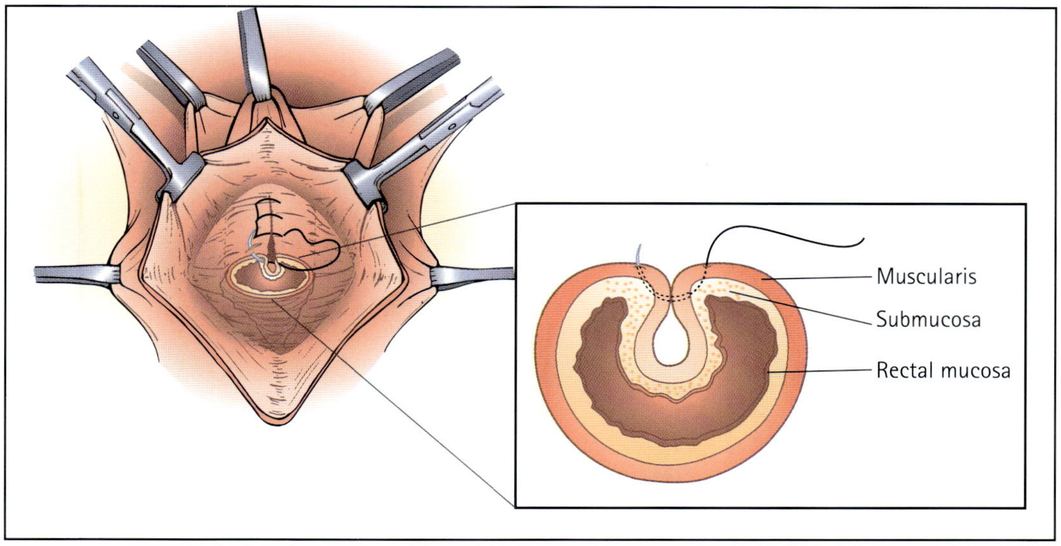

FIGURE 9-22.

Rectal wall imbrication [33,34]. Rectal wall imbrication has been reported in few series. A transvaginal or transanal approach may be used. This figure shows the transvaginal repair. A posterior midline incision into the rectovaginal space is made. The rectal muscularis and submucosa are plicated for the length of the rectocele with a running interlocking suture. The width of suture placement depends on the size of the rectocele. This results in a ridge of rectal mucosa and muscularis inverted into the rectal lumen, which purportedly undergoes necrosis narrowing the rectum. In the transanal approach, a running interlocking suture is placed through the rectal mucosa, submucosa, and superficial muscularis. The incorporated tissues slough and scarring results narrowing the rectal lumen.

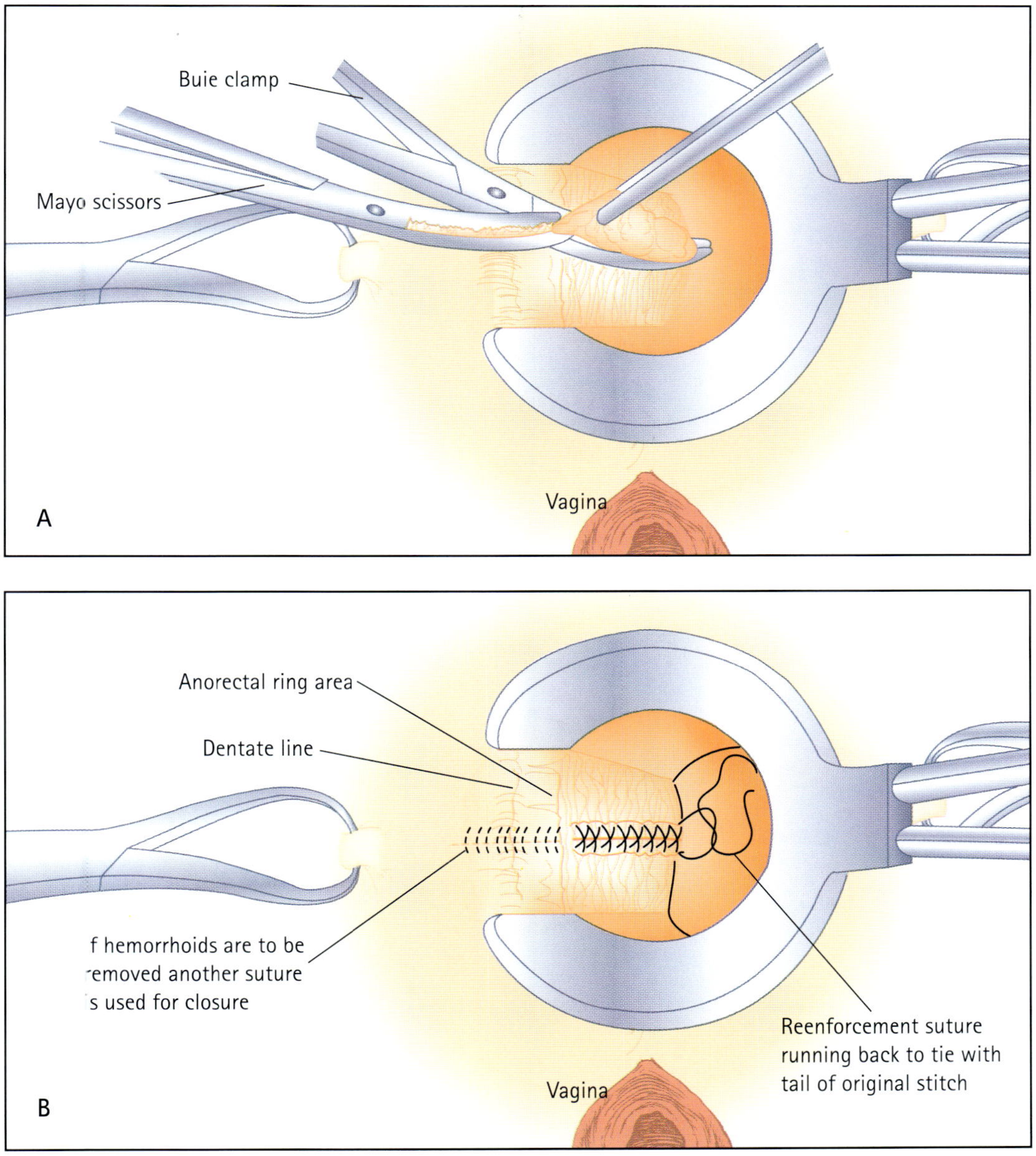

FIGURE 9-23.

Transanal repair [35,36]. The transanal rectocele repair is unfamiliar to many gynecologic surgeons; however, it is well known to colorectal surgeons. The patient is placed in the jackknife position. **A**, Lubricated rectal dilators are used to allow the passage of a Fansler speculum or Hill-Ferguson rectal retractors. Using a long slightly curved clamp, redundant rectal mucosa is pulled into the clamp. **B**, The excess mucosa is trimmed and a running suture is placed around the clamp from proximal to distal. A suture tail is left at the proximal end for tying later. The clamp is removed and the suture is run back from distal to proximal for reinforcement and tied. Excision is performed in from one to three quadrants depending on the amount of mucosal redundancy.

(*Continued on next page*)

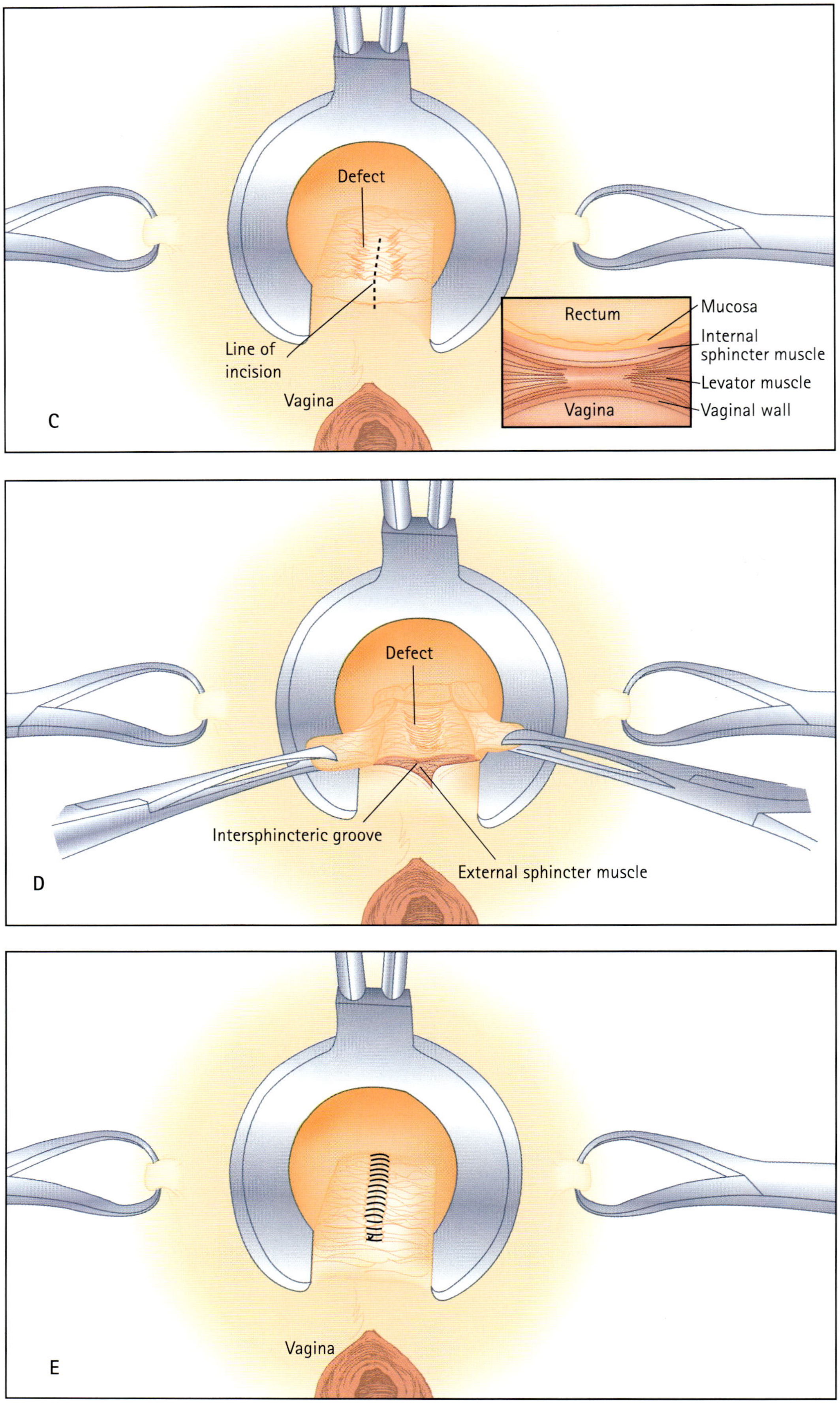

FIGURE 9-23. *(Continued)*

C, The anterior rectal wall is addressed. A mucosal incision is made superiorly from the dentate line 7 to 8 cm. **D**, The rectal mucosa is mobilized for 1 to 2 cm on each side of the midline incision. **E**, The rectal muscularis and rectovaginal septum are plicated with horizontal mattress sutures. The rectal mucosa is closed with a running suture. (*From* Sehapayak [36].)

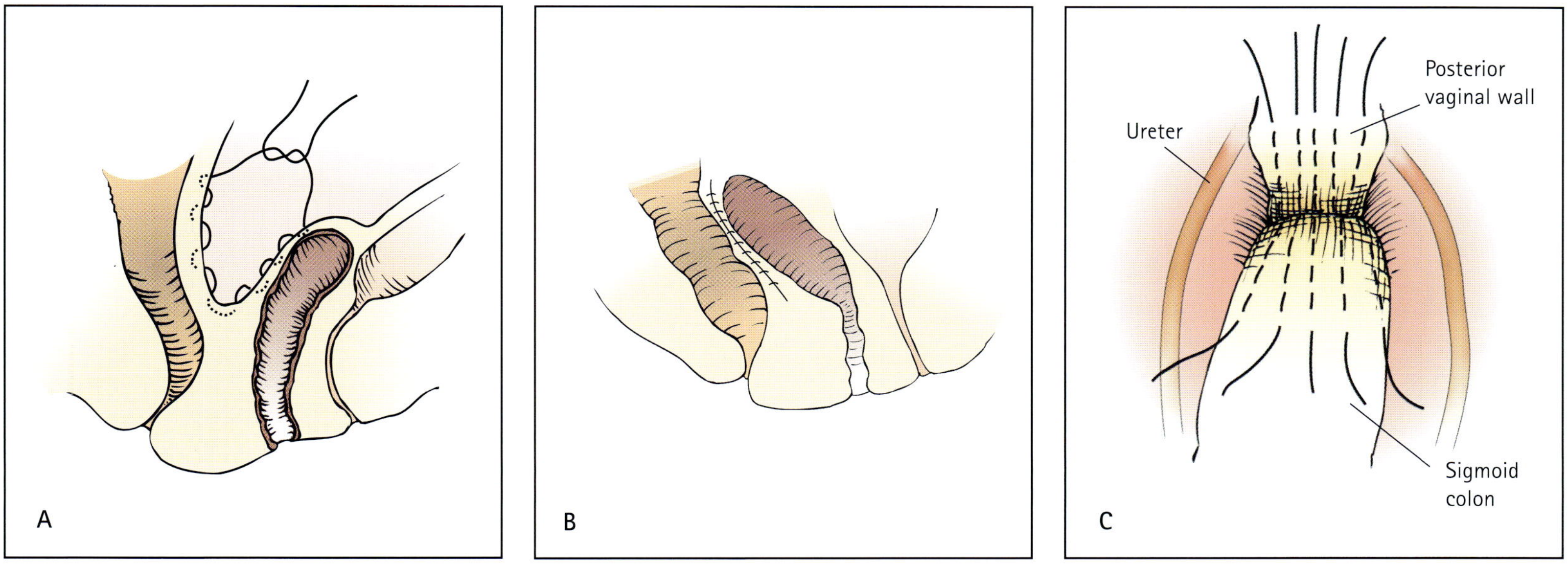

FIGURE 9-24.

Halban repair [37]. Cul-de-sac depth may have little to do with the finding of an enterocele. An enterocele is formed when the musculofascial tissue between the vaginal epithelium and the cul-de-sac peritoneum is interrupted allowing the peritoneum to come in direct contact with the vaginal epithelium. In any repair of enterocele the vaginal axis must be restored over the levator plate. **A**, In this abdominal approach, successive vertical sutures are used to obliterate the cul-de-sac. The repairis begun at the S2 to S3 level of the serosa overlying the sigmoid colon continuing on across the cul-de-sac and finally up the posterior vaginal wall. The first suture serves as the midline with the remaining being place to the right and left. **B**, Sutures should be placed about 1cm apart and end 1cm medial to the ureters. The sutures should also taper in as the posterior vaginal wall is approached to avoid crossing the ureter as it dives below the cardinal ligament. **C**, Appropriate apical support should be restored as needed and the Halban sutures tied down.

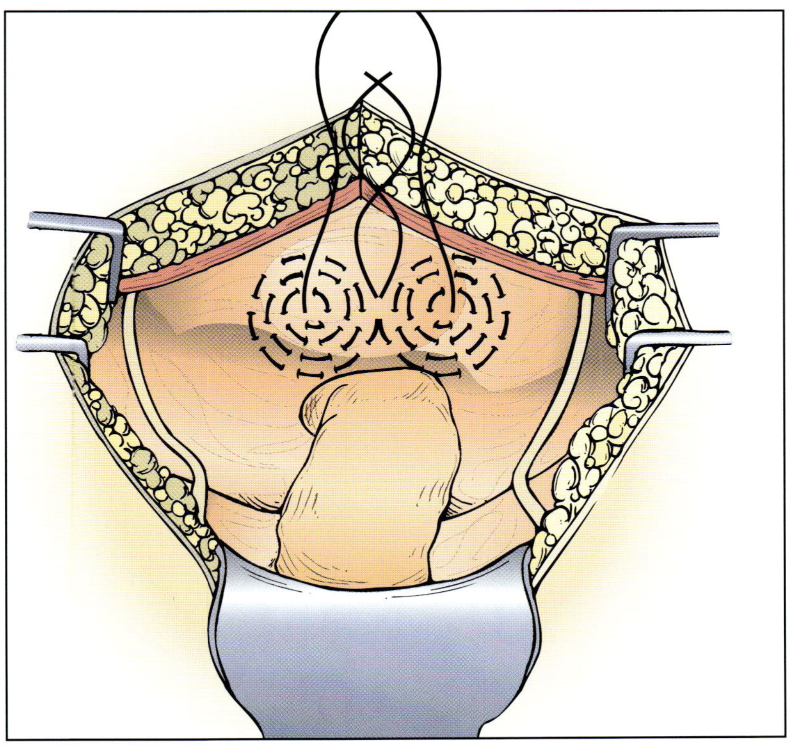

FIGURE 9-25.

Moschowitz repair [38]. The Moschowitz repair involves successive pursestring sutures placed around the cul-de-sac through the peritoneal and serosal surfaces only. The most superior suture should be 1 cm below the ureter to prevent kinking. Moschowitz sutures can be placed on either side of the sigmoid as shown or across the sigmoid as a single suture. The Halban and Moschowitz procedures possess little intrinsic strength themselves. Vaginal axis restoration over the levator plate is needed for these to be successful.

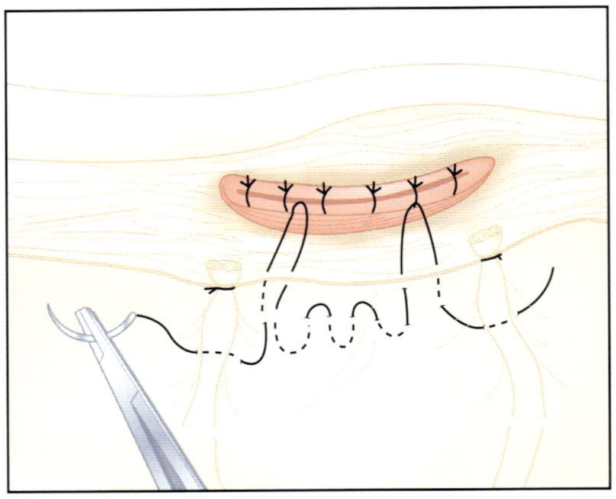

FIGURE 9-26.

McCall culdoplasty [39]. Originally described for vaginal approach cul-de-sac closure, this technique may also be modified for an abdominal approach. The uterosacral ligament is appropriately shortened, brought through the ipsilateral posterior vaginal wall, reefed across the cul-de-sac, through the contralateral posterior vaginal wall, and lastly through the contralateral uterosacral ligament. Excessive bunching of tissue in the midline should be avoided because it can lead to dyspareunia. An internal McCall suture can be placed above this suture to help further occlude the cul-de-sac. The internal suture does not enter the posterior vaginal wall.

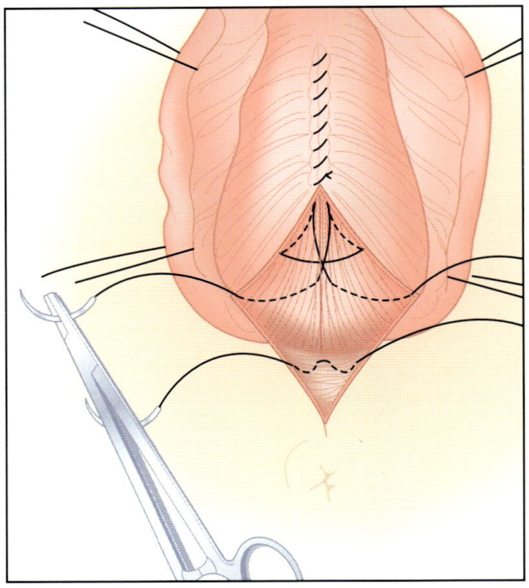

FIGURE 9-27.

Perineorrhaphy. An enlarged introitus and perineal body disruption often accompanies pelvic organ prolapse. Allis clamps are placed laterally on the introital opening so that when brought together they approximate the new opening. A diamond-shaped incision is made incorporating the perineal body and posterior vaginal wall and the epithelium removed. After completing other vaginal repairs, the perineorrhaphy is begun. At about the level of the hymen, the transversus vaginae muscle is approximated along with the inferior parietal fascia of the pubococcygeus. A modified crown suture is used to join the bulbocavernosus muscle and introital epithelium. The rectovaginal septum and anterior capsule of the anal sphincter are placed together followed by the superficial transverse perinei muscle. A subcuticular stitch is used to close the epithelium.

REFERENCES

1. Olsen A, Smith VJ, Bergstrom JO, *et al.*: Epidemiology of surgically managed pop and urinary incontinence. *Obstet Gynecol* 1997, 89:501–506.
2. Bureau of Census 1996. National Center for Health Statistics. www.census.gov/population/www/projections/natproj.html
3. Wall LL, DeLancey JOL: The politics of prolapse: a revisionist approach to disorders of the pelvic floor. *Perspect Biol Med* 1991, 34:486–496.
4. Maglinte DDT, Kelvin FM, Fitzgerald K, Hale DS, Benson JT: The association of compartment defects in pelvic floor dysfunction in 100 women. *AJR Am J Roentgenol* 1998, in press.
5. Benson JT, Lucente V, McClellan E: Vaginal versus abdominal reconstructive srugery for the treatment of pelvic support defects: a prospective randomized study with long-term outcome evaluation. *Am J Obstet Gynecol* 1996, 175:1418–1422.
6. DeLancey JOL: Anatomic aspects of vaginal eversion after hysterectomy. *Am J Obstet Gynecol* 1992, 166:1717–1728.
7. Webber AM, Walters MD: Anterior vaginal prolapse: review of anatomy and techniques of surgical repair. *Obstet Gynecol* 1997, 89:311–318.

7a. Maloney JC, Dunton CJ, Smith K: Repair of vaginal vault prolapse with abdominal surgery. *J Repro Med* 1990, 35(1):6–10.

7b. Beck RP, McCormick RN, Nordstrom L: The fascia lata sling procedure for treating recurrent genuine stress incontinence of urine. *Obstet Gynecol* 1988, 72(S): 699–703.

8. Iglesia CB, Fenner D, Brubaker L: The use of mesh in gynecologic surgery. *Int Urogynecol J* 1997, 8:105–115.
9. Richardson AC: Pelvic support defects in women (urethrocele, cystocele, uterine prolapse, enterocele, and rectocele). In *Hernia: Surgical Anatomy and Technique.* Edited by Skandalakis J, Gray S, Mansberger A Jr, Colborn G, Skandalakis L. New York: McGraw-Hill; 1989:238–263.

9a. Benson JT, McClellan E: The effect of vaginal dissection on the pudendal nerve. *Obstet Gynecol* 1993, 82:387–389.

9b. Zivkovic F, Tamussino K, Ralpit G, Schiad G, *et al.*:Long-term effects of vaginal dissection on the innervation of the striated urethral sphincter. *Obstet Gynecol* 1996, 87(2):257–260.

10. Cundiff GW, Harris RL, Coates K, *et al.*: Abdominal sacral colpoperineopexy: a new approach for correction of posterior compartment defects and perineal descent associated with vaginal prolapse. *Am J Obstet Gynecol* 1997, 177:1345–1355.
11. Fischer JR, Hale DS, Benson JT *et al.*: Combined rectocele repair and abdominal sacralcolpopexy. A new method for repair of Denovillier's fascia. Presented at the AUGS 18th Annual Scientific Meeting, Tuscon, Arizona; 1997.
12. Timmons MC, Addison WA, Addison SB, *et al.*: Abdominal sacral colpopexy in 163 women with posthysterectomy vaginal vault prolapse and enterocele, evolution of operative techniques. *J Reprod Med* 1992, 37:323–327.

13. Randal CL, Nichols DH: Surgical treatment of vaginal inversion. *J Obstet Gynecol* 1971, 38:327–332.
14. Nichols DH: Sacrospinous fixation for massive eversion of the vagina. *Am J Obstet Gynecol* 1982, 142:901–904.
15. Morley GW, DeLancey JOL: Sacrospinous ligament fixation for eversion of the vagina. *Am J Obstet Gynecol* 1988, 158:872–881.
16. Barksdale PA, Gasser RF, Gauthier CM, *et al.*: Intraligamentous nerves as a potential source of pain after sacrospinous ligament fixation of the vaginal apex. *Int Urogynecol J* 1997, 8:121–125.
17. Sharp TR: Sacrospinous suspension made easy. *Obstet Gynecol* 1993, 82:873–875.
18. Lind LR, Choe J, Bhatia NN: An in line suturing device to simplify sacrospinous vaginal vault suspension. *Obstet Gynecol* 1997, 89:129–132.
19. Veronikis DK, Nicols DH: Ligature carrier specifically designed for transvaginal sacrospinous colpopexy. *Obstet Gynecol* 1997, 89:478–481.
20. Watson JD: Sacrospinous ligament colpopexy: new instrumentation applied to a standard gynecologic procedure. *Obstet Gynecol* 1996, 88:883–885.
21. Miyazaki FS: Miya hook ligature carrier for sacrospinous ligament suspension. *Obstet Gynecol* 1987, 70:286–288.
22. Shull BL, Capen CV, Riggs MW, *et al.*: Bilateral attachment of the vaginal cuff to iliococcygeus fascia: an effective method of cuff suspension. *Am J Obstet Gynecol* 1993, 168:1669–1677.
23. Zaccharin RF: Abdomino-perineal repair of large pulsion enterocele. In *Pelvic Floor Anatomy and the Surgery of Pulsion Enterocele. Edited by Zaccharin RF. New York: Springer-Verlag; 1985:135–155.*
24. Williams BFP: Surgical treatment for uterine prolapse in young women. *Am J Obstet Gynecol* 1966, 95:967–971.
25. Kovac SR, Cruikshank SH: Successful pregnancies and vaginal deliveries after sacrospinous uterosacral fixation in five of nineteen patients. *Am J Obstet Gynecol* 1993, 168:1778–1786.
26. Arthure HE, Savage D: Uterine prolapse and prolapse of the vaginal vault treated by sacral hysteropexy. *J Obstet Gynaecol Br Emp* 1957, 64:355–360.
27. Durfee RB: Suspension operations for treatment of pelvic organ prolapse. *Clin Obstet Gynecol* 1966, 9:1047–1061.
28. DeLancey JOL, Morley GW: Total colpocleisis for vaginal eversion. *Am J Obstet Gynecol* 1997, 176:1228–1235.
29. Richardson AC: The rectovaginal septum revisited: its relationship to rectocele and its importance in rectocele repair. *Clin Obstet Gynecol* 1993, 36:977– .
30. Kuhn RJP, Hollyock VE: Observations on the anatomy of the rectovaginal pouch and septum. *Obstet Gynecol* 1982, 59:445–447.
31. Jeffcoate TNA: Posterior colpoperineorrhaphy. *Am J Obstet Gynecol* 1959, 77:490–502.
32. Kahn MA, Stanton SI: Posterior colporrhaphy: its effects on bowel and sexual function. *Br J Obstet Gynecol* 1997, 104:82–86.
33. Benson JT: Rectocele, descending perineal syndrome, enterocele. In *Female Pelvic Floor Disorders: Investigation and Management*. Edited by Benson JT. New York: Norton; 1992:384.
34. Block IR: Transrectal repair of rectocele using obliterative suture. *Dis Colon Rectum* 1986, 11:707–711.
35. Sullivan ES, Leqverton GH, Hardwick CE: Transrectal perineal repair: an adjunct to improved function after anorectal surgery. *Dis Colon Rectum* 1968, 11:106–114.
36. Sehapayak S: Transrectal repair of rectocele: an extended armamentarium of colorectal surgeons, a report of 355 cases. *Dis Colon Rectum* 1985, 28:422–433.
37: Halban J: *Gynakologische Operationslehre*. Berlin: Urban and Schwarzenberg; 1932.
38. Moschcowitz AV: The pathogenesis, anatomy, and cure of prolapse of the rectum. *Surg Gynecol Obstet* 1912, 15:7.
39. McCall ML: Posterior culdoplasty; surgical correction of enterocele during vaginal hysterectomy: a preliminary report. *Obstet Gynecol* 1957, 10:595.

Vesicovaginal Fistula, Urethrovaginal Fistula, and Urethral Diverticulum

CHAPTER 10

Jack R. Robertson

As the millenium approaches, a brief review of the 20th century reveals great progress in the treatment of vesicovaginal fistulas. Problems, however, persist with urethral diverticula. The complication rate of diverticulectomy has risen to nearly 20% [1].

In 1845, Frederick Diffenbach wrote, "It is a shame we must still acknowledge that the lucky cure of a vesicovaginal fistula must always be reckoned among the rarest of occurrences" [2]. Marion Sims, the "Father of Gynecology," was the first to successfully close vesicovaginal fistulas. In 1851, he reported a successful closure in 230 of 312 patients [2]. Despite Sims' success, the gloomy prospect of curing fistulas by the vaginal operation prevailed. In 1872, Sir James Young Simpson wrote, "A urinary fistula is an infirmity which is beyond all relief and all hope" [3].

The advances in obstetrics during the 20th century have made obstetric fistulas a rarity except in third world countries. A fistula now is most commonly the result of a complication of hysterectomy. These fistulas are best closed by the Latzko procedure, which was first reported in 1942 [4]. More widespread use of recent hysteropscopic technology should cut the rate of 600,000 hysterectomies a year in the United States.

Diagnosing a vesicovaginal fistula was never a problem, especially if it were obstetric in origin. There was, and still is, a problem in diagnosing urethral diverticula. Successful treatment remains a problem as well. In 1953, Novak stated that urethral diverticulum was a relatively rare condition and that no gynecologist would see more than a few [5]. Davis and Cain, in 1955, at the same institution, Johns Hopkins, reported positive pressure urethrography and diagnosed more diverticula in 1 year than in the pervious history of Johns Hopkins Hospital [6].

Magnetic resonance imaging and perineal ultrasound have added greatly to advances in diagnosis. Ultrasound is preferred because it is less expensive. A recent and most promising advance is three-dimensional ultrasound.

The problem is physician awareness. Fantle reviewed 100 urology charts and noted there was a record of urethral palpation in every one. However, in 100 gynecology charts, there was no record of urethral palpation (A. Fantle, personal communication). The time factor in medical practice of today, unfortunately, adds to this problem.

URETHRAL DIVERTICULUM

ANATOMY AND DIAGNOSIS

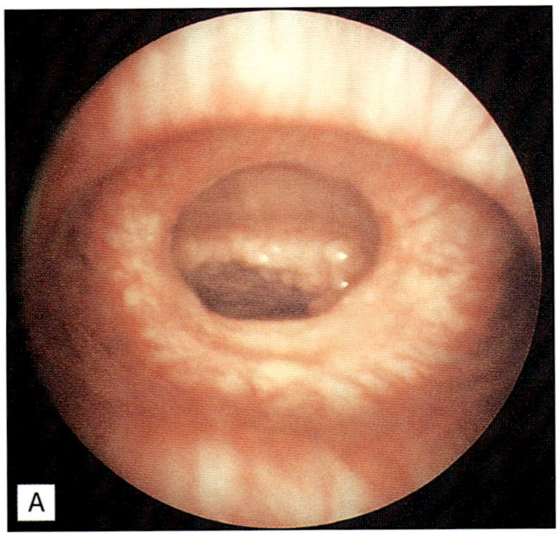

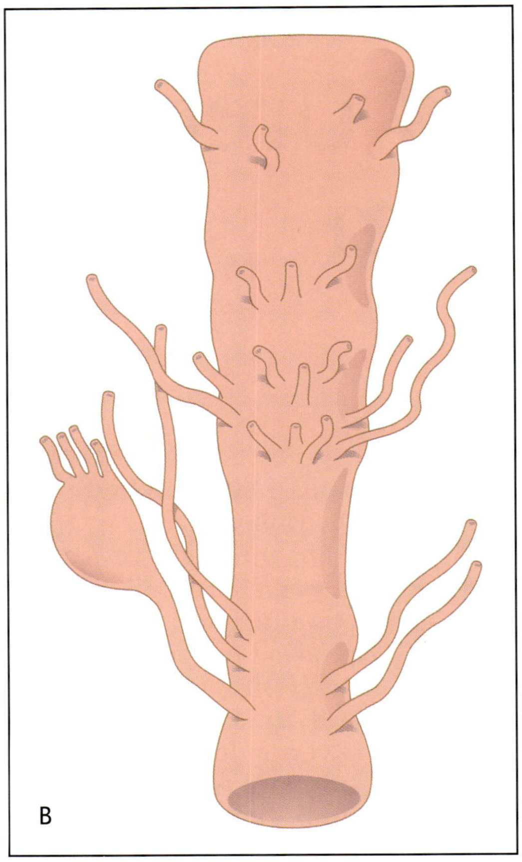

FIGURE 10-1.
Anatomy. **A**, The female urethra is only a little over an inch in length, but it is the key to the continence mechanism [7]. This view is looking back at the bladder neck from the distal urethra. The urethral sphincter (circular) is clearly outlined at the midurethra. **B**, The submucosa has periurethral and paraurethral glands. Gynecologists and urologists disagreed about whether glands were present in the urethra. Huffman, a gynecologist, settled this by injecting female cadaver urethras with paraffin wax. Sectioning of the urethras demonstrated multiple glands, primarily at midurethra. Most diverticula are found at midurethra and usually are located above the striated voluntary sphincter. Their location is important for treatment.

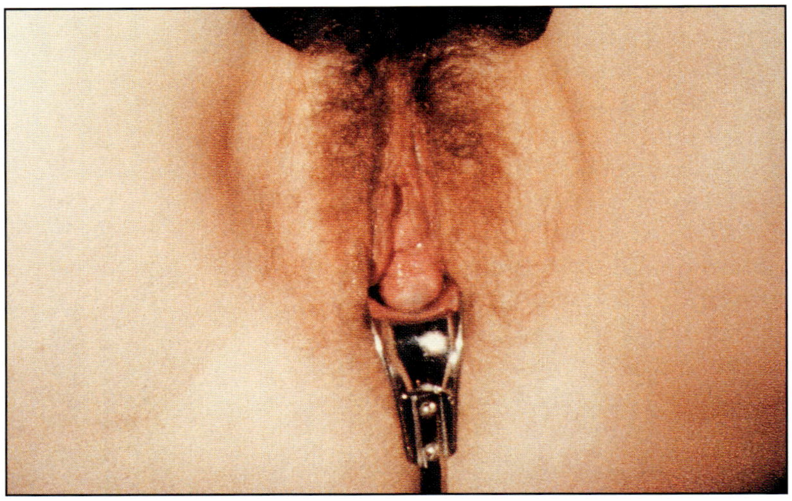

FIGURE 10-2.
Masses. A suburethral mass is seldom seen and may be palpated in about 50% of cases. However, urethral palpation is usually neglected in pelvic examinations. Also, if the urethra is palpated, pus is seldom seen unless urethroscopy is done at the same time.

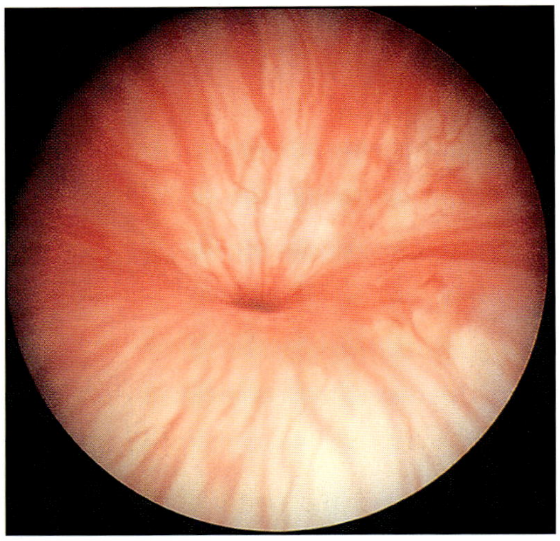

FIGURE 10-3.
Normal urethral epithelium. Note the vascularity. The urethra is sensitive to hormonal changes. One-third of the intrinsic pressure in the urethra is secondary to its vascularity, which is secondary to estrogen.

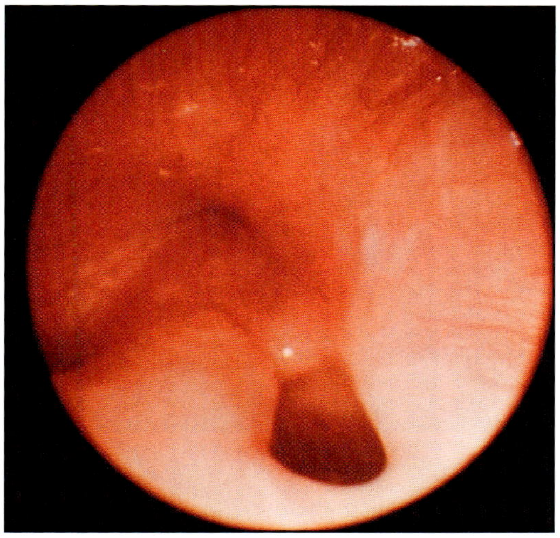

FIGURE 10-4.

Urethral diverticulum. In 1953 Novak reported, "This is a relatively rare condition and no gynecologist would see more than a few in a lifetime." [5] The urology department at Charity Hospital in New Orleans reported 9 cases at their huge institution and found 79 cases in the world's literature [8].

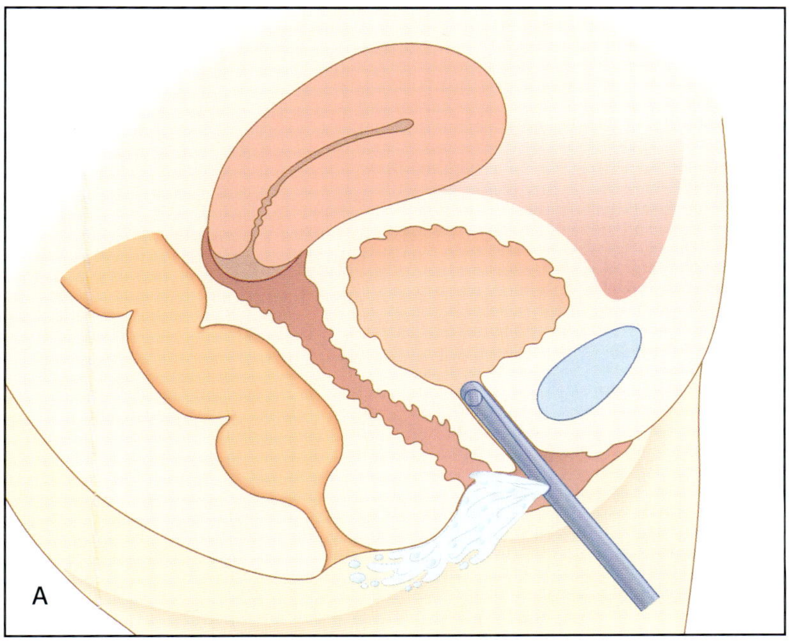

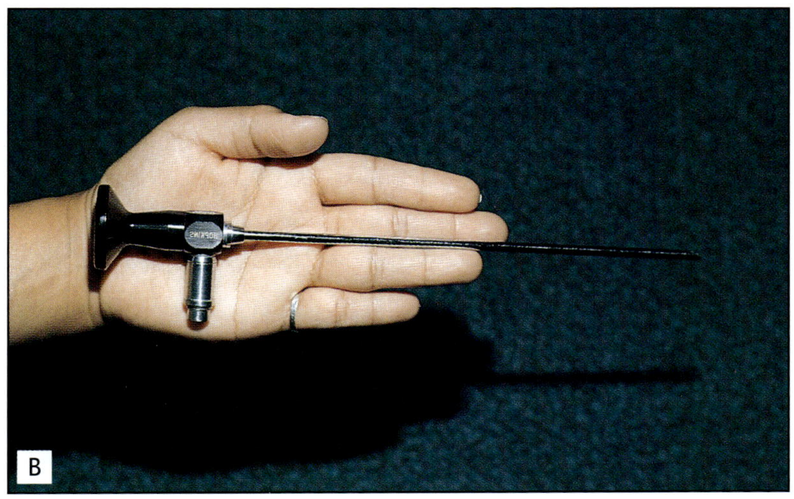

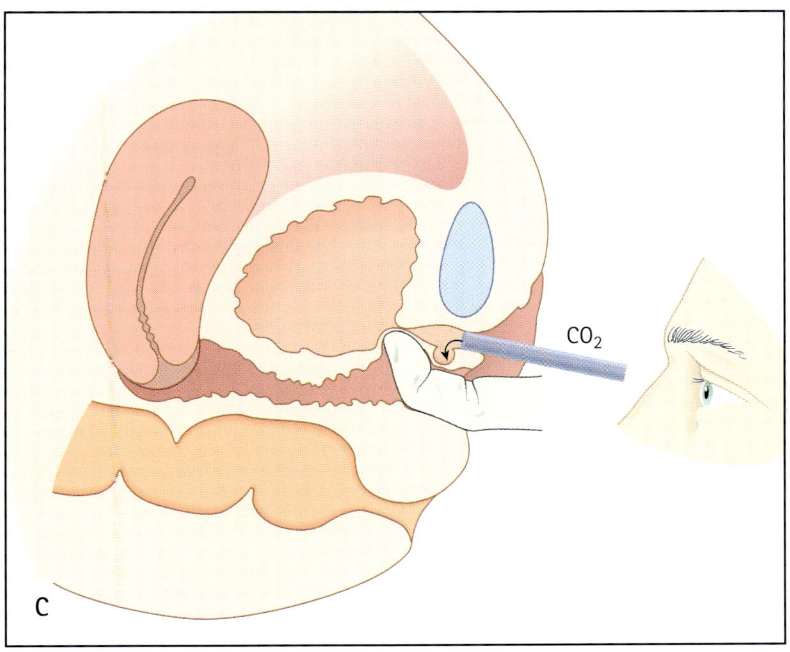

FIGURE 10-5.

Cystoscopic examination. **A**, Most women are examined with a male cystoscope. The patient gets a mini douche, a very good perineal wash, but at best the examiner sees only about 20% of the female urethra. Fifty percent of the diverticula examined by the author had been previously examined once or many times without the diagnosis having been made. **B**, A female urethroscope is essential for examination. It is half the length of the cystoscope and has a direct view. All of the pictures in this segment were taken with the female urethroscope. Also, they were taken using carbon dioxide as the distending medium. It is an optical principal that you can see better through gas than through water. **C**, Urethroscopy is essential for diagnosis. Carbon dioxide is preferred to water for insufflation. The examiner's fingers in the vagina push the vesical neck against the symphysis to trap the gas and expand the urethra [9].

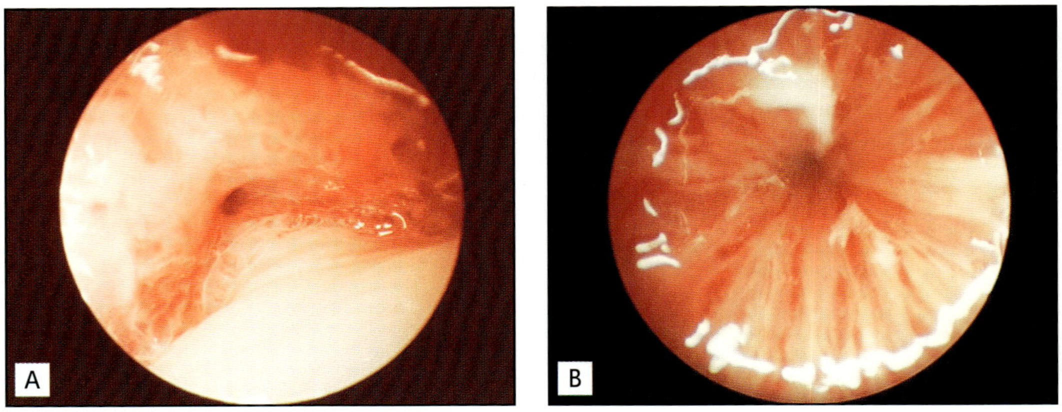

FIGURE 10-6.
Vaginal massage. **A**Under direct vision and with vaginal massage, the entire urethra may fill with pus. **B**, Pus exudes from the orifice.

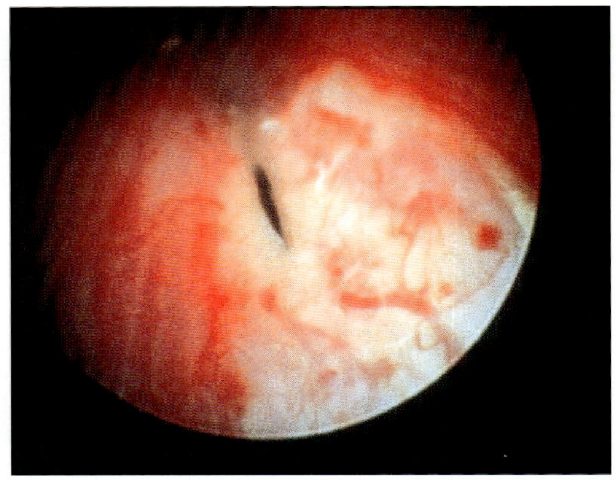

FIGURE 10-7.
Urinary tract infection. This patient has recurrent urinary tract infection. Urethroscopy reveals a diverticulum with infection. Urinary tract infections are commonly secondary to urethral diverticula.

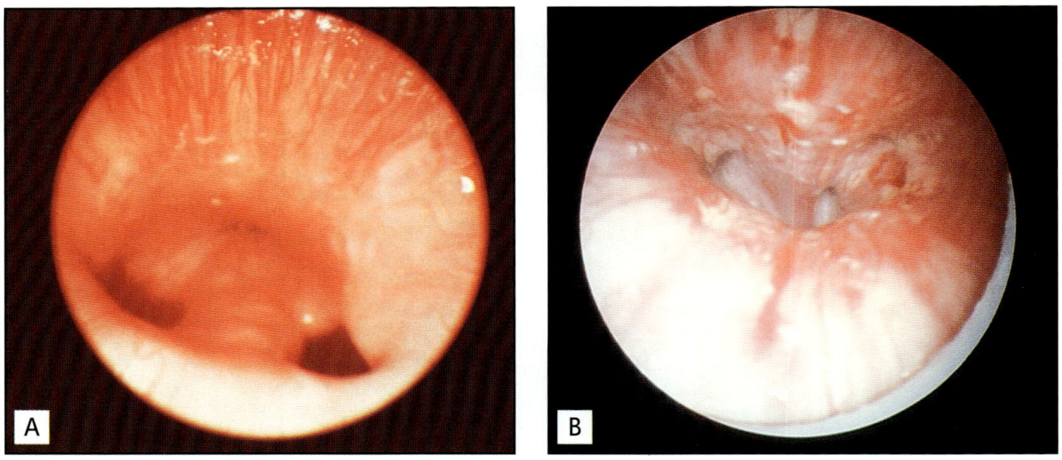

FIGURE 10-8.
Multiple diverticula. **A**, Two diverticula are not uncommon. These are above the voluntary sphincter seen at six o'clock. It will be difficult to resect these and not get a urethrovaginal fistula. **B**, This patient has multiple diverticula. With treatment she is at risk for urethrovaginal fistula. The risk of fistula complications is the same as that in **A**.

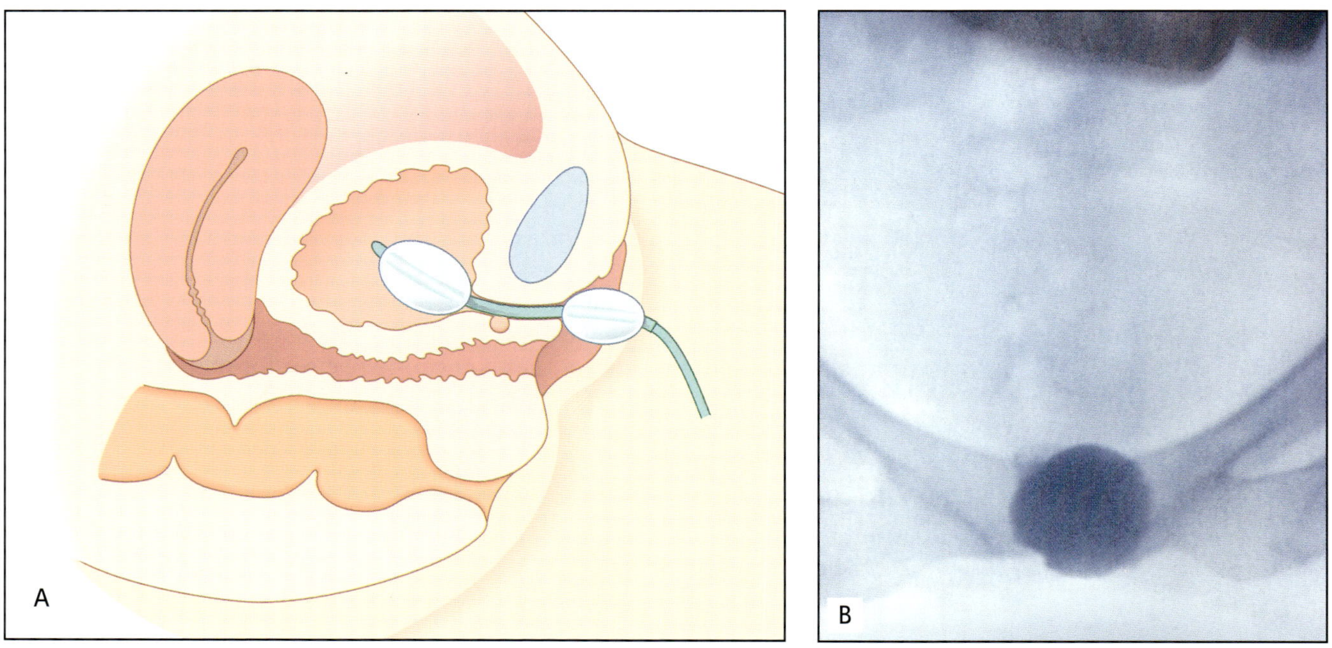

FIGURE 10-9.
Catheterization. **A**, Double balloon urethral catheters isolate the urethra. Injection of radio-pague dye makes the diagnosis [9]. This was a major diagnostic advance. The procedure is uncomfortable for the patient and is now replaced by perineal ultrasound. **B**, This x-ray is the typical picture obtained with a double balloon catheter.

A. SYMPTOMS IN PATIENTS WITH SUBURETHRAL DIVERTICULUM

Symptoms	Percent,%
Frequency	62
Urgency	31
Recurrent cystitis	57
Dribbling	37
Dysuria	49
Pain	25
Hematuria	15
Dyspareunia	17
Incontinence	29
Vaginal discharge	12
Urinary retention	2
Mass	49
Asymptomatic	5

Data from Davis and TeLinde (1958), Hoffman and Adams (1965), Ward, Draper and Tovell (1967), Davis and Robinson (1970), Pathak and House (1970).

B. URETHRAL DIVERTICULA: INCIDENCE

		Percent,%	No.
Wharton and Kearns	1950	0.4	1/2300
Bruning	1959	0.6	3/500
Adams	1965	4.7	6/129
Andersen	1967	3	9/300
Davis and Robinson	1970	1.8	120/648
LAC-USC	1978	5.5	49/900

FIGURE 10-10.

Symptoms and incidence. **A**, Practically any lower urinary tract symptom may be associated with a urethral diverticulum. There is a common saying that any pain within 2 feet of the urethra may be due to the urethra. **B**, The incidence of urethral diverticula is variable. The 5.5% incidence was from a urogynecology clinic. The principal method of diagnosis was with use of a female urethroscope.

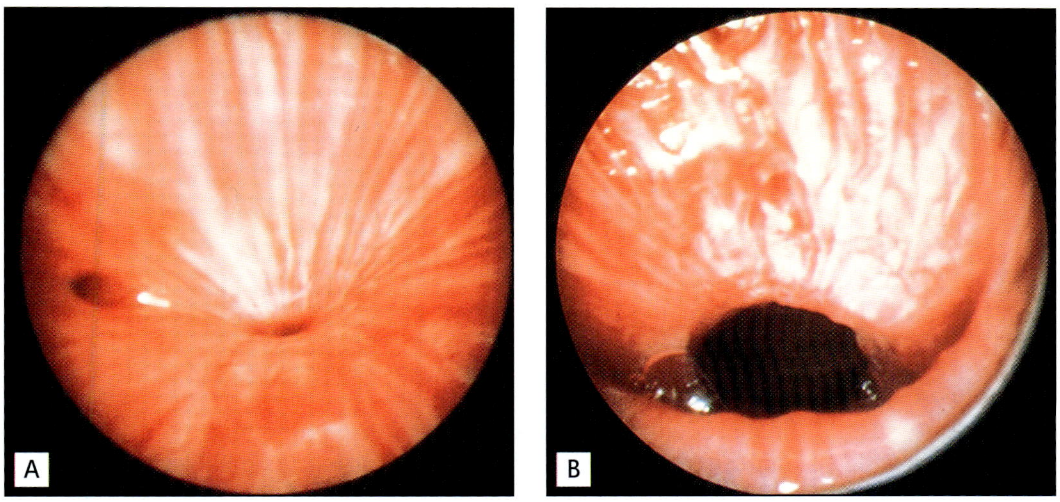

FIGURE 10-11

Location. **A**, This diverticulum is at midurethra. **B**, A vesical contraction shows the diverticulum is clearly located above the sphincter. The location of a urethral diverticulum in relation to the sphincter may be questionable. Stimulation of a vesical contraction during endoscopy clearly showed the diverticulum to be above the sphincter.

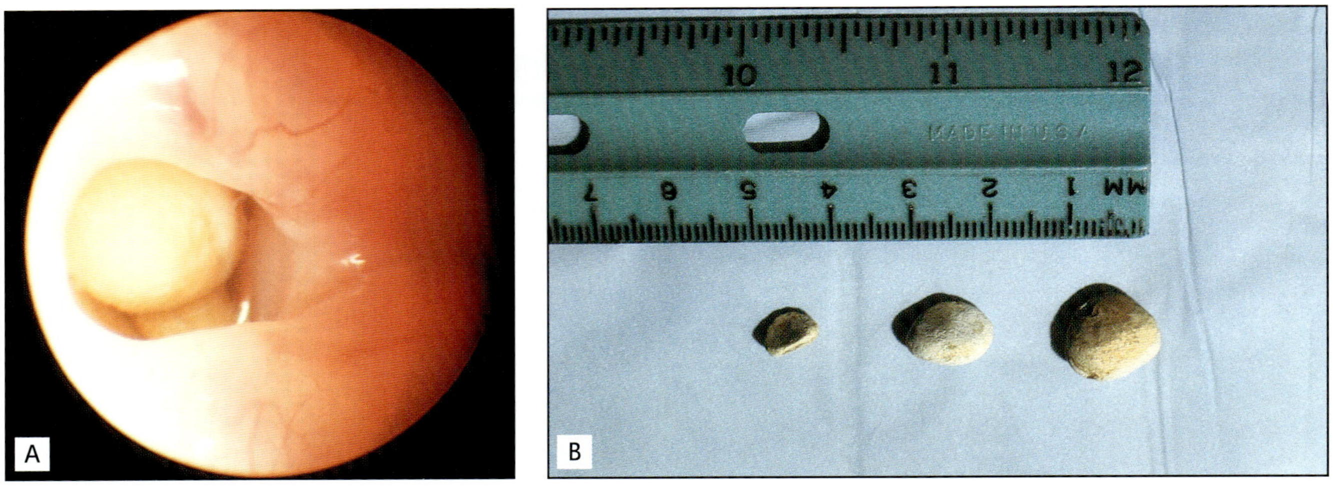

FIGURE 10-12.
Urethral calculus. **A**, Diverticular calculi form only after many years of recurrent infection. **B**, Urethral palpation of the patient felt like a chicken's craw. Urethroscopy revealed large calculi. This patient was the mother of 20 children. She had innumerable recurrent urinary tract infections before this diagnosis was made.

Treatment

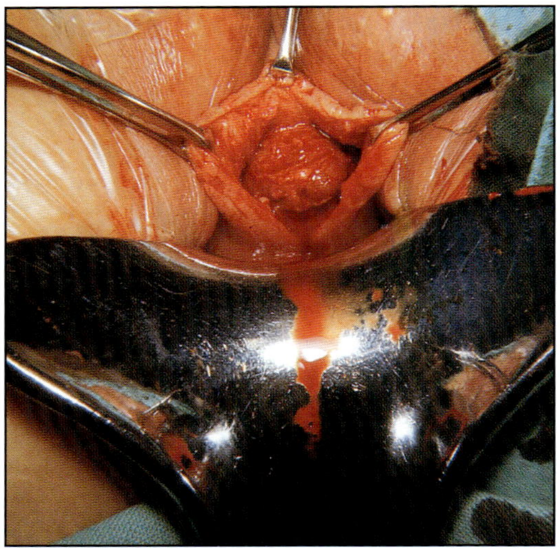

FIGURE 10-13.
Surgical enucleation. This is plastic surgery; not cut, clamp, and ligate. Closure of diverticulectomy must be done in three layers. Postoperative catheter drainage is necessary. The author prefers a suprapubic catheter to keep the catheter off the suture site. Surgical enucleation should be done only by experienced surgeons.

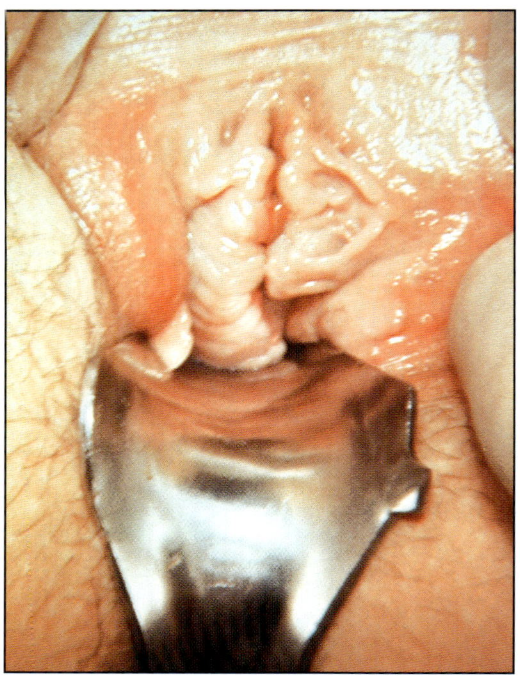

FIGURE 10-14.
Spence procedure. If the diverticulum is located distal to the sphincter, a Spence procedure may be accomplished, a simple procedure similar to marsupialization of a Bartholin's gland. Postoperatively, it looks gruesome, but in 6 months it epithealizes and resembles a generous meatotomy [10].

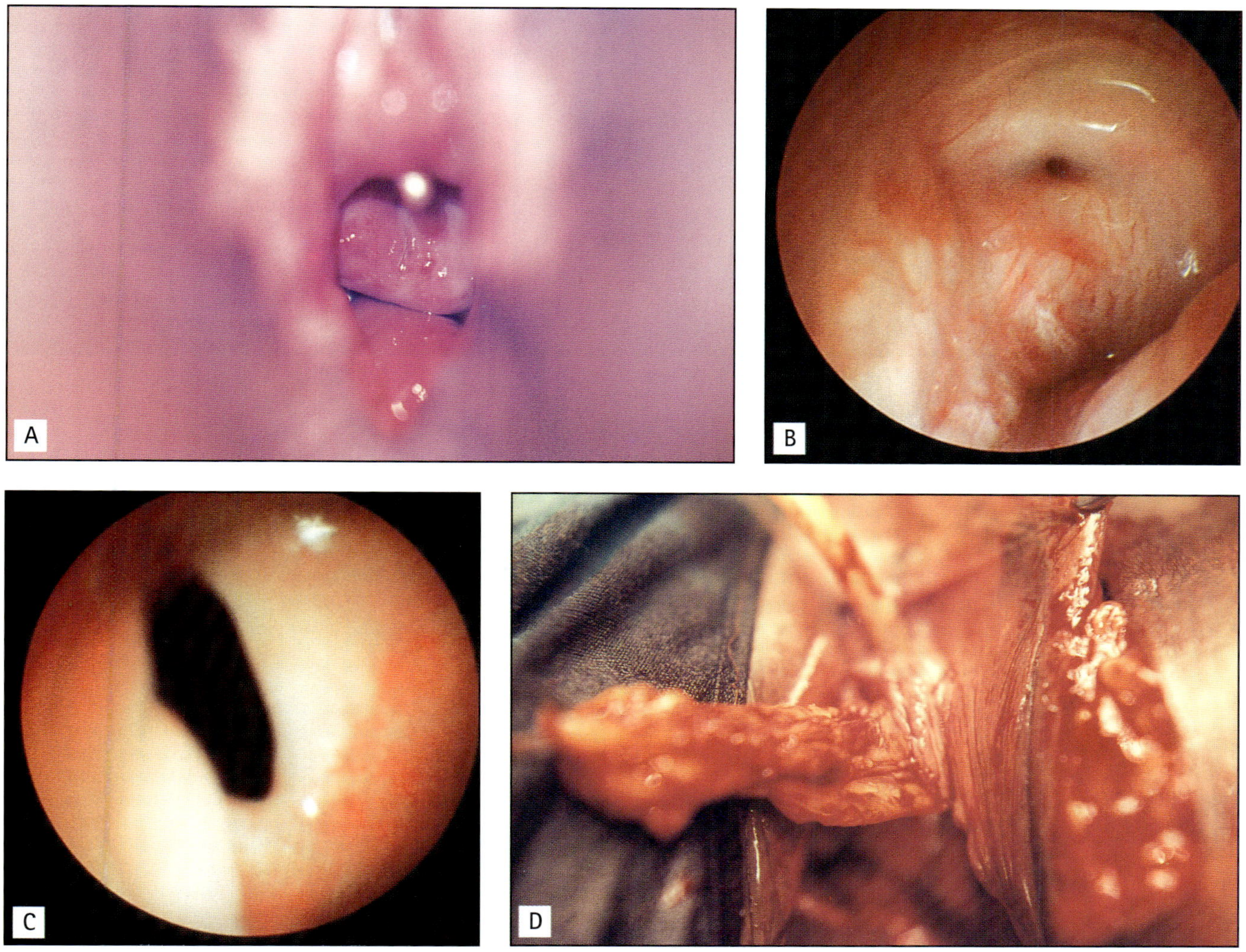

FIGURE 10–15. Fistula formation. **A**, The sound extends from the urethra into the vagina, demonstrating a urethrovaginal fistula. **B**, Nearly 20% of urethrodiverticulectomies are complicated by urethrovaginal fistulas. **C**, This large urethrovaginal fistula involves the vesical neck. **D**, These fistulas may require a bulbocavernosis flap for support and blood supply.

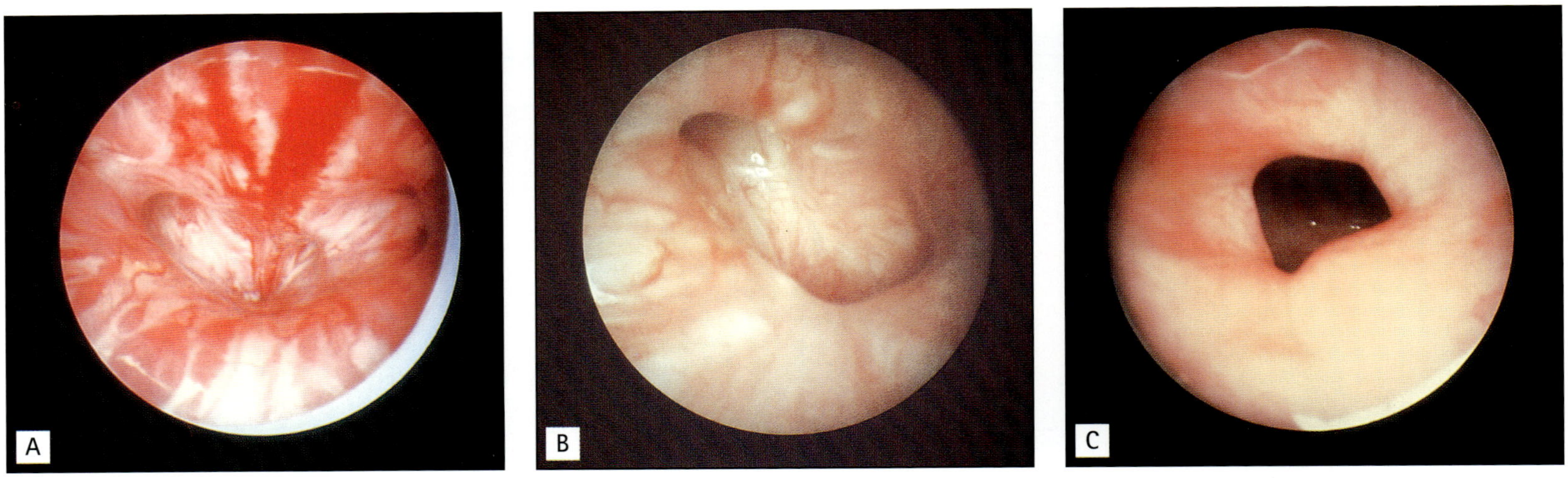

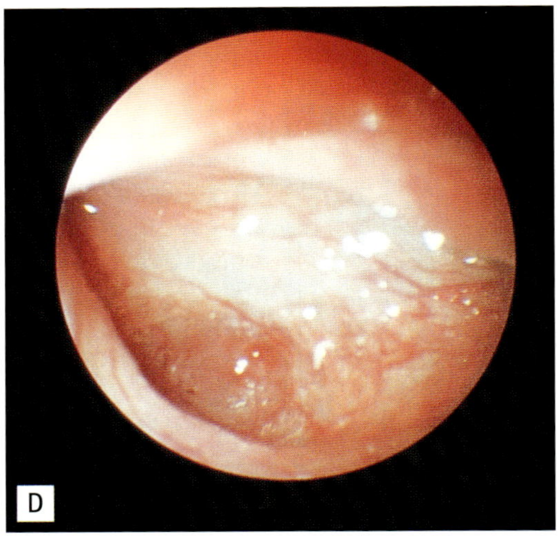

FIGURE 10-16.

Incomplete resection of diverticula. **A**, Further surgery is required with the risk of fistula formation. **B**, Incomplete dissection of a diverticulum is a common problem that may require further surgery and carries the risk of fistula formation. **C**, In this patient the first operation was a diverticulectomy combined with a needle procedure for incontinence. The second procedure was necessary to resect the incomplete dissection in the first operation. **D**, In this patient the diverticulum was resected but the urethra was compromised. Her sphincter was intact. Treatment must be carefully explained to patient because the complication rate is high. Kegel's exercises are recommended over further surgery.

CONCLUSIONS

- The urethral diverticulum is a surgical disease and requires surgery for correction
- The *best procedure* depends on three factors primarily
  - Location of the urethral diverticula stomata on the urethra
  - Presence or absence of other urinary tract or pelvic pathology
  - Amount or type of previous vaginal or pelvic surgery

FIGURE 10-17.

Conclusions. Urethral diverticula require surgery, based on the three factors listed.

FISTULAS

DIAGNOSIS

A. FISTULAS OF THE LOWER URINARY TRACT

- Urethrovaginal
- Urethrovesicovaginal
- Vesicovaginal
- Vesicocervical
- Vesicocervicovaginal

B. CAUSES OF FISTULAS

Obstetric	Surgical
Labor	Hysterectomy
Forceps	Colporrhaphy
Cesarean section	Urethral Surgery
	Radiation
	Miscellaneous

FIGURE 10-18.
Fistulas of the lower urinary tract. Types (**A**) and causes (**B**) of urinary fistulas in industrialized countries are listed. Vesicovaginal fistulas are common in third world countries, where practically all are related to unattended labor and childbirth.

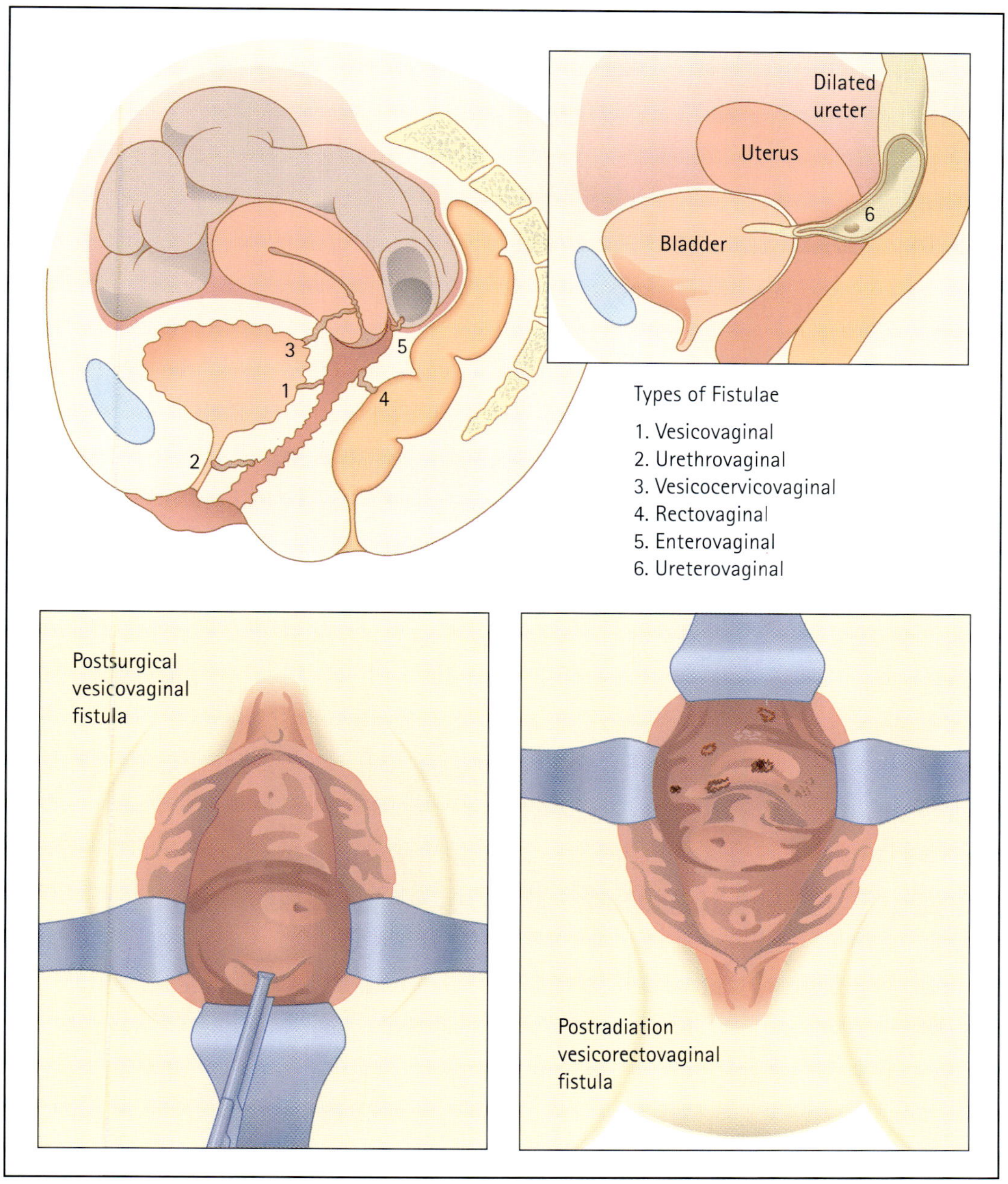

FIGURE 10-19.
Diagram of fistulas. In the industrialized world most fistulas are vesicovaginal, secondary to hysterectomy. On the vaginal side, the fistula is just above the scar, and on the vesical side, it is just above the interureteric ridge. For 35 years the author did office video endoscopy. You can show diagrams, such as this one, but it is preferable to show the patient a picture of her own problem. Also, still shots can be taken for reference in her chart with a copy to the referring physician.

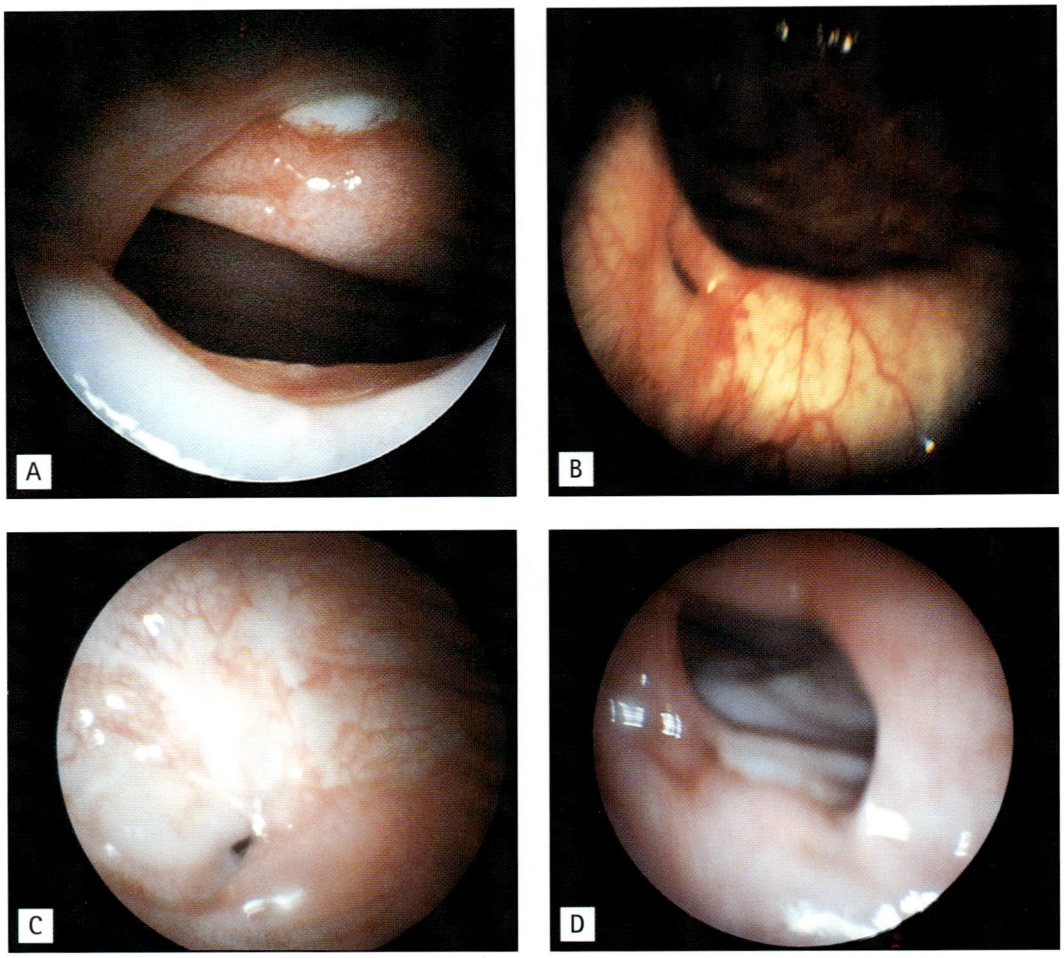

FIGURE 10-20.

Vesicovaginal fistulas. **A**, This fistula is seen from the vaginal side. **B**, This vesicovaginal fistula is seen from the vesical side. **CB**, This is an intravesical view of small vesicovaginal fistula that was secondary to a hysterectomy.

The patients in **B** and **C** reside in third world nations. The patients are devastated; families shun them; all but a very few hospitals cannot treat them. In Africa, many young women commit suicide as a result of this diagnosis. **D**, This is an intravesical view of a large vesicovaginal fistula. In Africa, India, and China unattended births are common. If the infant cannot deliver, the uterus ruptures and the woman is left with a huge hole in her bladder.

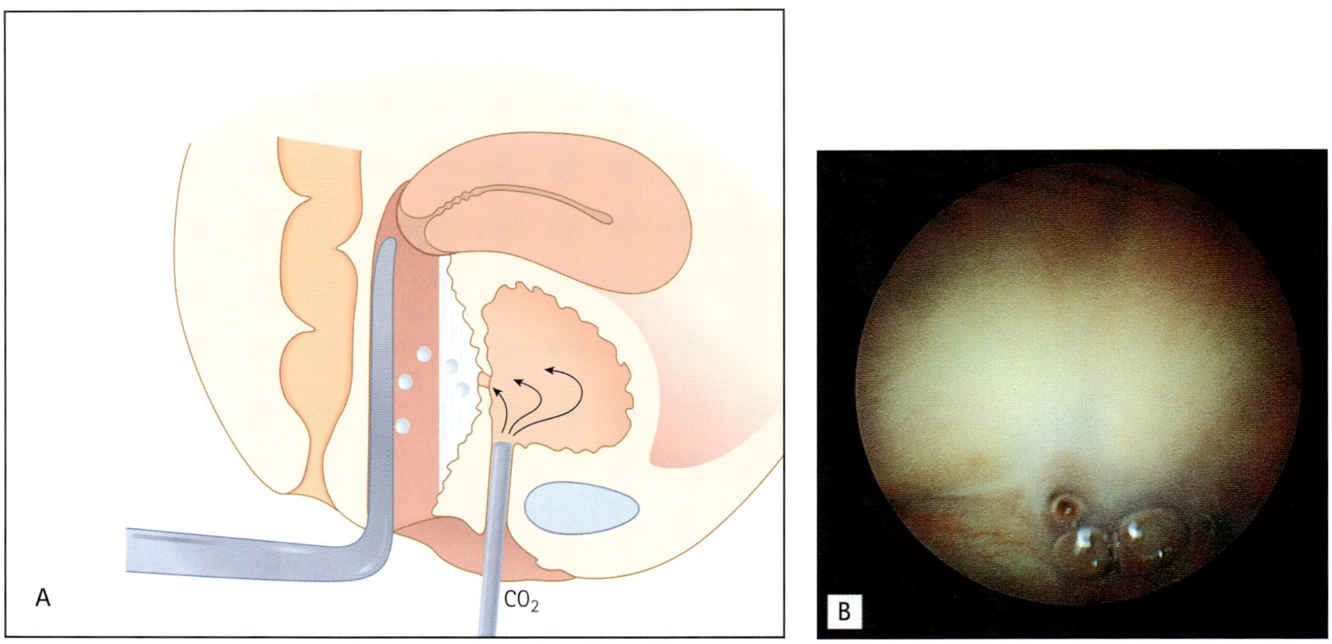

FIGURE 10-21.

Flat tire technique. **A**, Small fistulas may be difficult to find. The flat tire technique is recommended for diagnosis. The patient is placed in the knee-chest position and the vagina is filled with water. Carbon dioxide gas is insufflated into the bladder [9]. **B**, The fistula is noted to open, and gas bubbles through the water.

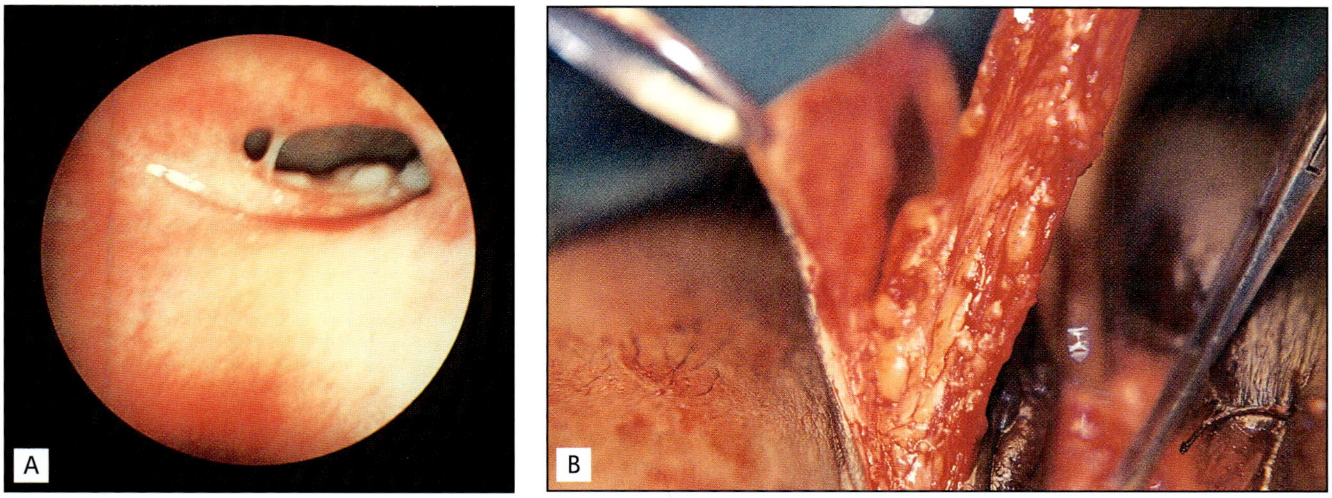

FIGURE 10-22.
Repair of a vesicovaginal fistula. **A**, Note the scarring in this failed repair of a vesicovaginal fistula. **B**, The fistula in **A** and in Figure 10-20**D** may require a bulbocavernosis flap for support and blood supply. This procedure is available in very few third world countries.

POSTOPERATIVE MANAGEMENT

Urinary Drainage
Antibiotics
Position, ambulation
Acidify urine
Irrigations
Examinations

FIGURE 10-23.
Postoperative management. The author still prefers suprapubic catheter drainage despite the fact this requires placing another hole in the bladder [9]. The patient is more comfortable, and a 14 F catheter is adequate.

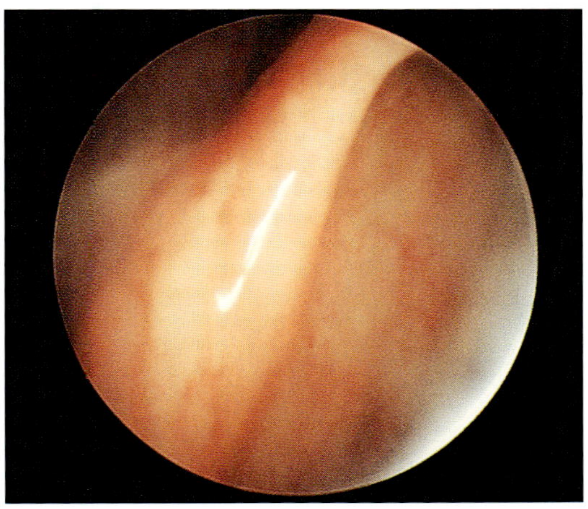

FIGURE 10-24.
Cortisone treatment. Preoperative cortisone may allow closure in 3 weeks instead of waiting months. An endoscopic view of the fistula after cortisone treatment shows the clean edge of the fistula [11]. If the edges are not clean, then it is necessary to wait until they are. This is preferable to having a set time for repair, such as 3 months.

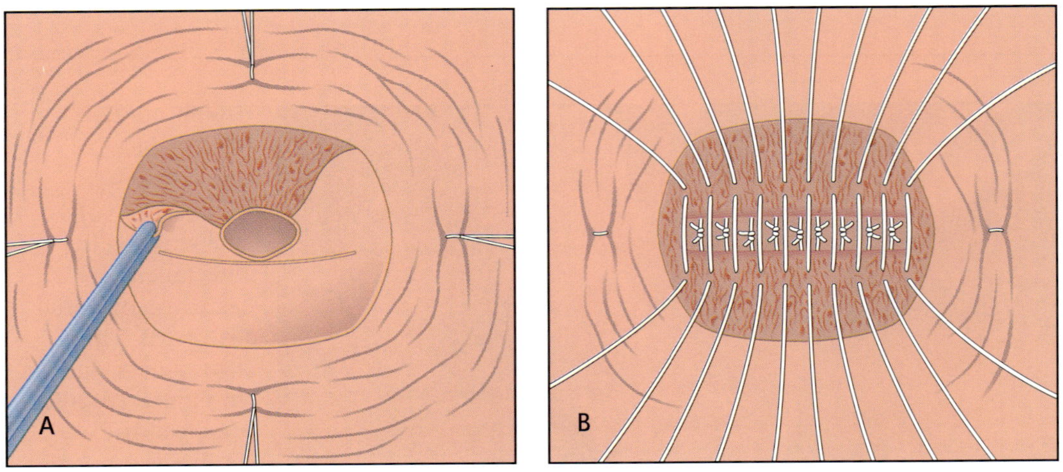

FIGURE 10-25.
Latzko procedure. Most vesicovaginal fistulas can be repaired vaginally, using the Latzko procedure. Pelvic examination should be delayed because it will become obvious if the fistula has not been closed. **A**, Start of the incision. **B**, The closure is in three layers.

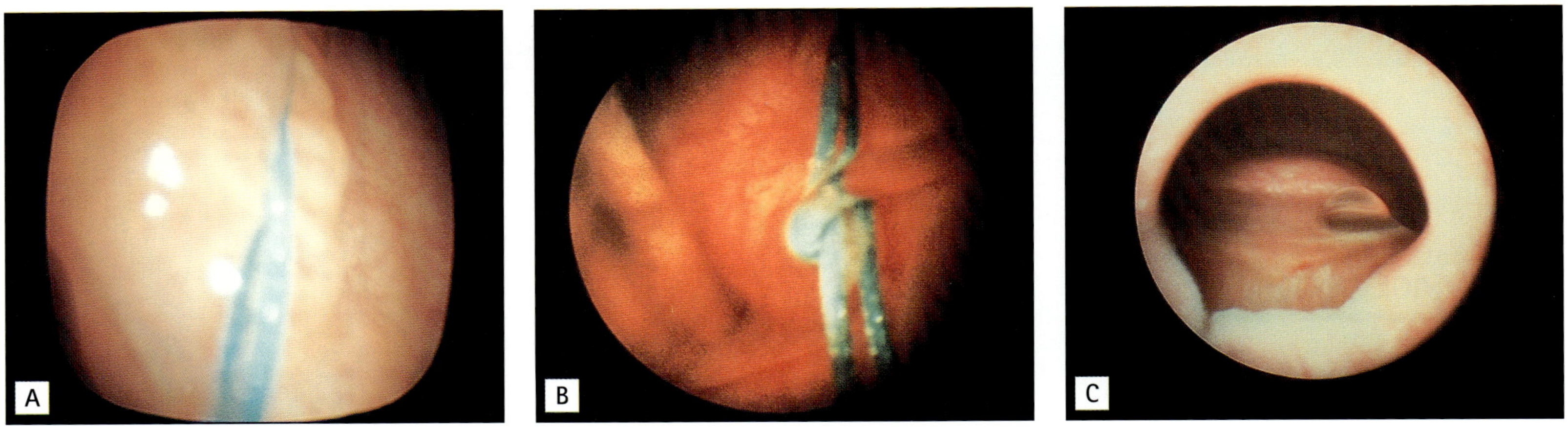

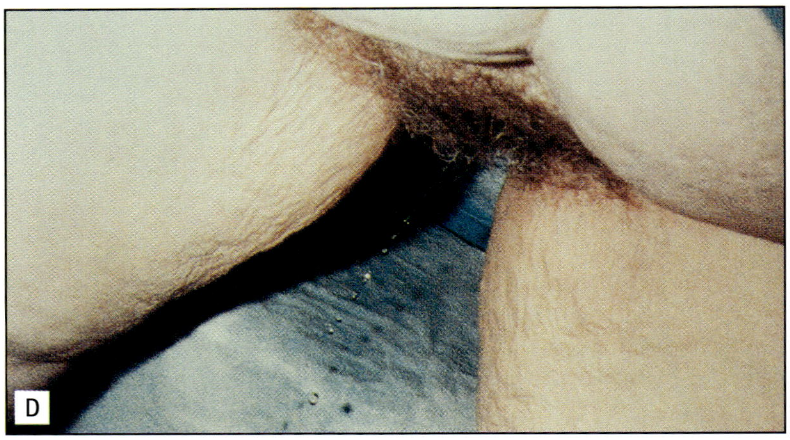

FIGURE 10-26.
Suture through the bladder wall. **A**, Cystoscopy at the end of surgery is important to ensure that postoperative problems will not develop.**B**, This postoperative problem would not have occurred if cystoscopy had been accomplished before the patient left the operating room. **C**, An important reason for cystoscopy at the end of surgery is to know that the ureters are intact and functioning. If ureteral damage is discovered in the operating room, these patients do well. This is true even if the ureter has to be transplanted. **D**, A common problem is that the diverticulum has been closed, but the patient is incontinent because she had undiagnosed stress incontinence. The author starts these patients on Kegel's exercises preoperatively and continues postoperatively.

REFERENCES

1. Lichtman A, Robertson J: Suburethral diverticula treated by marsupialization. *Obstet Gynecol* 1976, 47:203.
2. Sims J: On the treatment of vesico-vaginal fistula. *Am J Med Sci* 1852, 23:50.
3. Simpson JY: *Clinical Lectures on Diseases of Women.* Philadelphia: 1872:21.
4. Latzko W: Postoperative vesicovaginal fistulas: genesis and therapy. *Am J Surg* 1942, 58:211.
5. Novak E. Editorial comment. *Obstet Gynecol Surv* 1953, 8:423.
6. Davis J, Cain L: Positive pressure urethrography: a new diagnostic method. *J Urol* 1856, 75:753.
7. Huffman, J. The detailed anatomy of the paraurethral ducts in the adult human female. *Am J Obstet Gynecol* 1948, 55:86.
8. Johnson C: Diverticula and cyst of female urethra. *J Urol* 1938, 39:506.
9. Robertson J: *Genitourinary Problems in Women.* Springfield, IL: Charles C. Thomas; 1978:69.
10. Spence H, Duckett J: Diverticulum of the female urethra: clinical aspects and presentation of a single operative technique for cure. *J Urol* 1970, 104:432.
11. Collins C, Pent D, Jones F: Results of early repair of vesicovaginal fistula with preliminary cortisone treatment. *Am J Obstet Gynecol* 1960, 80:1005.

CHAPTER 11

Rectovaginal Fistula

Marc I. Brand and Theodore J. Saclarides

Diseases of the anogenital region may be accompanied by significant psychosocial and sexual dysfunction; this is especially so with rectovaginal fistulas where "contamination" of the vulva by intestinal waste can be devastating for women and their sexual partners. In addition to the physical symptoms of vaginitis, dyspareunia, and vulvar skin excoriation, patients often have significant reduction of self-esteem. The patient is often worried that despite whatever efforts to keep the area clean, the smell of gas and stool will not be controlled and her companions will know she has a problem. Of more concern is the worry the patient may have regarding the reaction of her sexual partner.

Various conditions may cause rectovaginal fistulas. In addition, there may be wide variation in the location of the fistula as well as which adjacent organs are involved. Consequently, the etiology and management of rectovaginal fistula can be complex. It is crucial that a surgeon treating a patient with rectovaginal fistula understand the distress to the patient, the etiology of the fistula, as well as associated conditions, and be able to offer several options for the management of each particular fistula. This chapter details the etiology, evaluation, and techniques of local repair of rectovaginal fistulas. Diligence and persistence provide a more optimistic future for patients with rectovaginal fistulas than was previously available.

DEFINITIONS AND PATIENT EVALUATION

DEFINITIONS

Fistula: Abnormal communication between two epithelial-lined surfaces

Anovaginal fistula: Fistula arising in the anal canal, usually at or below the dentate line, communicating with the distal vagina

Rectovaginal fistula: Fistula arising in the rectum (above the anorectal ring, below the sacral promontory), communicating with the vagina

FIGURE 11-1.
Definitions. The pertinent definitions are listed.

ETIOLOGY OF RECTOVAGINAL FISTULA

Category	Condition	Mechanism
Truamatic		
Obstetric	Prolonged 2nd stage of labor	Pressure necrosis of rectovaginal septum
	Midline episiotomy	Extension directed into rectum
	Perineal lacerations	
Foreign body	Vaginal pessaries	Pressure necrosis
	Violent coitus	Mechanical Perforation
	Sexual abuse	Mechanical perforation
Iatrogenic	Hysterectomy	Injury to anterior rectal wall
	Stapled colorectal anastomosis	Staple line includes vagina
	Transanal excision of anterior rectal tumor	Deep margin of resection into vagina
	Enemas	Mechanical perforation
	Anorectal surgery such as incision and drainage of intramural abscesses	Mechanical perforation
Inflammatory	Crohn's disease	Transmural inflammation/perforation
	Pelvic radiation	Early-tumor necrosis
	Pelvic abscess	Late-transmural inflammation
	Perirectal abscess	
Neoplastic	Rectal	Local tumor growth into neighboring structure
	Cervical	
	Uterine	
	Vaginal	
	Primary or recurrent tumors	

FIGURE 11-2.
Etiology. The etiology of a rectovaginal fistula (RVF) greatly affects its management and prognosis and may provide clues to associated conditions that need to be addressed (e.g., coexisting sphincter injury or tumor recurrence requiring further treatment) as well as health of the surrounding tissue. Acquired RVFs may be caused by multiple conditions; obstetric injuries are by far the most common cause, accounting for 50% to 90%, depending on the referral patterns of the institution [1]. It is estimated that 0.1% of vaginal births will result in a RVF [2]. An RVF caused by an obstetric injury is frequently associated with an anal sphincter injury and fecal incontinence [3]. This must be considered when planning operative repair. The surrounding tissues are generally healthy in the setting of a traumatic RVF; consequently, a higher success rate for primary repair can be expected. In contrast, inflammatory and neoplastic RVFs are usually associated with diseased neighboring tissue, which can adversely affect the results of repair. Proximal fecal diversion may be necessary either as definitive treatment or as an adjunct to local reconstruction. Congenital RVFs are associated with imperforate anus and are beyond the scope of this chapter.

CLASSIFICATION OF RECTOVAGINAL FISTULA

	Simple	Complex
Size	< 2.5 cm diameter	> 2.5 cm diameter
Level of vaginal opening	Low or mid vaginal septum	High vaginal septum
Etiology	Trauma, infections	Crohn's, radiation, cancer
Repairs	Primary	Recurrent

FIGURE 11-3.

Classification. Several classification schemes have been used to describe rectovaginal fistula based on size, level, etiology, and whether the fistula is primary or recurrent. The utilities of a classification scheme are to aid in defining prognosis for successful outcome, planning the operative approach, and comparing results of different treatments on similar cases. All of the individual factors that have been used for classification are important and complete classification should include all of these factors.

PRESENTATION AND SYMPTOMS OF RECTOVAGINAL FISTULA

- Passage of gas per vagina
- Passage of stool per vagina
- Vaginal discharge with fecal odor
- Vaginitis, persistent
- Vulvar skin excoriation
- Dyspareunia
- Fecal incontinence

FIGURE 11-4.

Presentation and symptoms. The *sine qua non* of a rectovaginal fistula (RVF) is the passage of stool or gas or both through the vagina, which often results in a fecal odor. The stool that passes through the fistula is often loose and causes vaginitis and vulvar skin excoriation. Dyspareunia may be due to a rectovaginal septal abscess or to residual inflammation. Fecal soilage may be a presenting symptom; the patient may not be able to distinguish between vaginal discharge and anal drainage caused by the sphincter defect.

Associated symptoms will vary depending on the underlying cause. If caused by inflammatory bowel disease, an RVF may be accompanied by diarrhea, cramps, and additional anorectal problems such as fistulas and fleshy skin tags. If caused by cancer, vaginal and rectal bleeding as well as pain can be as distressing to the patient as the symptoms caused by the RVF itself.

GOALS IN THE EVALUATION OF RECTOVAGINAL FISTULA

- Determine etiology of RVF
- Define RVF tract (level, size)
- Evaluate surrounding rectal mucosa (indurated, radiated, acutely inflamed)
- Exclude coexisting rectovaginal septal abscess
- Identify associated sphincter injury

FIGURE 11-5.

Evaluation goals. Each of the several goals in the evaluation of a rectovaginal fistula (RVF) provides important information to guide subsequent management (timing, additional treatment, prognosis). The etiology of an RVF gives clues to potential associated conditions that require further evaluation and to the integrity of surrounding tissues; also knowing the cause of a fistula helps to guide the choice of management and affects prognosis. Definition of the fistula tract is critical in planning the operative approach. The status of the surrounding rectal mucosa may affect the timing of RVF repair, indicate additional therapy, or determine the operative approach. Coexisting rectovaginal septal abscess must be identified and treated before RVF repair to avoid an otherwise certain failure. Anal sphincter injury is common in obstetric tears, and concomitant sphincter repair is often necessary.

METHODS OF EVALUATION OF RECTOVAGINAL FISTULA	
History	Suggests etiology of RVF Defines symptoms, severity, distress to patient Role of stool frequency and consistency in symptoms May give clues to undiagnosed Crohn's disease
Physical examination	Inspection of perineum Digital rectal examination (assess sphincter, masses) Bimanual examination of rectovaginal septum Anoscopy/proctoscopy (identify fistula, quality of tissues) Vaginal speculum examination Tampon test
Examination under anesthesia	Better exposure than office examination Mark fistula tract with Seton suture Drain rectovaginal septal abscess
Contrast radiography	Barium enema Vaginogram Small bowel series (Crohn's or radiation enteritis)
Ultrasonography	May identify fistula tract Useful in assessing sphincter defects

FIGURE 11-6.
Evaluation methods. Several components of the evaluation of a rectovaginal fistula (RVF) are useful in reaching the goals. History and physical examination in the office are useful and can often identify the etiology of the RVF and define the tract. Inspection of the perineum may reveal a cloaca (common anorectal and vaginal canals), attenuated perineal body, anteriorly displaced anus, and asymmetric anal wink on active squeezing. Digital rectal and bimanual septal examinations are useful to assess sphincter tone, anal stricture, masses, or the presence of a dimple at the site of a fistula. Anoscopy or vaginal speculum examination is often useful in identifying the anal or vaginal orifice. Proctoscopy is particularly important if Crohn's disease or a rectal mass is suspected. A drop of methylene blue on the gloved examiner's index finger during the ano-rectal examination may sometimes be seen vaginally. Placement of a tampon in the vagina before administering a dilute methylene blue enema (held for several minutes) can often document the fistula and may act as a guide to its level. Examination under anesthesia is an extremely useful means to study the fistula tract. This may be the only way to properly examine a patient with significant tenderness, or it may be necessary when an office examination fails to disclose the tract. It has the advantages of better lighting and exposure and greater patient comfort. Lighted retractors (Hill-Ferguson, Pratt bivalve) can provide excellent exposure and lighting. If a septal abscess is identified, it can be drained at this time. If the orifice on only one side is found, it can be injected with hydrogen peroxide using a blunt needle or angiocatheter while the other orifice is sought. If neither orifice can be seen on inspection, a vaginal speculum examination under water with rectal air insufflation via a proctoscope may reveal air bubbles at the vaginal orifice. Once the fistula tract is identified, a Seton suture should be placed through it to mark it for identification at the time of definitive repair. Contrast radiography may be effective in defining the fistula tract when the above techniques have failed. The contrast may be administered transanally (barium enema) or transvaginally (vaginogram). These studies are particularly useful for the complex, high fistula, which is more difficult to find by examination and originates proximal to the mid or lower rectum. Endoluminal ultrasonography is an excellent tool for detecting occult anal sphincter defects associated with traumatic RVFs, and it may be able to identify the fistula tract as well.

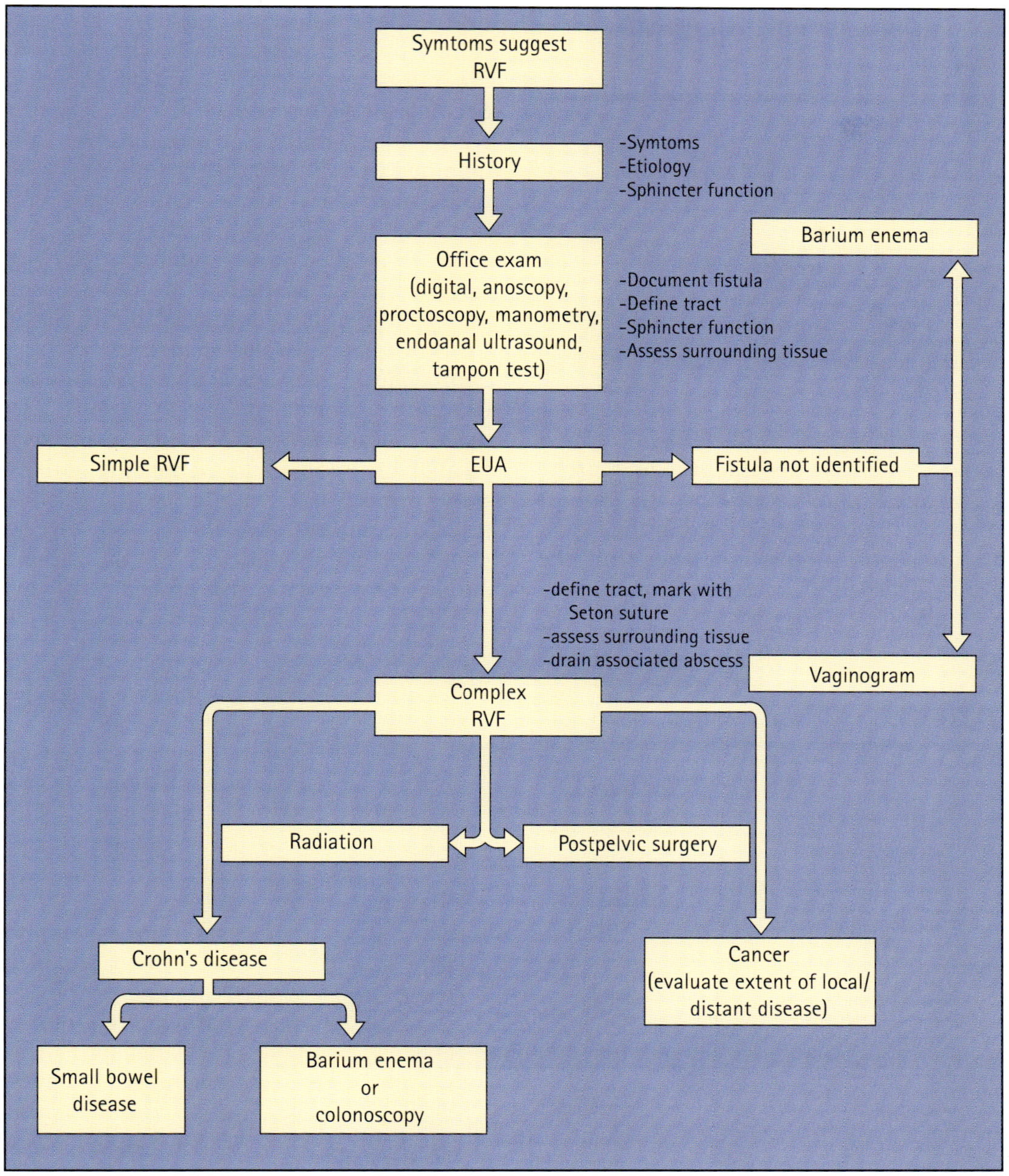

FIGURE 11-7.

Algorithm for evaluation of rectovaginal fistula (RVF). The initial evaluation of patients presenting with symptoms suggestive of an RVF is history and physical examination. The history is directed at defining the symptoms the patient is experiencing, as well as clues in the history that may disclose the etiology of the fistula. Therefore, questions regarding bowel function, obstetric history, and previous surgical or radiation treatments to the pelvis must be asked. Additionally, subjective evaluation of continence to gas and liquid or solid stool should be sought from the patient. Office examination is then carried out in an attempt to document the fistula as well as define its tract. The integrity of the anal sphincter may be assessed by digital examination, manometry, or endoanal ultrasound. The surrounding tissues are assessed by digital examination, anoscopy, and proctoscopy. Despite these measures, it is often difficult to perform an adequate examination in the office. In this situation, an examination under anesthesia (EUA) is useful. All of the maneuvers used in the office (with the exception of assessment of sphincter tone by digital examination and manometry) can and should be repeated to define the fistula tract. At the conclusion of the EUA, one of three outcomes is expected. If a simple RVF is identified (as previously described), the evaluation is complete and planning for repair of the fistula can begin. If a complex RVF is identified, further evaluation may be necessary based on the etiology. If Crohn's disease is the underlying cause, then evaluation of the small bowel and colon should be performed using a combination of a small bowel series and either barium enema or colonoscopy. If cancer is the cause of the fistula, the patient should be evaluated for the extent of local and distant disease to determine the feasibility and desirability of radical resection. Finally, after completion of an EUA, it is possible that the fistula tract is still not identified. In this case, a vaginogram followed by a barium enema is often useful in being able to disclose the fistula tract. The vaginogram is performed first because retained contrast following the study will not delay the ability to perform the barium enema. The converse is not true if a barium enema is performed initially.

SURGICAL PRINCIPLES

Timing	Surrounding inflammation quiescent Associated infection drained and resolved Tissue soft and mobile
Tissue interposition	Healthy tissue, well vascularized
Tailoring treatment to fistula	Local or transabdominal repair Need for diversion

FIGURE 11-8.

Surgical principles. Although rectovaginal fistulas (RVFs) represent a heterogenous group of conditions, several principles are applicable to the surgical treatment of all cases. First, the timing of the operation should be such that the tissue used in the repair is in its best possible condition. Thus, surgery is delayed until the inflammation of recent trauma, infection, or active Crohn's disease has subsided. A delay of 3 to 6 months is usually sufficient; however, repair may be considered sooner than this once the induration has settled and the tissues are soft and mobile. Second, the fistula tract should be excised and the space filled with healthy, well-vascularized tissue. This tissue may be obtained from a local source (external sphincter, levator ani, bulbocavernosus muscle). Third, the operative approach needs to be tailored to the circumstances of each RVF, that is, the choice between local or transabdominal repair is generally based on the level of the fistula (high RVF often needs transabdominal approach) and the etiology of the fistula (obstetric, infectious, and Crohn's-related fistulas are generally amenable to local approaches). Lastly, fecal diversion may be indicated for control of severe symptoms related to the fistula. The stoma is then left in place until the definitive fistula repair has healed. The need for fecal diversion to aid in the healing of the repair is controversial. Some authors use it routinely, whereas others reserve it for selected complex cases. Rarely, fecal diversion may be the only choice for symptomatic relief in the patient unfit for major surgery or with extensive cancer or radiation injury.

MANAGEMENT OPTIONS

Symptomatic Relief

- Bowel regimen
- Obturator [4]
- Fecal diversion

Curative

- Local
  - Transanal (CARF, LARF, ARS)
  - Transperineal
  - Transvaginal
- Transabdominal
  - Proctectomy with:
    - Colorectal anastomsis
    - Coloanal anastomosis
    - Turnbull-Cutout pull-through [5]
    - Abdominoperineal resection [5]

FIGURE 11-9.

Management options. Treatment regimens can be divided into those that are aimed at controlling the symptoms produced by the rectovaginal fistula (RVF) and those that are aimed at eliminating the RVF. The majority of symptoms related to an RVF are due to transvaginal passage of stool. In some cases, this is more problematic when the stool is liquid, particularly for small RVFs. As such, the addition of fiber supplements, antidiarrheal agents, and other methods to control diarrhea is often helpful. In other cases, stimulation of bowel action by enema at a defined time may be able to prevent transvaginal passage of stool at a socially embarrassing time. Patients with severe fecal incontinence or large RVF may need a special catheter to retain the enema. A recently described device for occluding the fistula tract [4] may gain a role in controlling the symptoms of RVF before definitive repair or in place of it when definitive repair is not feasible.

A wide array of options exists for definitive repair of RVF. The remainder of this chapter focuses on local techniques of RVF repair. Transanal approaches are preferred by most colorectal surgeons, whereas gynecologists generally prefer the transvaginal approach. This difference is largely based on specialist familiarity with a particular approach because success has been reported with both. The transanal approach has the theoretical advantages of direct access to and repair of the rectal opening of the fistula, which is considered by many to be the high-pressure side of the RVF. The transvaginal approach has the theoretical advantage of better exposure. Once the fistula tract has been excised, both approaches must use healthy, pliable tissue in the creation of a flap. A transperineal approach is also feasible. This is particularly useful when an anterior injury to the anal sphincter is associated with the RVF.

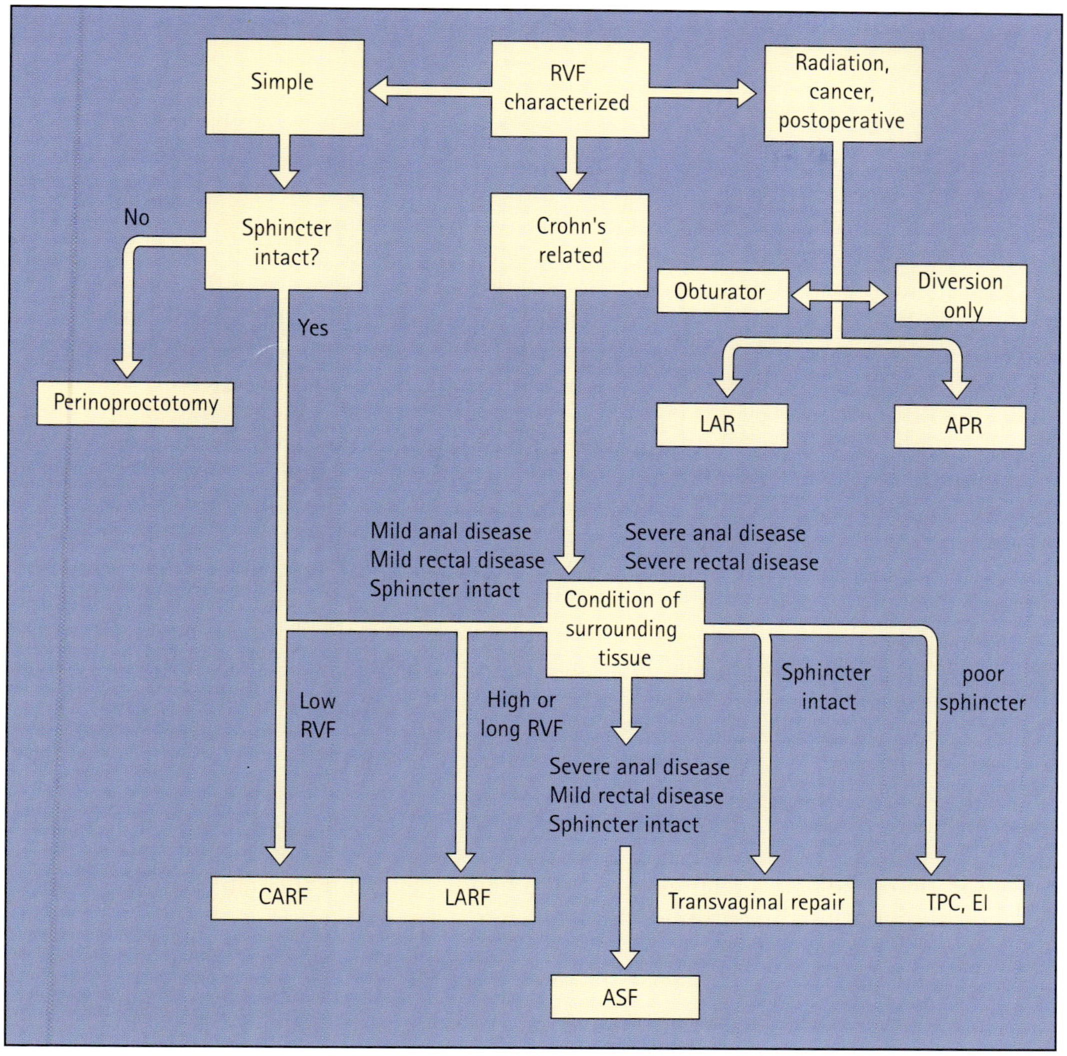

FIGURE 11-10.

Algorithm for the management of rectovaginal fistula (RVF). Once the RVF is characterized, a treatment strategy can be planned with the patient and expected outcomes discussed. If the fistula is identified as a simple RVF, the decision as to which repair should be used depends on the status of the anal sphincter. If the anal sphincter has been injured, then a perineoproctotomy is used. This procedure involves converting the RVF into a fourth degree perineal laceration. The fistula is excised, then the rectal mucosa, anal sphincter, and vaginal mucosa are repaired in layers thereby restoring normal anatomy and bulk to the perineal body. If the sphincter is found to be intact on preoperative evaluation, then local repair of the fistula alone can be performed. Our preference is the use of a curvilinear advancement rectal flap (CARF).

If the RVF is related to anorectal Crohn's disease, the choice of repair depends on the condition of the surrounding tissue and the integrity of the anal sphincter. For patients who have an intact anal sphincter, and have mild involvement of both the anus and rectum with Crohn's disease, local transanal repair can be performed. If the fistula is low in the anal canal and is easily accessible, a CARF can be performed. However, some fistulas related to Crohn's disease are either higher in the rectum or have a long vertical orientation. In these cases, a linear advancement rectal flap (LARF) is useful. For patients who have an intact anal sphincter, with severe anal Crohn's disease, but a relatively spared rectum, the advancement sleeve flap (ASF) can be used. For patients who have severe involvement of both the anus and rectum with Crohn's disease but still have an intact anal sphincter, a transvaginal repair may be used. This allows the surgeon to work with relatively healthy vaginal tissue and limits the manipulation of the diseased tissue in the anus and rectum. The transvaginal repair can also be used in any of the previously described conditions where a local flap is recommended. In addition, proximal fecal diversion should be considered in any patient with Crohn's disease undergoing local flap repair. Its use should be strongly considered in any patient in whom the repair is less than technically perfect, patients having failed previous attempts at local repair, and patients requiring a concurrent laparotomy for intestinal Crohn's disease. Finally, for the patient who has severe involvement of the anus and rectum by Crohn's disease and has poor sphincter function, the best option is a total proctocolectomy (TPC) and end-ileostomy (EI). The prospect for successful local repair in this situation is very low, and fecal incontinence will remain a significant problem after the procedure.

Patients who have a complex RVF (due to radiation injury, primary or recurrent cancer, or after prior pelvic surgery) will most likely require an abdominal approach for management of the RVF. Definitive cure requires proctectomy; control of symptoms may be achieved with less radical procedures such as fecal diversion alone or perhaps the placement of a newly described device for occluding the fistula tract [4]. With the exception of recommending resection for iatrogenic RVF due to previous pelvic surgery, decisions regarding optimal management of the RVF due to radiation or cancer are extremely complicated and must be highly individualized. APR—abdominoperineal resection; LAR— linear advancement rectal.

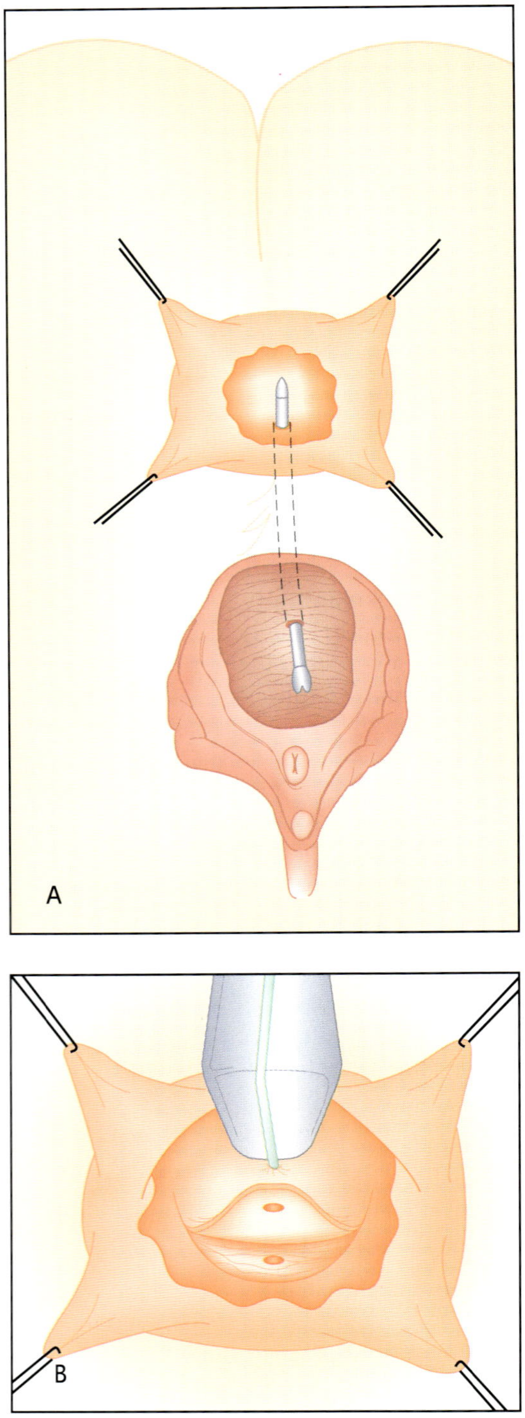

FIGURE 11-11.

Curvilinear advancement rectal flap (CARF). **A**, For this transanal procedure, the patient is placed in the prone jackknife position. Proctoscopy is performed to irrigate the lower rectum and remove any residue from the preoperative bowel preparation. The perineum and vagina are prepared with a povidone-iodine solution. Exposure of the low rectal mucosa can be enhanced by the placement of four effacement sutures at the anal verge and tied to the perianal skin about 2 to 3 inches from the verge. A Betadine-soaked gauze with a long heavy silk suture tied to it is placed in the rectum several centimeters above the fistula. This prevents contamination because rectal contents may be propelled distally should the patient strain during the procedure. **B**, The flap is elevated. Examination of the rectal side of the fistula is made using a lighted retractor. A curvilinear incision beginning at the dentate line and comprising one-third to one-half circumference of the anal canal is planned. A light touch of the cautery can be used to mark this planned flap. The mucosa of this area is then infiltrated with a dilute epinephrine solution (1:100,000). This provides hemostasis and aids in definition of the plane of dissection. The cutting current of the electrocautery is then used to create a curvilinear incision at the previously marked site. The most caudal aspect of the flap consists of mucosa and submucosa. The flap is thickened as it is extended cephalad to the fistula site. At this level, the superficial portion of the circular muscle fibers are included with the flap. As the flap is being raised, additional injection of saline into the plane of dissection will further delineate the plane of dissection and keep the flap thick, thereby ensuring adequate blood supply to the flap. This dissection is carried proximally until the entire flap can easily be advanced to cover the fistula tract without tension. The caudal-most portion of the flap is retained to act as a handle, allowing the flap to be grasped without traumatizing the portion to be used later.

(*Continued on next page*)

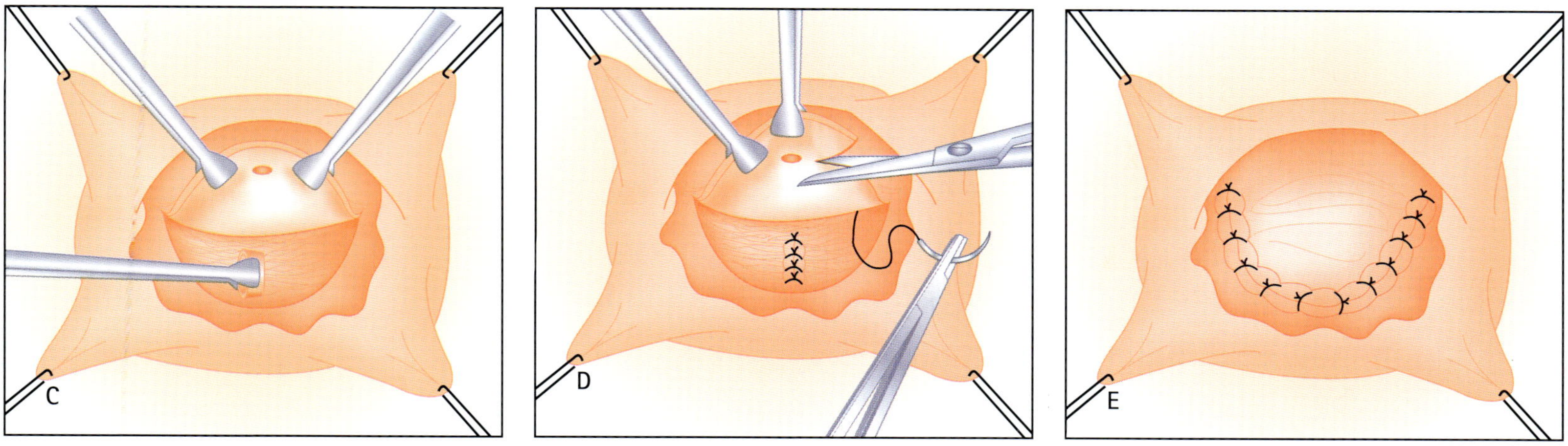

FIGURE 11-11. *(Continued)*

C, The lining of the fistula tract through the rectovaginal septum must be removed next. Although this may be performed with curettage, this is often inadequate, leaving tissue with poor blood supply and limited healing capacity in the tract. Although it is more difficult to excise the entire fistula tract, this is generally preferable. A small ellipse of tissue surrounding the fistula tract can be marked out with the cautery and then grasped with an Allis clamp. As the dissection around the fistula tract is carried deeper into the septum, regrasping of the tissue with the Allis clamp helps to elevate the plane of dissection up into the wound. This dissection is carried completely through to the posterior vaginal mucosa to excise the vaginal orifice. The defect is then closed in one or several layers. The layers of the sphincter being repaired are approximated using simple interrupted 2-0 long-lasting absorbable suture. A UR-6 needle is very helpful in closing this defect. The vaginal mucosa is left open for drainage. **D**, In preparing the flap for closure, hemostasis is obtained before suturing the flap in place. Use of the cautery should be precise, to avoid excessive eschar within the wound. The fistula component of the flap is excised at this point with scissors. The use of scissors allows one to visualize bleeding from the cut edge, ensuring viability of the flap at this level. If any tension is appreciated as the flap is being closed, one can elevate the flap more cephalad; alternatively, a flap of mucosa distal to the dentate line may be elevated in a cephalad direction. If the flap is thick enough, buried sutures between the under surface of the flap and the underlying muscle can be placed between the upper aspect of the flap and its most distal end to take tension off the suture line. **E**, The flap is sutured using a series of interrupted 3-0 long-lasting absorbable suture. Hemostasis must be excellent before closure of the flap because a hematoma beneath the flap will doom it to failure. Tension on the flap should be kept to a minimum as well because this will also cause failure of the flap. It should be remembered that once the anal effacement sutures are released, the distal mucosa will return to the anal canal and reduce some of the tension on the flap.

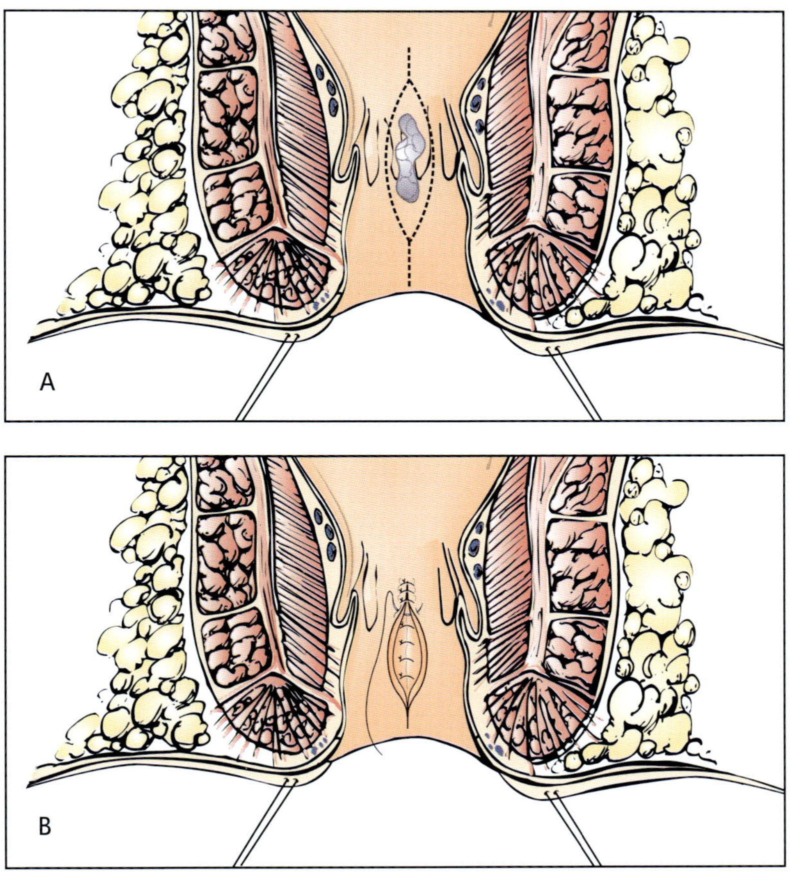

FIGURE 11-12.

Linear advancement rectal flap (LARF). For fistulas that are high and long, curvilinear advancement rectal flap (CARF) may be difficult to perform due to excessive tension in the flap at closure or due to the height of dissection necessary to minimize this tension. In these cases, LARF is a simple alternative. The patient is prepared and positioned as described as for the CARF procedure. A dilute epinephrine solution is injected in the submucosa in an elliptical fashion surrounding the fistula tract. An elliptical incision surrounding the fistula tract is then made, perpendicular to the dentate line. This may be extended proximally or distally to add sufficient length and mobility to the flap. Lateral flaps are then made in each direction, elevating the mucosa and submucosa off the underlying muscle (internal sphincter or circular muscle layer of the low rectum). The fistula tract is then excised down to the level of the vaginal mucosa. Hemostasis is secured using the pinpoint electrocautery tip. **B**, The muscular defect following fistulectomy is closed in layers, oriented perpendicular to the dentate line. A 2-0 long-lasting absorbable suture on a UR-6 needle is used and the vaginal mucosa is left open for drainage. The mucosa and submucosa are then closed over the muscular repair, using interrupted 3-0 long-lasting absorbable suture.

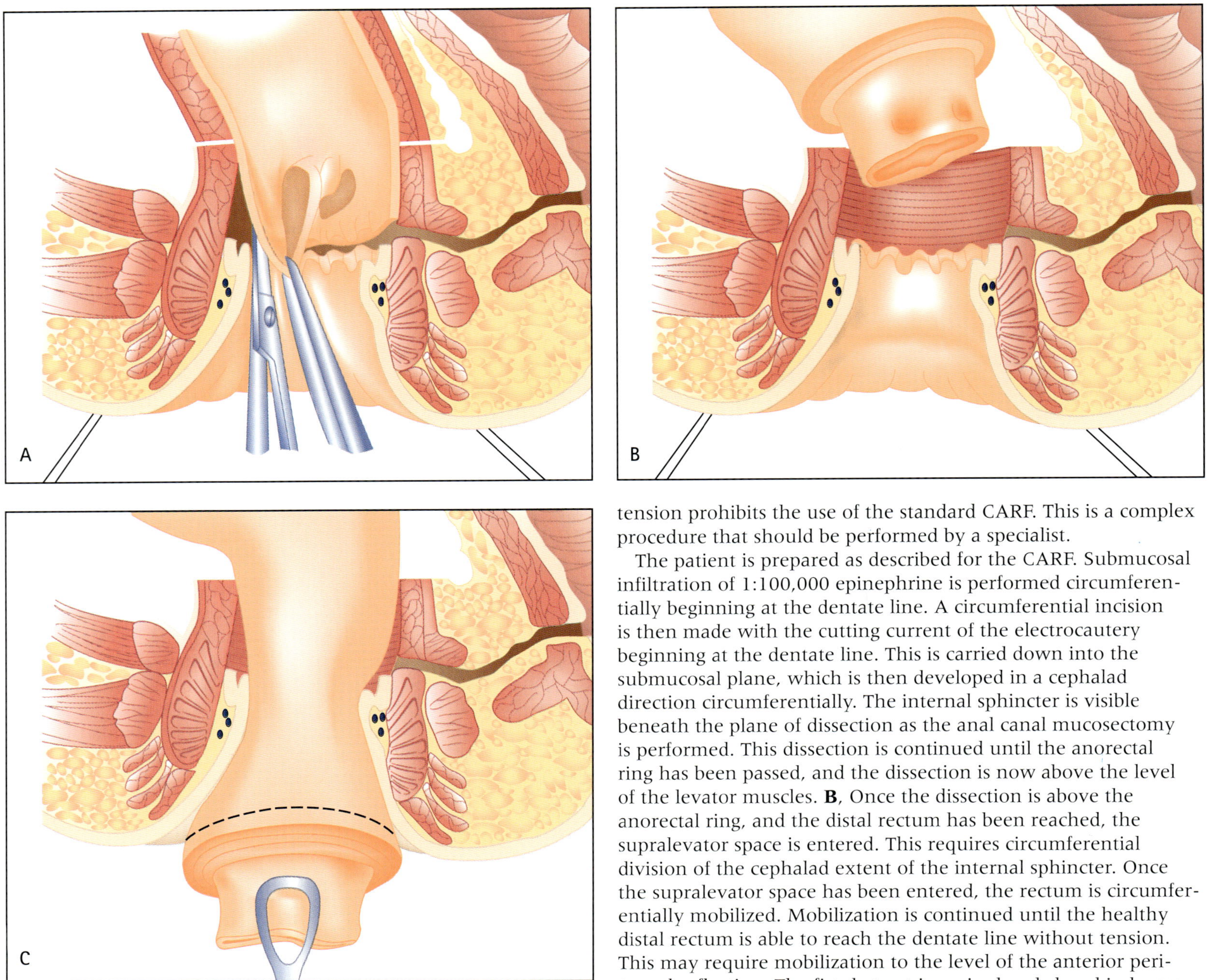

FIGURE 11–13.

Advancement rectal sleeve (ARS). **A**, The ARS procedure involves circumferential mobilization of the distal rectum and removal of the anal mucosa. This procedure is ideally suited for the patient who has significant anal Crohn's disease (prohibits use of a curvilinear advancement rectal flap [CARF]) but has a relatively spared rectum and the patient who has concomitant anal canal stenosis from Crohn's disease. Because of the excellent mobility the procedure provides, it is also useful when significant tension prohibits the use of the standard CARF. This is a complex procedure that should be performed by a specialist.

The patient is prepared as described for the CARF. Submucosal infiltration of 1:100,000 epinephrine is performed circumferentially beginning at the dentate line. A circumferential incision is then made with the cutting current of the electrocautery beginning at the dentate line. This is carried down into the submucosal plane, which is then developed in a cephalad direction circumferentially. The internal sphincter is visible beneath the plane of dissection as the anal canal mucosectomy is performed. This dissection is continued until the anorectal ring has been passed, and the dissection is now above the level of the levator muscles. **B**, Once the dissection is above the anorectal ring, and the distal rectum has been reached, the supralevator space is entered. This requires circumferential division of the cephalad extent of the internal sphincter. Once the supralevator space has been entered, the rectum is circumferentially mobilized. Mobilization is continued until the healthy distal rectum is able to reach the dentate line without tension. This may require mobilization to the level of the anterior peritoneal reflection. The fistula tract is excised and closed in layers as previously described. The vaginal mucosa is left open for drainage. **C**, The rectum is delivered through the anal canal and the diseased anal mucosa is amputated by sharp division across the full thickness of the lower rectum. The distal rectum is then sutured to the dentate line where the mucosectomy began. This is done using interrupted 2-0 long-lasting absorbable suture. Because this is a complex procedure that often involves patients with anorectal Crohn's disease, a temporary diverting proximal stoma is frequently used.

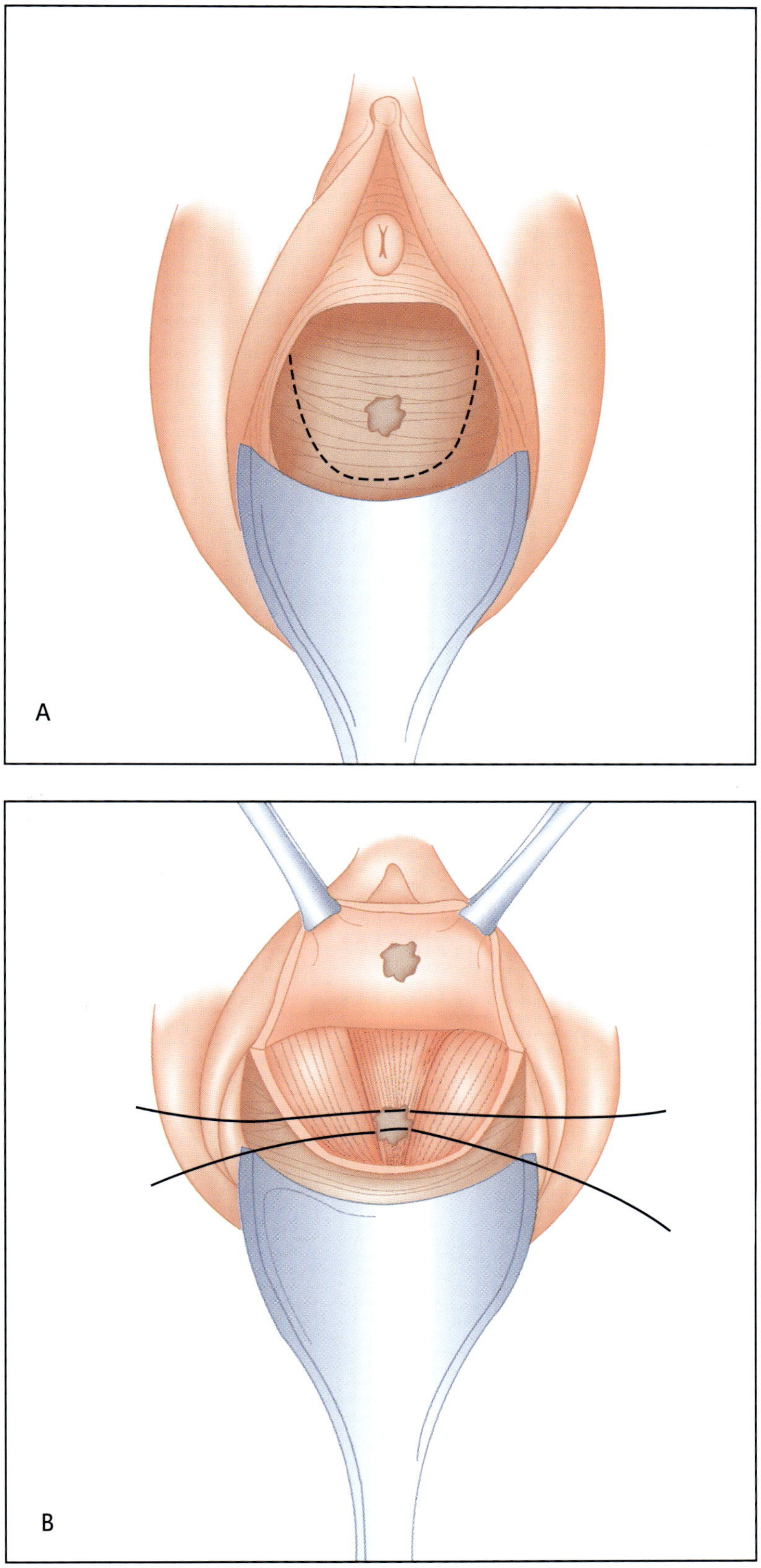

FIGURE 11-14.

Transvaginal repair. **A**, Patient preparation for transvaginal repair of a rectovaginal fistula (RVF) is similar to that for transanal RVF repair. However, the patient is positioned in the lithotomy position. The fistula tract is identified. The submucosal plane of the posterior vaginal wall is infiltrated with 1:100,000 epinephrine solution for hemostasis. A curvilinear incision beginning caudal to the fistula orifice on the posterior vaginal wall is made with the cutting current of the electrocautery. The flap is raised with a broad curvature that is extended laterally and posteriorly to the ischial tuberosities. This will provide adequate mobility. **B**, After the fistula tract is debrided and meticulous hemostasis is achieved, the rectal orifice of the fistula is closed using simple interrupted 3-0 long-lasting absorbable suture.

(*Continued on next page*)

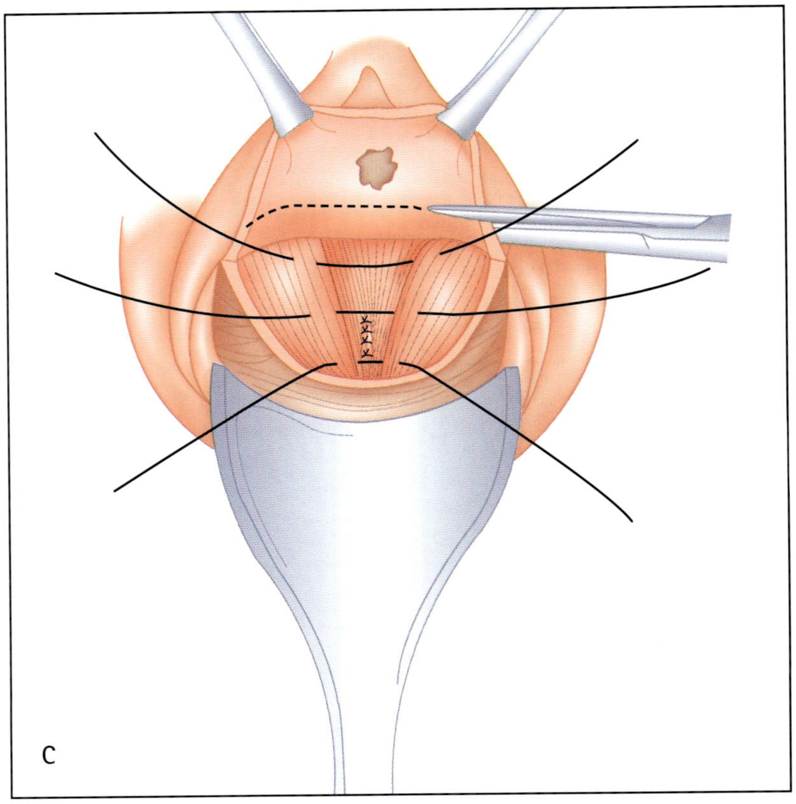

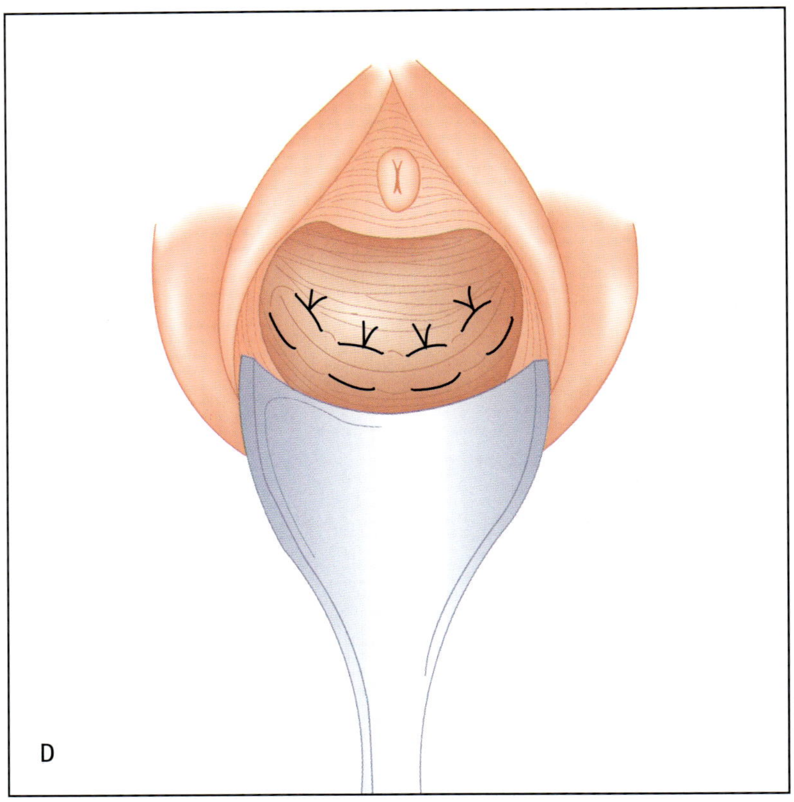

FIGURE 11-14. *(Continued)*

C, The levator ani muscles are closed next. These muscles are recognized as fibers that are oriented in a near vertical direction. Interrupted sutures of #0 long-lasting absorbable suture are used to approximate the levator ani muscles. In this way, they are interposed between the rectal and vaginal mucosal repairs and add layers to the repair. Approximation of the levator ani muscles becomes increasingly difficult as the suture line is moved distally. **D**, For flap closure, the distal aspect of the vaginal mucosal flap is then excised sharply to include the vaginal orifice of the fistula. The vaginal flap is then sutured to the distal incision line in the vaginal mucosa using interrupted 2-0 long-lasting absorbable suture. If this procedure is performed for a complex RVF, proximal fecal diversion is often necessary.

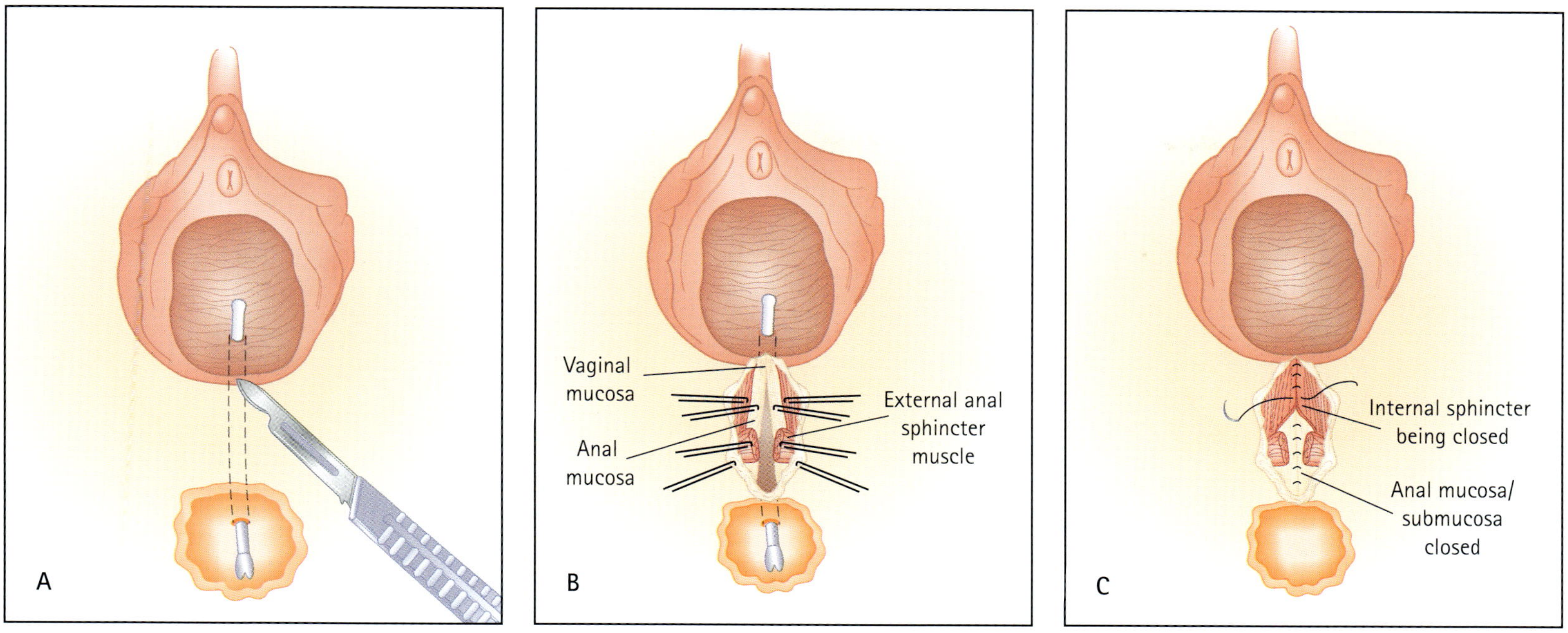

FIGURE 11-15.

Perineoproctotomy. **A**, Perineoproctotomy is a useful procedure for the patient with both a rectovaginal fistula (RVF) and an associated sphincter defect. The patient is prepared as previously described for transanal repair. The patient is then placed in the lithotomy position and a probe is passed through the RVF. The perineum, anal sphincter, and fistula tract are then sequentially opened, using the knife. As each layer is divided, the corresponding edges are secured with stay sutures. The fistula tract is then excised or curetted to healthy tissues. **B**, Four layers are prepared by dissecting them from surrounding tissues to both the right and left sides of the perineoproctotomy. These four layers from anterior to posterior are a vaginal mucosa, external anal sphincter and perineal body, internal anal sphincter, and anal canal mucosa and submucosa. Separation of the individual layers allows for tension-free repair and accurate tissue apposition. **C**, The perineoproctotomy is repaired in layers from posterior to anterior. Each layer is repaired using 2-0 long-lasting absorbable suture in an interrupted fashion. The anal mucosa and submucosa are repaired first. The internal sphincter is approximated next. The external sphincter and perineal body are approximated, and this layer may also include the levator ani at the cephalad extent of the repair. Finally, the vaginal mucosa and then perineal skin are repaired.

REFERENCES

1. Tsang CBS, Rothenberger DA: Rectovaginal fistulas: therapeutic options. *Surg Clin North Am* 1997, 77:95–114.
2. Venkatesh KS, Ramanujam PS, Larson DM, Haywood MA: Anorectal complications of vaginal delivery. *Dis Colon Rectum* 1989, 32:1039–1041.
3. Tsang CB, Madoff RD, Wong WD, *et al.*: Anal sphincter integrity and function influences outcome in rectovaginal fistula repair (review). *Dis Colon Rectum* 1998, 41:1141–1146.
4. Lee BH, Choe DH, Lee JH, *et al.*: Device for occlusion of rectovaginal fistula: clinical trials. *Radiology* 1997, 203:65–69.
5. Turnbull RB, Cuthbertson A: Abdominal pull-through resection for cancer and for Hirschsprung disease. *Cleve Clin Q* 1961, 28:109–115.

CHAPTER 12

Lower Urinary Tract Injury: Prevention, Recognition, and Management

W. Glenn Hurt

In the female, the close embryologic and anatomic relationship between the reproductive tract and the lower urinary tract predisposes the lower urinary tract to involvement by gynecologic disorders and places it at risk for injury during pelvic surgery and radiation therapy. The majority of surgical injuries to the lower urinary tract occur as a result of gynecologic surgery. It is inevitable that radical surgical procedures and pelvic radiation therapy performed to cure gynecologic malignancies will be associated with a low incidence of injuries to the urinary tract. But, regrettably, the gynecologic procedure most often associated with lower urinary tract injury is an abdominal or vaginal hysterectomy preformed for the treatment of a benign and otherwise uncomplicated condition. Therefore, most of these injuries should be preventable.

The incidence of lower urinary tract injury at the time of major gynecologic surgery is 0.5% to 2.5%; it is the same whether the procedure is performed by laparotomy or laparoscopy. Of concern is the fact that the majority of these injuries are not recognized at the time of surgery. If these injuries were recognized and appropriately managed at the time of surgery, postoperative morbidity could be significantly reduced. Therefore, emphasis must be placed on the prevention, recognition, and management of lower urinary tract injuries associated with gynecologic surgery [1–4].

Preoperatively, the history and physical examination, urinalysis, urine culture, and blood chemistries may give important information about the condition of the urinary tract and its involvement by pathologic conditions. Preoperative intravenous urograms are helpful in detecting congenital anomalies of the urinary tract and in documenting involvement by pelvic tumors, pelvic inflammatory disease, or invasive processes such as endometriosis or cancer. Imaging studies may be used to document the integrity and function of the urinary tract, but they have not been shown to lower the incidence of operative injures to the urinary tract [5]. Ureteral catheters may be used to assist in the identification and dissection of the ureters, but their need cannot always be predicted and their use can contribute to ureteral injury. For these reasons, many surgeons prefer to insert ureteral catheters when they are needed intraoperatively rather than preoperatively.

Intraoperatively, certain surgical principles contribute to the safety of all pelvic procedures. When surgery is performed within the peritoneal cavity, it is important that the anatomy be restored and the course of the ureters be identified. In dissecting retroperitoneally, the attachment of the ureters to the pelvic peritoneum should be preserved and the adventitial blood supply to the ureters should not be damaged. Most ureteral injuries that are the result of gynecologic surgery occur in the distal 4 to 5 cm of each ureter; the types of injury vary and are sometimes difficult to recognize. Intraoperatively, when ureteral injury is suspected, a number of procedures can be used to determine the location and extent of the injury. Bladder injuries are also more likely to occur in specific locations; partial-thickness injuries of the bladder wall may rupture postoperatively if the bladder becomes overdistended. When bladder injury is suspected, it is important to distend the bladder with a sterile solution to determine the integrity of its wall.

Postoperatively, unrecognized lower urinary tract injuries or unsuccessful repairs should be suspected when oliguria or anuria, fever, chills, or flank pain develops. Intraperitoneal or retroperitoneal leakage of urine may cause abdominal distention, ileus, and urinoma formation. Ultimately, a urinary fistula may develop or there may be ureteral obstruction with loss of renal function. Operative injuries to the lower urinary tract that are recognized within days of surgery should be repaired immediately if the patient's condition permits. The timing of the repair of injuries diagnosed later in the postoperative period or that are discovered in patients whose physical condition will not permit surgery must be individualized [6]. During the waiting period, urinary leakage may be managed with retrograde placement of ureteral catheters or by percutaneous nephrostomy catheter placement; bladder catheter drainage, either transurethral or suprapubic, and in the case of genitourinary fistulas also by vaginal drainage devices.

PREVENTION OF LOWER URINARY TRACT INJURY

PELVIC CONDITIONS PREDISPOSING TO LOWER URINARY TRACT INJURY

Large pelvic tumors
Cervical leiomyomas
Endometriosis
Ovarian remnants
Pelvic inflammatory disease
Pelvic malignancies
Pelvic organ prolapse
Diverticulosis
Congenital anomalies
Pregnancy
Prior pelvic surgery
Prior radiation therapy

FIGURE 12-1.

Pelvic conditions predisposing to lower urinary tract injury. Although these findings may predispose to surgical injury of the lower urinary tract, most injuries occur at the time of hysterectomy performed for a benign condition in which none of them is a complicating factor. Injury is more likely to occur with abdominal hysterectomy than with vaginal hysterectomy. Most lower urinary tract injuries are not recognized at the time of surgery [1].

SURGICAL PRINCIPLES FOR PROTECTION OF PELVIC ORGANS

- Before surgical entry
  - Bowel Preparation
  - Positioning in universal stirrups
  - Draping for abdominal and vaginal access
  - Bladder drainage
  - Examination under anesthesia
- After surgical entry
  - Adequate exposure of surgical field
  - Adequate light within surgical field
  - Adequate suction for surgical field
  - Restoration of anatomic relationships
  - Traction and countertraction to expose adjacent structures
  - Dissection of extraperitoneal "spaces"
  - Dissection along tissue planes
  - Maintaining hemostasis
  - Clamping, cutting, and suturing under direct vision
  - Avoidance of mass ligation of tissues

FIGURE 12-2.

Surgical principles for protection of pelvic organs. These principles are helpful in preventing injury to the lower urinary tract and bowel. When a difficult pelvic dissection is anticipated, the bowel should be prepared beginning 24 to 48 hours before surgery by prescribing a liquid diet, an oral bowel cleansing agent (e.g., citrate of magnesia, GoLYTELY™), and enemas. Positioning the patients for surgery in universal stirrups; prepping their abdomen, vulva, vagina, inner thighs; and draping them with a drape that provides abdominal and vaginal access will simplify intraoperative vaginal manipulation and cystoscopy. For most major gynecologic surgery, it is best to provide continuous bladder drainage by inserting a balloon catheter and connecting it to a closed drainage system. This is usually done using a double-lumen catheter; but if the need for bladder filling can be anticipated, it can be made easier by inserting a triple-lumen catheter and connecting it to a closed drainage system and to a bag containing a suitable sterile irrigating solution.

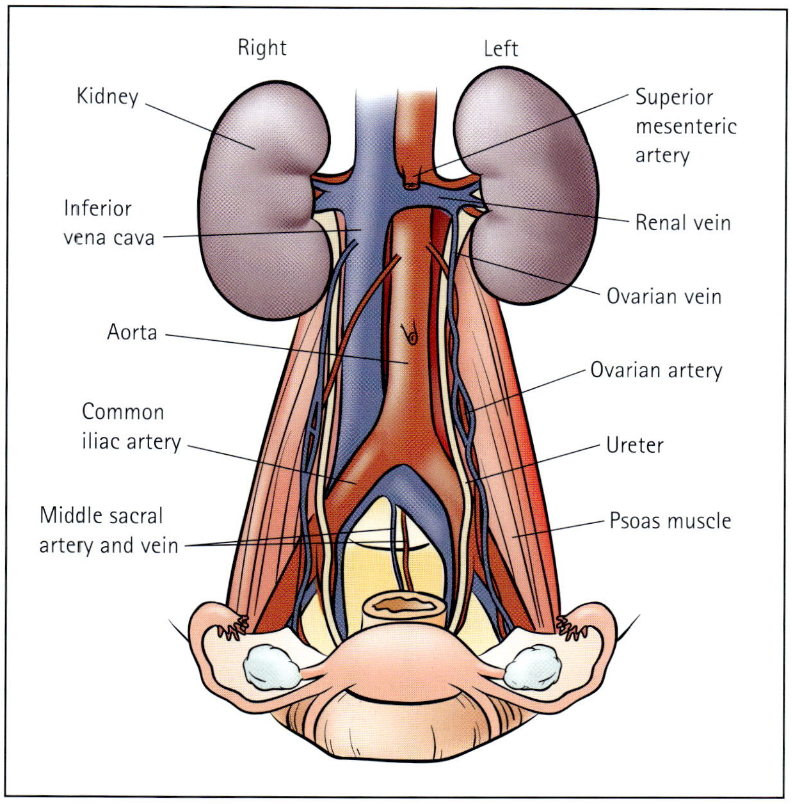

FIGURE 12-3.

Anatomy of the kidneys, ureters, and great vessels. The upper pole of each kidney lies on a level with the upper border of the 12th thoracic vertebra, their lower pole on a level with the third lumbar vertebra; the right kidney is usually slightly lower than the left; the renal arteries arise from the aorta at right angles at the level of the disk between L1 and L2 vertebrae, with the left renal artery slightly above the right. The ureters originate from the renal pelvis at the level of the spine of L1; they are 25 to 30 cm long. Each ureter is anatomically subdivided into abdominal ureter and pelvic ureter by crossing the pelvic brim; the abdominal and pelvic segments are about of equal length. The abdominal ureters descend along the anterior surfaces of the psoas muscles, posterior to the ovarian vessels, to the pelvic brim. The right ureter lies lateral to the inferior vena cava; the left ureter lies lateral to the aorta and passes beneath the inferior mesenteric artery, ovarian vessels, and colon. The ureters pass over the bifurcations of the common iliac arteries; descend along the posterolateral pelvic sidewalls lateral to the sacrum, anterior to the external iliac arteries; and each ureter passes under the uterine arteries 1 to 2 cm lateral to the internal cervical os after which they pass through the cardinal ligaments, then medially and anteriorly about the lateral vaginal fornices to enter their corresponding bladder tunnel to open onto the bladder trigone.

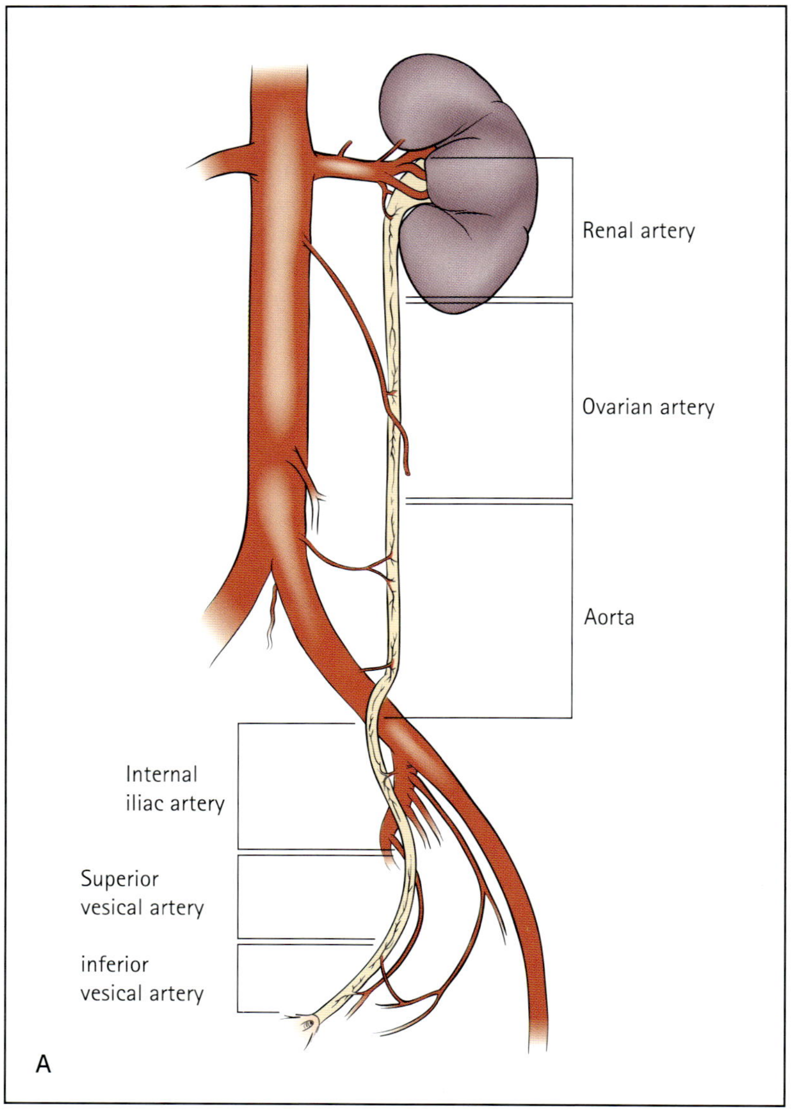

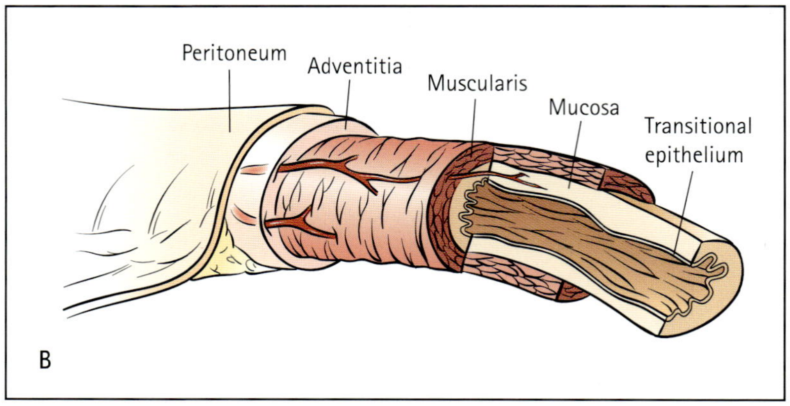

FIGURE 12-4.

Blood supply to and anatomy of the ureter. **A**, The blood supply to the ureters is unpredictable. Normally, in their course from the kidneys to the bladder, the ureters receive ureteral branches from the renal arteries, ovarian arteries, aorta, internal iliac arteries, and the superior and inferior vesical arteries. The veins follow the correspondingly named arteries and terminate in the correspondingly named veins. **B**, The wall of each ureter is comprised of three layers: mucosa, muscularis, and adventitia. Their major blood supply forms a rich anastomotic network within the adventitia and gives small branches to the inner muscularis and mucosa.

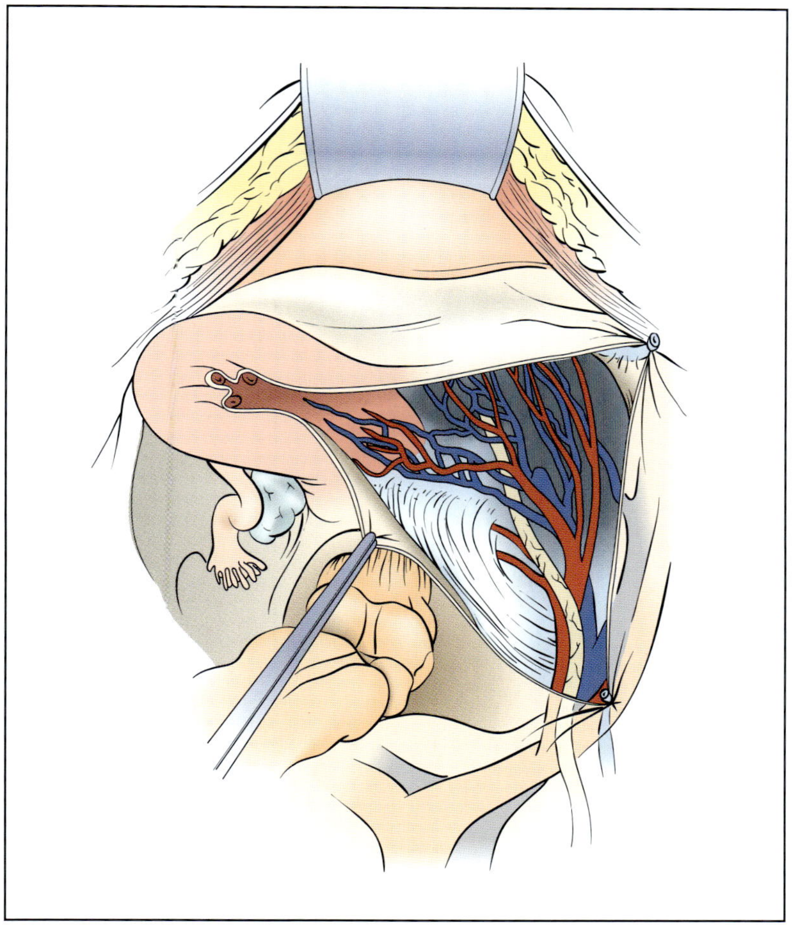

FIGURE 12-5.

Identifying and dissecting the course of the ureters during abdominal procedures. The best method of preventing ureteral injury is to demonstrate the course of each ureter at the time of laparotomy or laparoscopy and then to keep them out of harm's way. The pelvic ureters are most easily identified as they enter the pelvis by passing over the bifurcations of the common iliac arteries. An alternative method of identification is to locate the external iliac arteries and to follow them toward their corresponding common iliac artery; the first structure crossing the external iliac artery will the be ureter [7]. The ureter is best identified by direct visualization of its characteristic peristalsis. During palpation, when the ureter is allowed to pass between the index finger and thumb it will sometimes provide an audible "click" and impart a snapping sensation to the palpating fingers. On occasion, both of these findings may be rendered by palpating pelvic vessels or some other structure making this a less reliable way of positively identifying the ureters. When dissecting the ureters, it is important to preserve their attachment to the overlying peritoneum and to perform the dissection outside of their adventitial sheaths to avoid injuring their blood supply. Routine dissections of each ureter usually do not go much below the level of the uterine arteries. Circumstances may require dissection of the distal ureter.

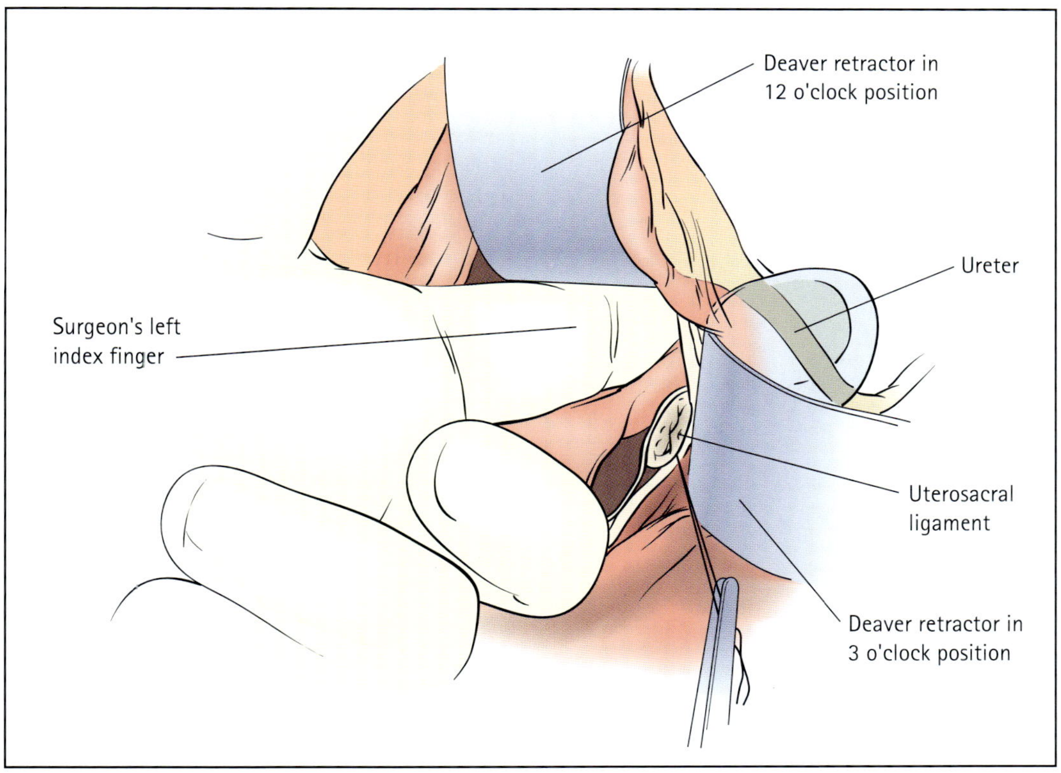

FIGURE 12-6.

Identifying the ureters during vaginal procedures. The distal ureter can be palpated through a colpotomy incision against a Deaver or similar retractor placed with its tip in the lateral vaginal fornix and with the assistance of another retractor lifting the trigone and base of the bladder [8]. Vaginal dissection of the ureter for purposes of identification has been described, but the dissection itself is tedious and may predispose the ureter to injury [9]. (*From* Lee [8]; with permission.)

RECOGNITION OF LOWER URINARY TRACT INJURY

A. TYPES OF URETERAL INJURY

- Angulation
- Devascularization
- Crushing
- Ligation
- Penetration
- Laceration, partial or complete
- Loss of segment

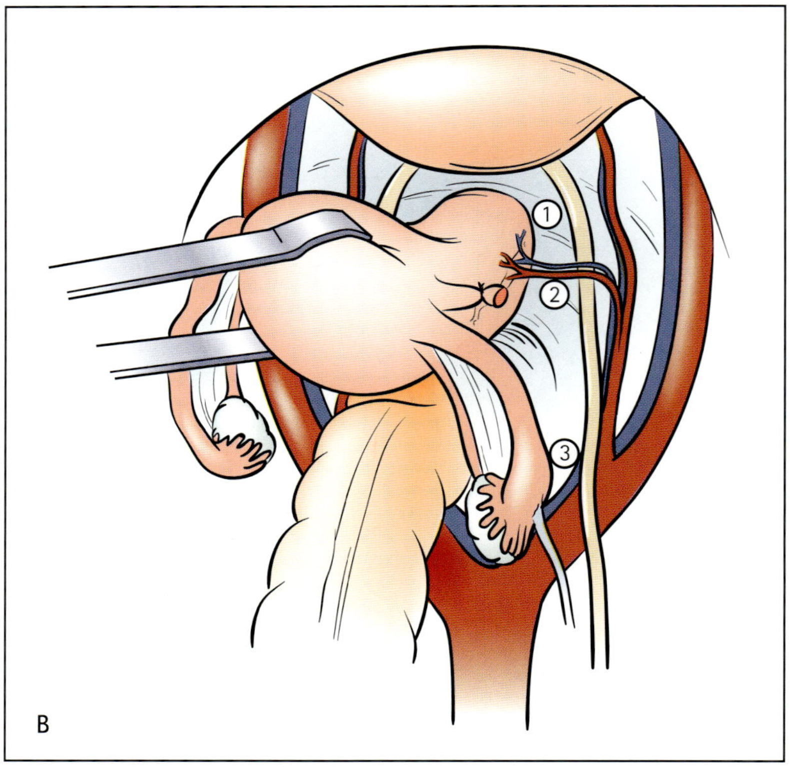

FIGURE 12-7.

Types and sites of ureteral injury. **A**, Ureteral injuries may be direct or indirect. **B**, During gynecologic surgery, the most frequent sites of ureteral injury are at the level of (*1*) the cardinal ligaments, (*2*) the uterine vessels, and (*3*) the infundibulopelvic ligaments.

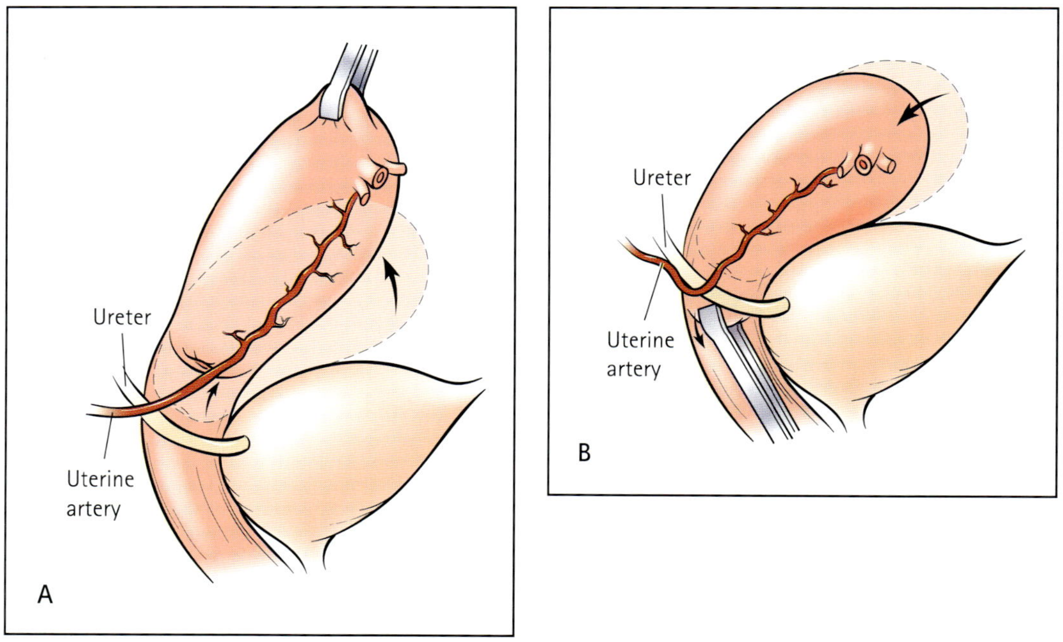

FIGURE 12-8.

Effect of traction on relationship of uterus to ureter. **A**, Upward countertraction on the uterine fundus during an abdominal hysterectomy normally increases the distance between the cervix and ureter at the level of the uterine vessels. **B**, Downward traction on the cervix during a vaginal hysterectomy decreases the distance between the cervix and ureter at the level of the uterine vessels. Remembering this is important in preventing ureteral injury.

METHODS OF DETECTING INTRAOPERATIVE URETERAL INJURY

- Dissection of course of ureter
- Ureteral dye injection
- Intravenous dye injection
- Ureteral catheterization
- Intravenous urography
- Cystoscopy or cystotomy

FIGURE 12–9.

Methods of detecting intraoperative ureteral injury. If intraoperative ureteral injury is suspected, one or more of these procedures may be used to prove the condition and function of a ureter.

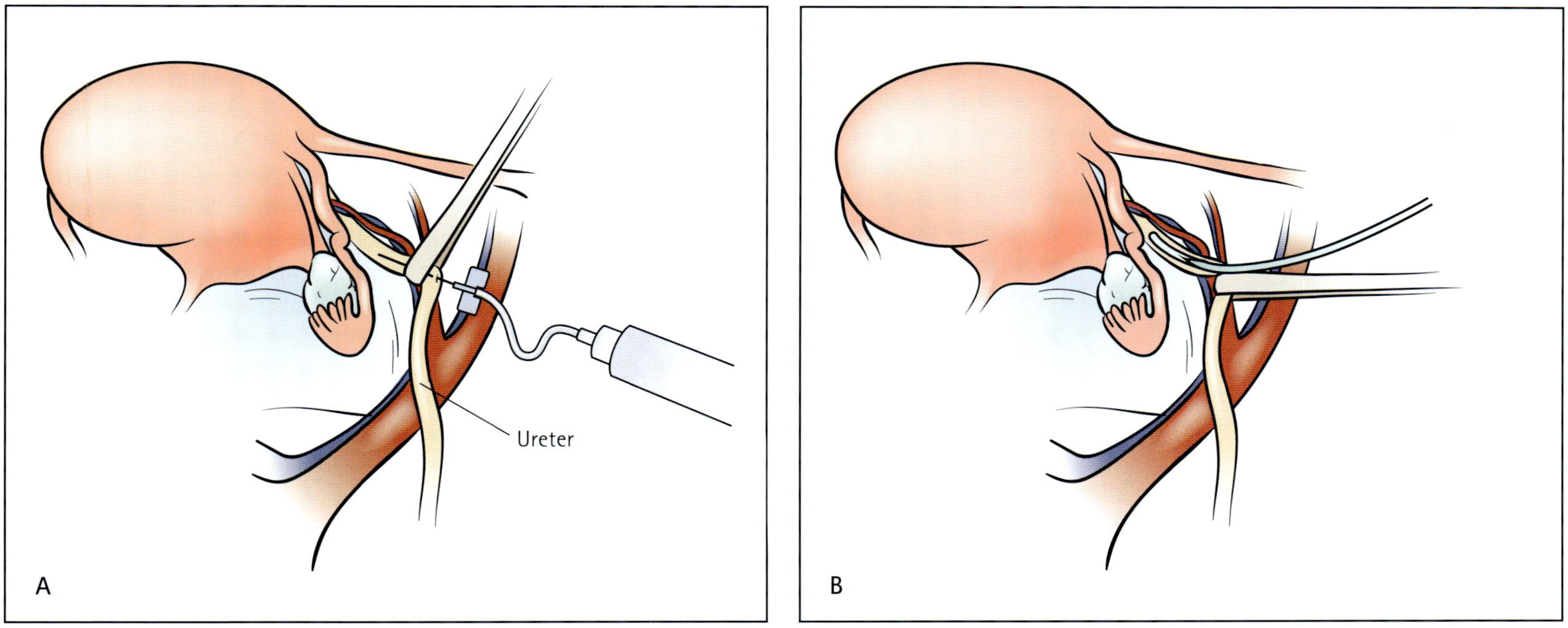

FIGURE 12–10.

Dye injection. **A**, Intraoperatively, the lumen of a ureter may be injected with indigo carmine or methylene blue. Isolate and stabilize a segment of ureter above the site of suspected injury with a Penrose drain or Babcock clamp. Use a butterfly needle (22 gauge) with tubing and a syringe containing 5 mL of indigo carmine or methylene blue to inject the lumen of the ureter in the direction of the bladder. Leakage of dye into the operative field suggests damage to the wall of the ureter. No leakage of dye into the operative field and passage of blue urine suggests an intact and patent ureter on the side of the injection. **B**, Intravenous injection of indigo carmine (5 mL) or methylene blue (5 mL) should be followed by renal excretion of blue urine within 5 to 10 minutes. To document that both kidneys and ureters are functioning, it is necessary to visualize the ureteral excretion of urine by cystoscopy.

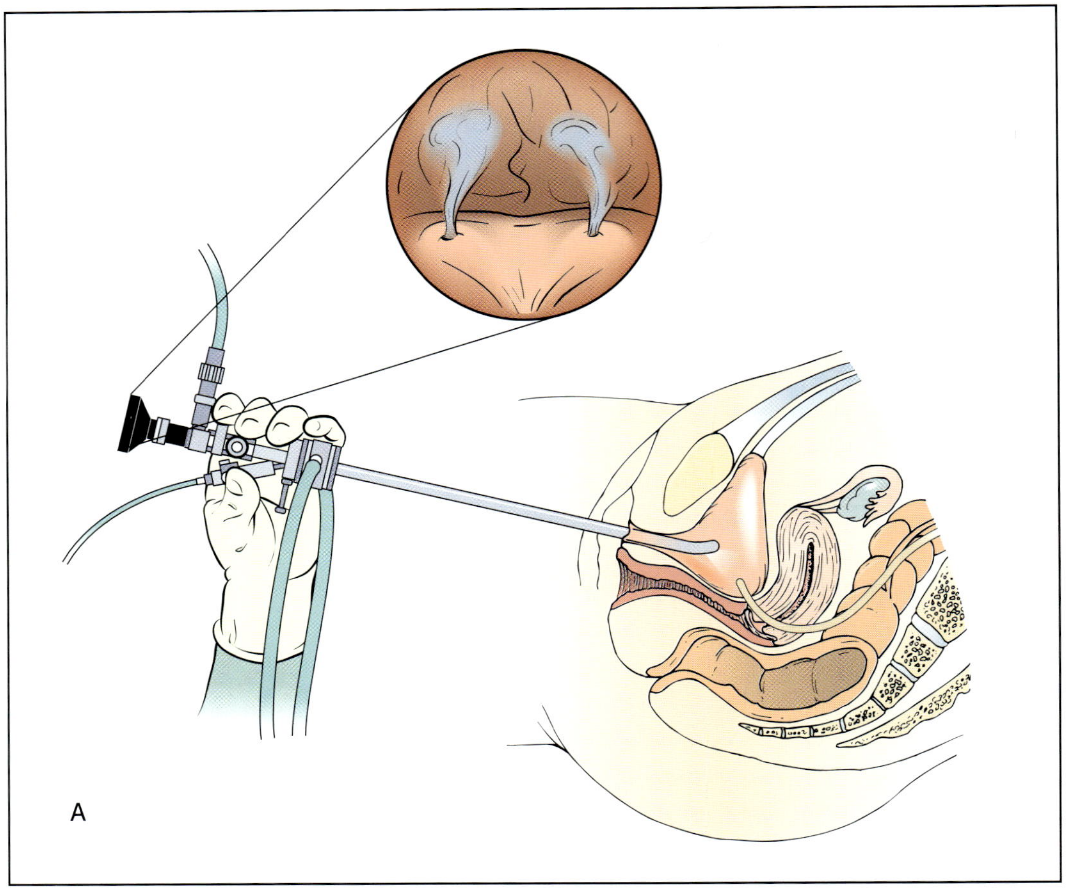

A

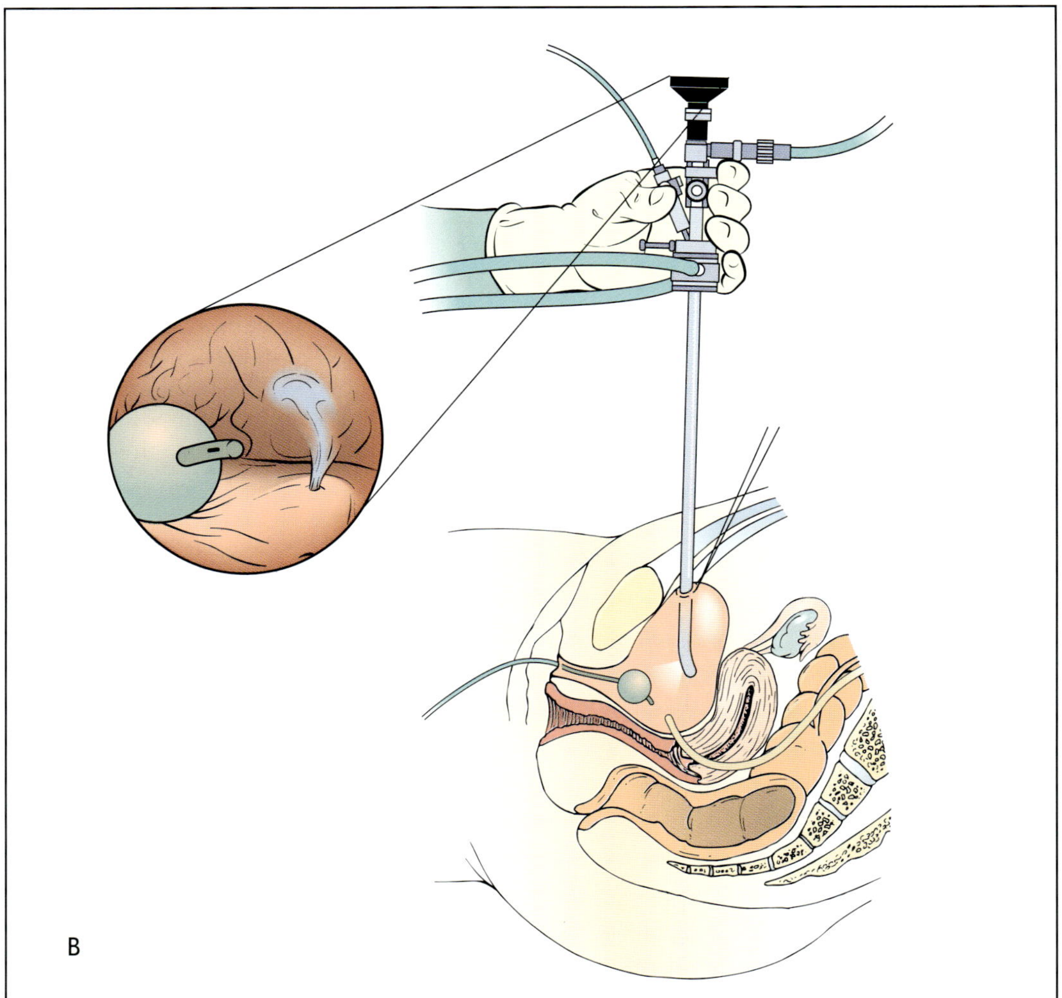

B

FIGURE 12-11.

Cystoscopy. **A**, Transurethral cystoscopy is facilitated by having the patient placed in the universal stirrups, positioned in the low lithotomy position, and draped with a drape that provides vaginal access [10]. **B**, Suprapubic cystoscopy, sometimes referred to as teloscopy, is performed by distending the bladder with sterile water or normal saline, placing a pursestring suture of absorbable or delayed-absorbable suture about what is to be a puncture site in the extraperitoneal dome of the bladder, puncturing the bladder, and inserting an endoscopic telescope to view the inside of the bladder [11]. The balloon of the transurethral catheter will usually have to be displaced upward to see the ureteral orifices to document ureteral function. Normally, the administration of intravenous indigo carmine (5 mL) or methylene blue (5 mL) will be followed by the excretion of blue urine from the ureteral orifices within 5 to 10 minutes. Failure of both ureters to excrete the blue urine must be explained.

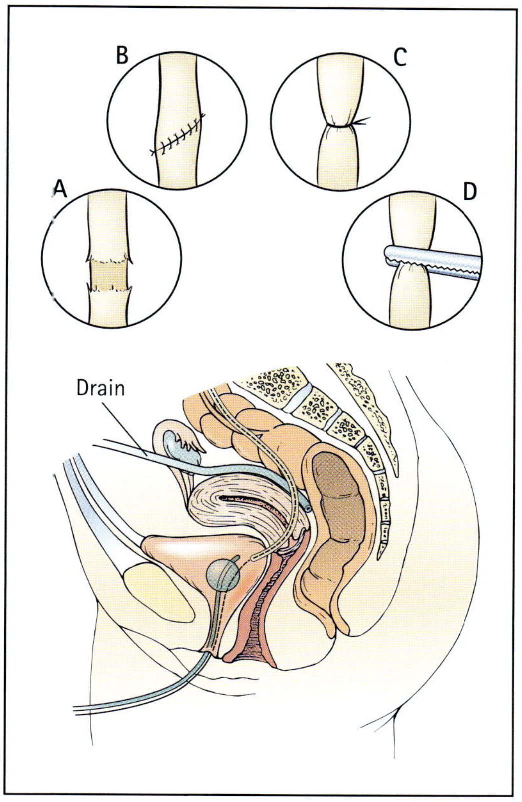

FIGURE 12-12.

Ureteral stenting or catheterization. Placement of ureteral stents or catheters should be considered when there are ureteral sheath injuries (**A**), partial or complete transections (**B**), ligations (**C**), or crushing injuries (**D**). Ureteral catheters may be passed up the affected ureter by cystoscopy or intentional cystotomy. Occasionally, a linear ureterotomy will be performed and a stent will be passed through the distal ureter into the bladder; or ureteral catheters will be passed through either end of a transected ureter into the renal pelvis proximally and the bladder distally.

When the stiffness of a ureteral catheter interferes with its placement, a small silicone pediatric feeding (5 F) tube may be substituted. If this is done, it is important to know the location of openings within the end of the tube and to confirm that it is placed at a location within the upper renal tract, which will ensure the drainage of urine.

When linear stents or catheters are left in place for urine drainage, they may be brought out of the body alongside a transurethral or suprapubic catheter. The urethral stent or catheter should be anchored to the transurethral or suprapubic catheter to maintain its position within the urinary tract. Urethral and bladder catheters will require separate closed drainage urine collection systems. Rarely, a ureteral catheter will be brought out directly through the skin as a temporary method of urinary drainage.

Sometimes it is helpful to have ureteral catheters or stents placed to help identify the course of one or both ureters during surgery. This may be done preoperatively or intraoperatively by cystoscopy or cystotomy. Ureteral catheterization is not without hazard. The placement of ureteral stents or catheters may cause ureteral injury resulting in hematuria, edema, and perforation. Surgeons who dissect ureters containing stents or catheters should be aware that the catheters or stents may impart a stiffness to the ureter, which may predispose it to injury.

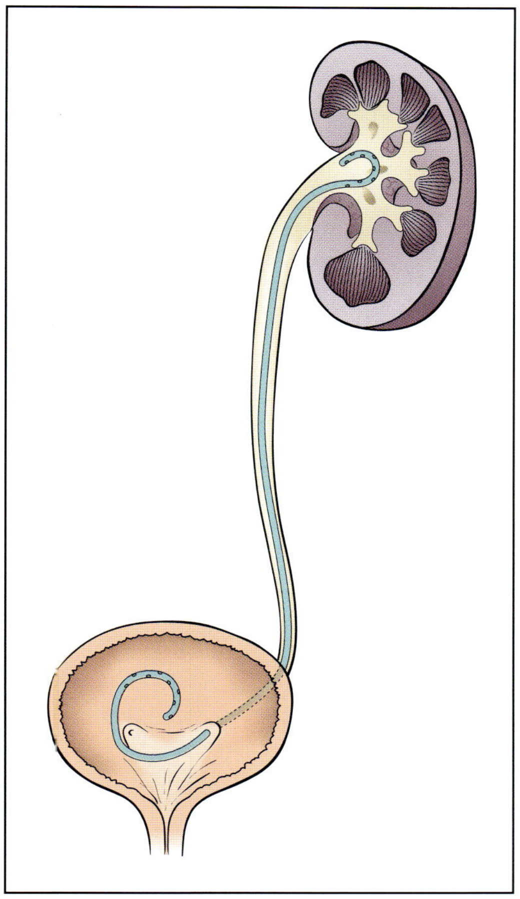

FIGURE 12-13.

Double-J catheters. These are positioned to have one end within the renal pelvis and one end within the bladder. Ureteral catheters must be positioned to allow the drainage of urine from the renal pelvis through the catheter and into the bladder. The curled ends of the double-J catheter maintain their position within the urinary tract.

MANAGEMENT OF LOWER URINARY TRACT INJURY

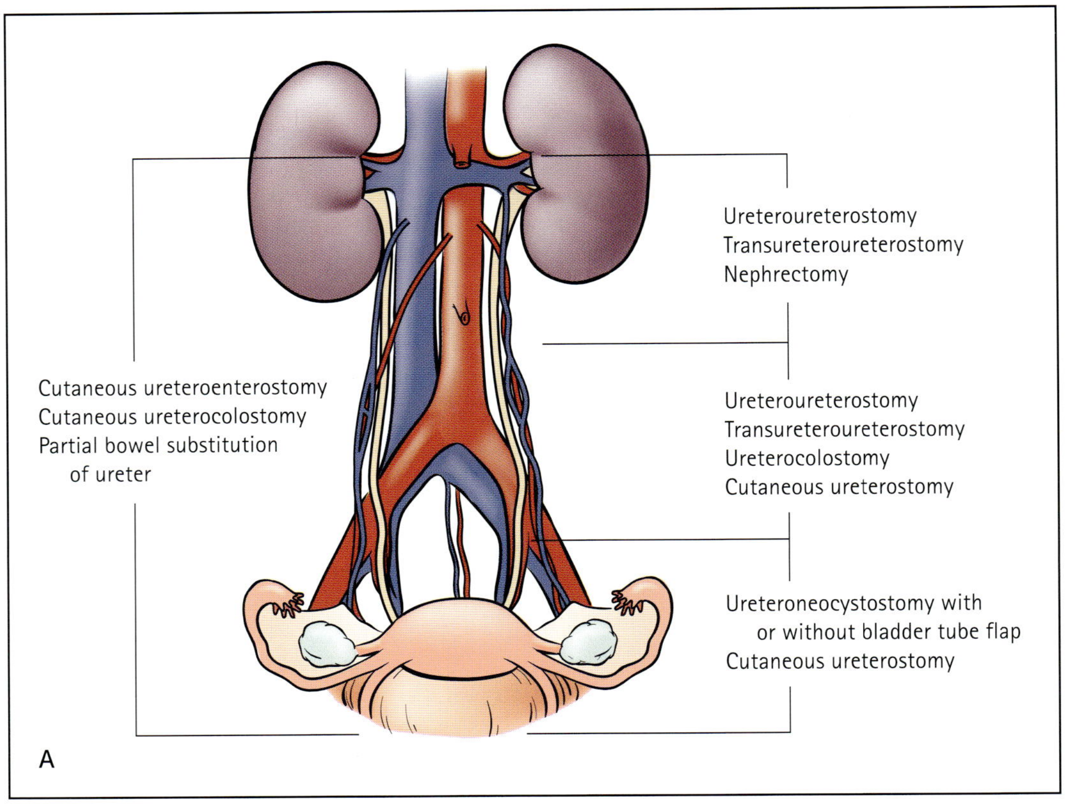

B. PRINCIPLES FOR SUCCESSFUL URETERAL REPAIR

Perform meticulous ureteral dissection using atraumatic instruments.

Preserve ureteral blood supply by leaving peritoneal attachments and dissecting outside of adventitial sheath.

Perform a tension-free anastomosis.

Use minimal amount of smallest absorbable suture needed to obtain watertight anastomosis.

Surround anastomosis with retroperitoneal fat or omentum to assist healing.

Drain retroperitoneal anastomotic site to prevent accumulation of urine.

Consider proximal urinary diversion, with or without stenting.

FIGURE 12-14.

Surgical procedures and principles for repair of ureteral injuries. **A**, The selection of a reparative procedure depends on the location and extent of the injury [2]. Other factors that must be considered are cause of injury, condition of the tissues, renal function, patient's prognosis, and surgeon's experience. Significant ureteral injuries that are the result of gynecologic surgery or radiation therapy usually involve the distal 4 to 5 cm of the ureter and are best treated by ureteroneocystostomy. **B**, The principles for successful ureteral repair are listed [12]. (*Part B* is modified from Schlossberg [12]; with permission.)

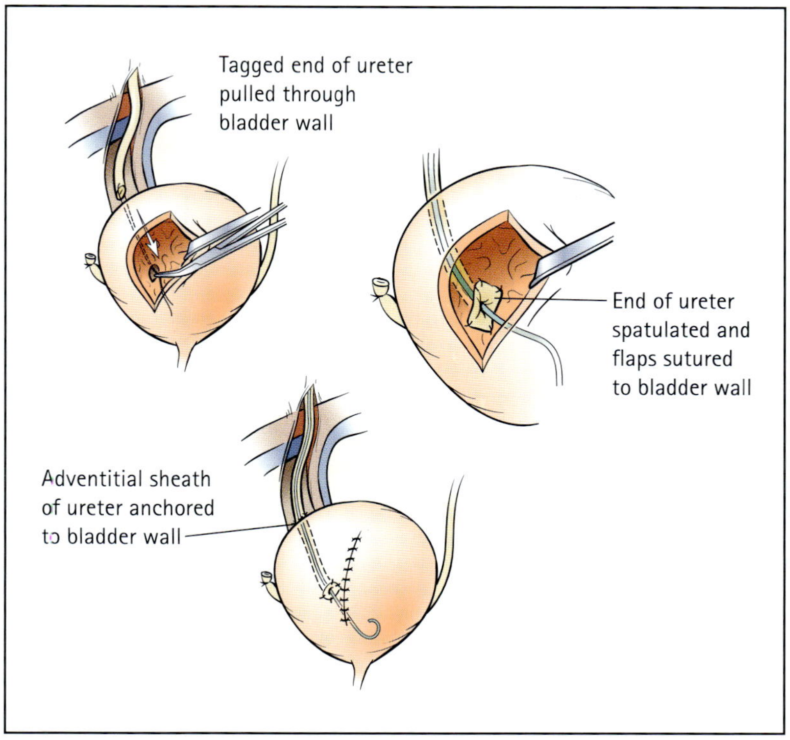

FIGURE 12-15.

Abdominal ureteroneocystostomy. This procedure is recommended for injuries to the lower 4 to 5 cm of either ureter. The pelvic ureter is meticulously dissected to prevent damage to its adventitial sheath and blood supply. The distal end of the ureter is ligated with permanent suture at the ureterovesical junction. Any damaged ureteral segment is excised. A 3-0 suture on an atraumatic tapered needle is passed through the diameter of the proximal ureter about 0.5 cm from its end. The needle is removed and the long ends of the suture are tagged with small forceps.

An extraperitoneal cystotomy is performed in the dome of the bladder, and the ureteral orifices are identified. A finger is placed inside the fundus of the bladder, which is displaced toward the cut end of the ureter to determine the best site for a tension-free reimplantation. For direct reimplantation, the entire thickness of the bladder wall is perforated with a right-angled or Adson forceps from within the bladder at the site of the reimplantation. The tips of the forceps are opened about 1 cm to enlarge the hole in the bladder wall and to grasp the tagged suture. The end of the ureter is drawn into the bladder for a distance of 1.0 cm. The end of the ureter is spatulated about 0.5 cm on opposite sides of its circumference, and the tagging suture is removed. Four 3-0 absorbable sutures are placed to secure the distal ureteral flaps to the inside of the bladder wall. Several 3-0 delayed-absorbable sutures are used to anchor the adventitial sheath of the ureter to the outside of the bladder wall. The need for placing a ureteral catheter will have to be determined. The bladder is drained with a transurethral or suprapubic catheter.

If there is physiologic compromise of renal function, the ureter may be reimplanted via a submucosal tunnel created within the wall of the bladder to prevent vesicoureteral reflux [13]. The tunnel is created by passing closed Metzenbaum scissors or small tapered forceps obliquely through the muscular layer of the bladder. The distal half of the tunnel should be submucosal before its entry into the bladder. The tagged ureter is drawn into the tunnel by traction on the tagging suture. The end of the ureter is spatulated and secured to the mucosal and muscular layers of the bladder by several 4-0 absorbable sutures. Several 3-0 delayed-absorbable sutures are used to anchor the adventitial sheath of the ureter to the outside of the bladder wall.

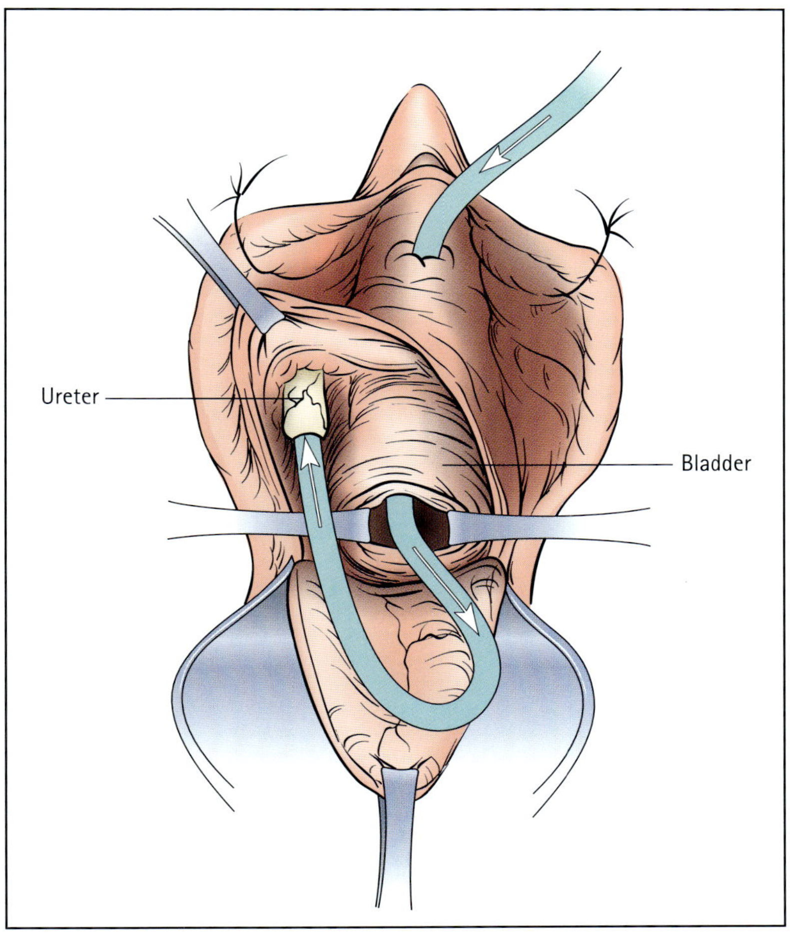

FIGURE 12-16.

Vaginal ureteroneocystostomy. This technique may be used for injuries of the terminal 3 cm of either ureter [14]. The distal end of the ureter is identified and ligated with permanent suture at the ureterovesical junction. The proximal end of the ureter is identified, trimmed, mobilized, spatulated bilaterally for a distance of about 0.5 cm, and catheterized. The catheter is passed through a cystotomy incision and brought out of the urethra. The spatulated end of the ureter is drawn into the bladder through a cystotomy and sewn to the inside of the bladder with two 4-0 absorbable sutures. The adventitial sheath is anchored to the external surface of the base of the bladder with two or three 3-0 interrupted delayed absorbable sutures.

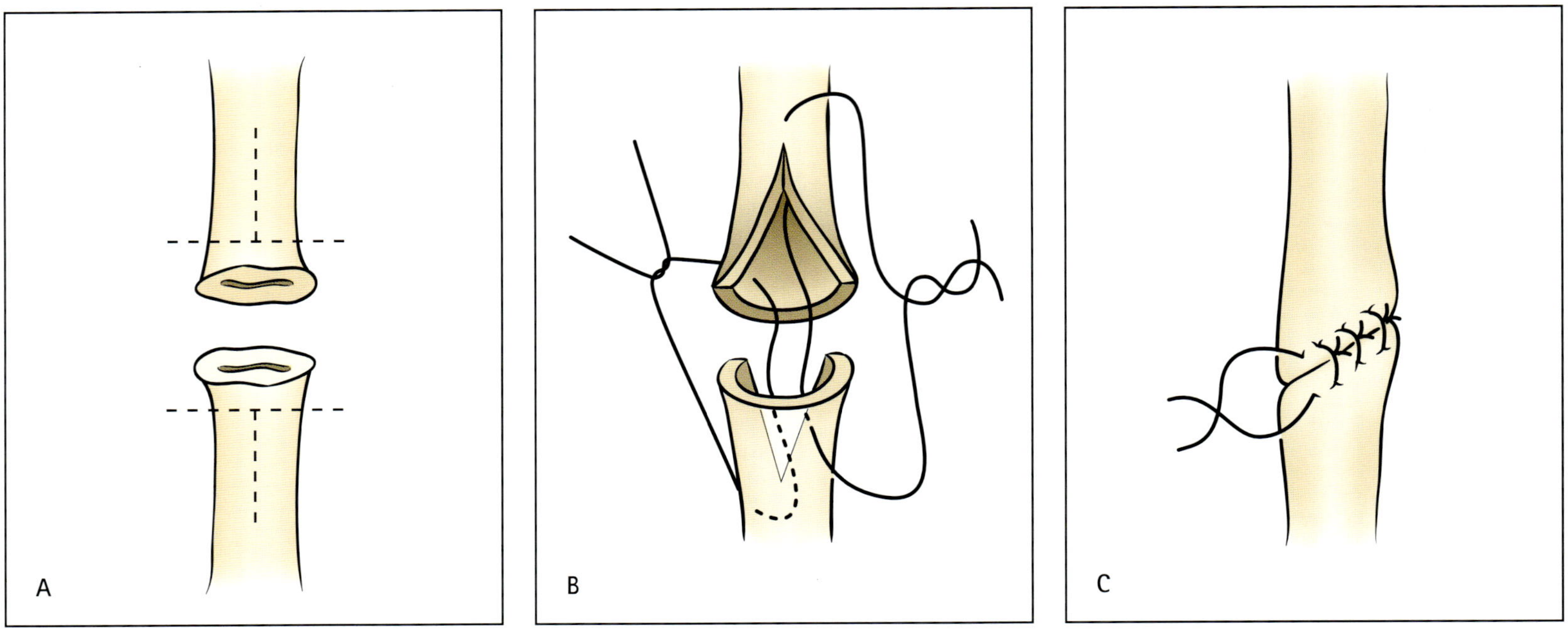

FIGURE 12-17.
Ureteroureterostomy. This is recommended for significant ureteral injuries above and just below the pelvic brim. In performing an end-to-end anastomosis of a ureter, trim the cut ends to healthy tissue (**A**), spatulate both ends to allow an oblique anastomosis and reduce the incidence of stenosis (**B**), and approximate the ends over a properly placed ureteral catheter using interrupted 4-0 chromic catgut or delayed absorbable suture (**C**). The anastomosis should be watertight, but not ischemic. The anastomotic site should be drained by an extraperitoneal suction drain. The end of the drain should be adjacent to but not in contact with the ureteral anastomosis.

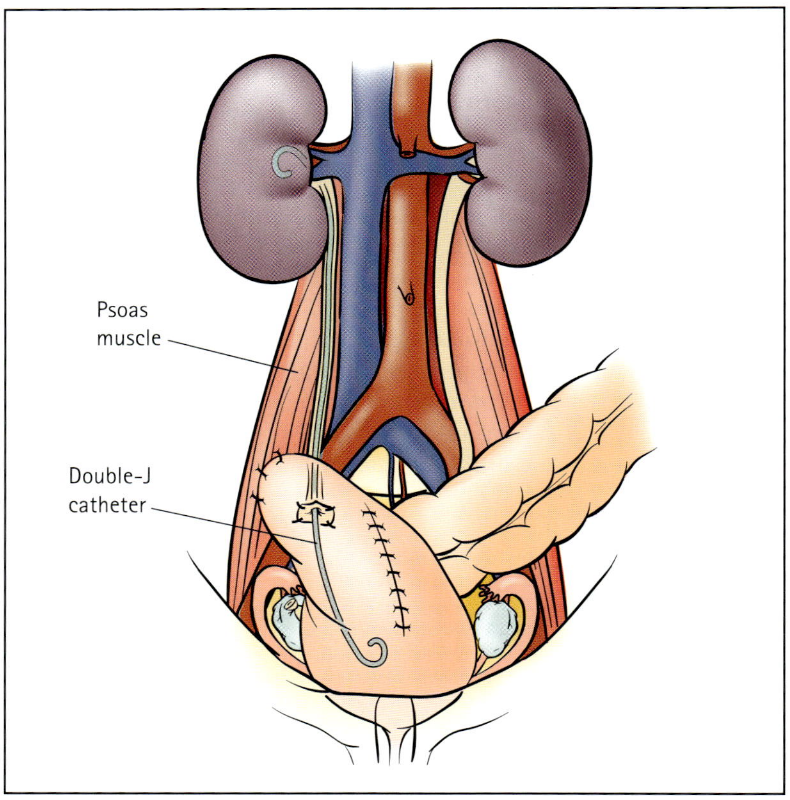

FIGURE 12-18.
Vesicopsoas hitch. A vesicopsoas hitch is recommended when performing a ureteroneocystotomy or ureteroureterostomy to ensure a tension-free ureteral anastomosis. The upward mobility of the bladder may be increased by freeing the dome of the bladder from its loose attachments to the retrosymphysis. The vesicopsoas hitch is performed by placing one or two fingers through an anterior extraperitoneal cystotomy in the dome of the bladder and displacing the bladder toward the end of the damaged ureter. The leading point of the outer wall and muscular layer of the bladder is sutured to the psoas major fascia with several interrupted 2-0 or 1-0 delayed absorbable sutures.

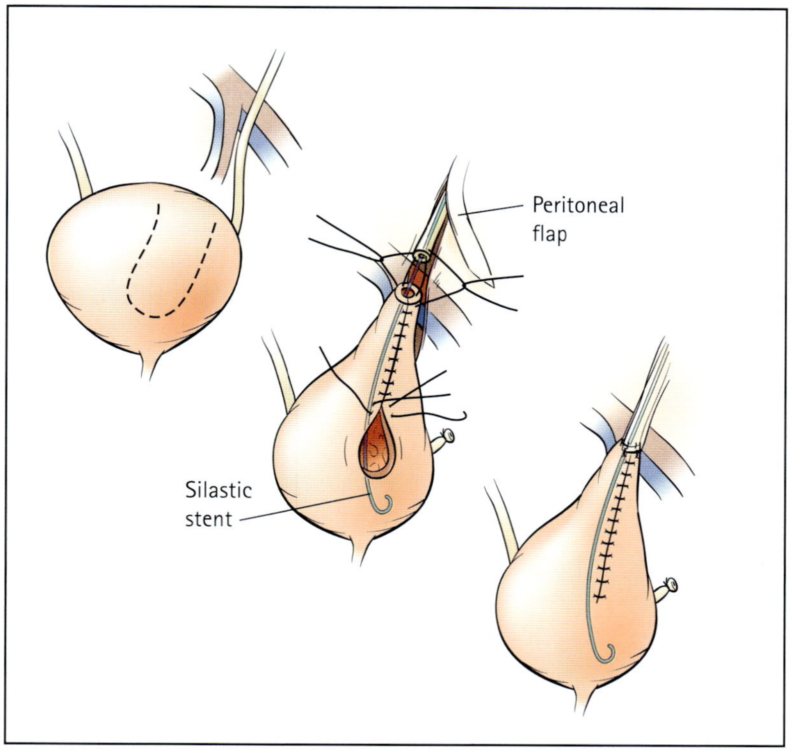

FIG 12-19.

Boari-Ockerblad bladder flap. A Boari-Ockerblad bladder flap is used to extend the bladder a greater distance toward a shortened ureter than is possible by using a vesicopsoas hitch [15]. The bladder is mobilized by freeing its attachments to the retrosymphysis. A vesicopsoas hitch is performed on the side that the ureter is to be reimplanted. A full-thickness, wide-based bladder flap is cut out of the anterior bladder wall. The distal ureter is reimplanted directly or by way of a submucosal tunnel into the upper end of the bladder flap with 4-0 interrupted absorbable or delayed-absorbable sutures. The cut edges of the flap are approximated with one layer of interrupted 4-0 or 3-0 absorbable or delayed-absorbable sutures.

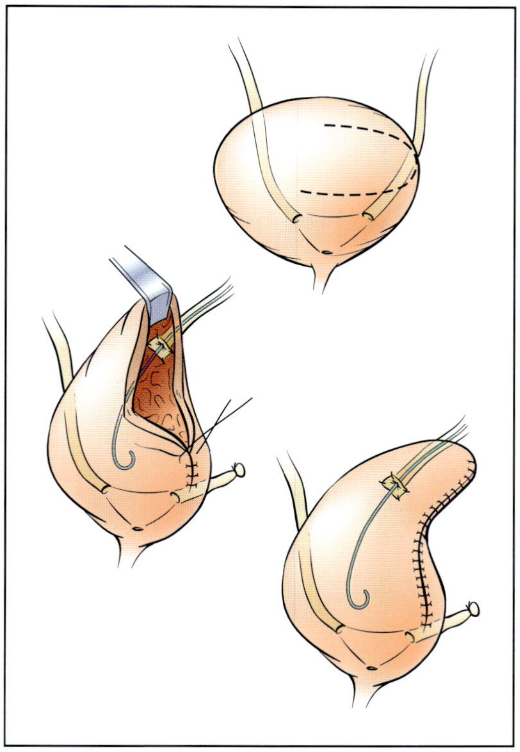

FIGURE 12-20.

Demel bladder flap. The Demel bladder flap differs from the Boari-Ockerblad bladder flap only in that the incision for the bladder flap is made about the anterolateral wall of the bladder on the side of the ureteral reimplantation [16].

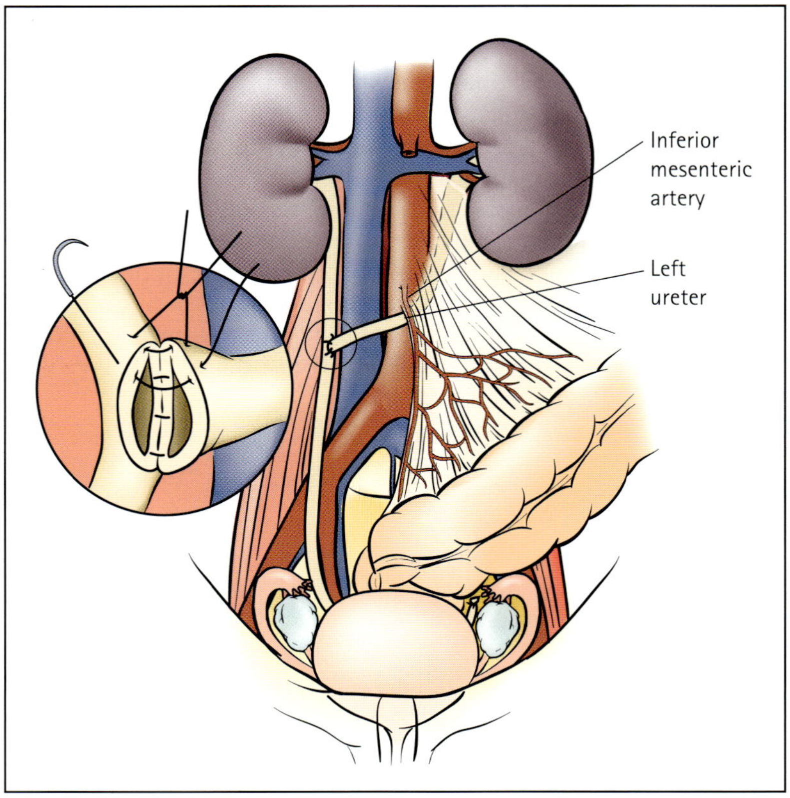

FIGURE 12-21.

Transureteroureterostomy. A transureteroureterostomy is performed when there is loss of a significant portion of one of the lower ureters. The distal end of that ureter is tied with permanent suture at its ureterovesical junction. The proximal end is mobilized and carried retroperitoneally below the inferior mesenteric artery and in front of the great vessels to meet the opposite ureter. The recipient ureter is longitudinally incised and an end-to-side anastomosis is performed using interrupted 4-0 delayed absorbable sutures through the adventitial and muscular layers of both ureters. The anastomosis should be watertight, but not ischemic. The anastomotic site should be drained by an extraperitoneal suction drain.

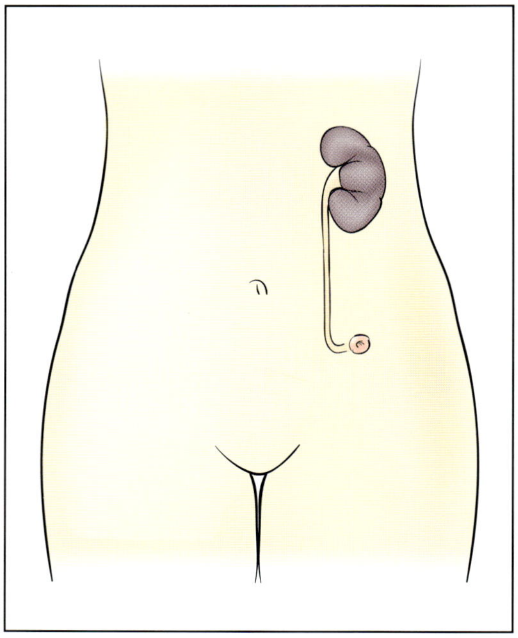

FIGURE 12-22.

Cutaneous ureterostomy. This procedure is recommended in patients whose chances of survival are limited or in those in whom the surgeon is not prepared to perform a definitive repair. The distal end of the ureter is tied with permanent suture at its ureterovesical junction. The cut end of the ureter is bought out retroperitoneally, and a ureter-to-skin anastomosis is performed. Ureteral catheterization or stent placement may not be necessary.

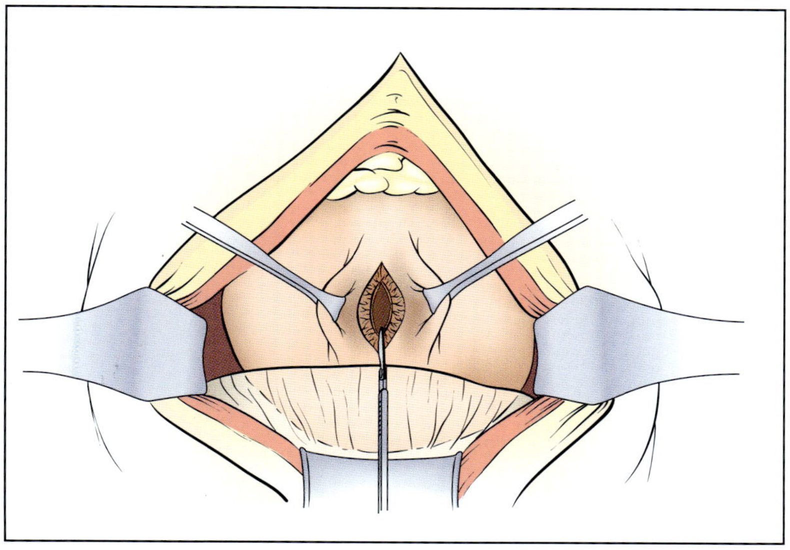

FIGURE 12-23.

Cystotomy. A cystotomy for inspection of the bladder, ureteral catheterization, or ureteroneocystostomy is best performed in the extraperitoneal portion of the dome of the bladder. A cystotomy for the repair of a genitourinary fistula may have to be placed through that portion of the bladder that is covered by peritoneum. Cystotomies should be closed in two layers with absorbable or delayed-absorbable suture. It is helpful to cover transperitoneal cystotomies and those in the base of the bladder with an intact layer of peritoneum or a flap of omentum. A suprapubic or transurethral catheter should be placed for postoperative bladder drainage.

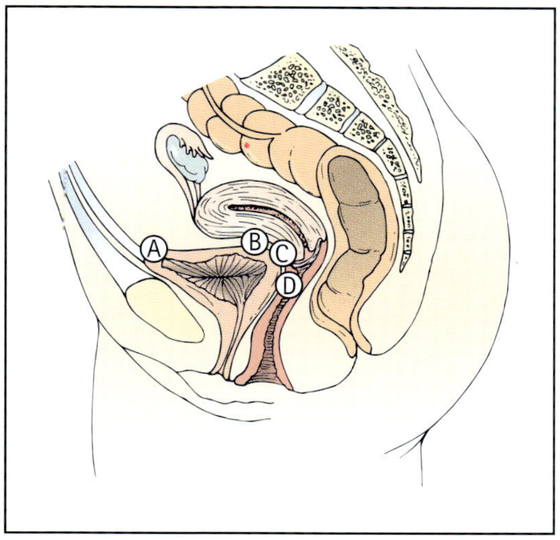

FIGURE 12-24.

Frequent sites of bladder injury. The dome of the bladder is the site of most frequent injury; this is often done at the time of entry into the abdomen. The base of the bladder is subject to injury when dissecting the bladder from the cervix during abdominal or vaginal hysterectomy and when clamping and suturing the vaginal cuff.

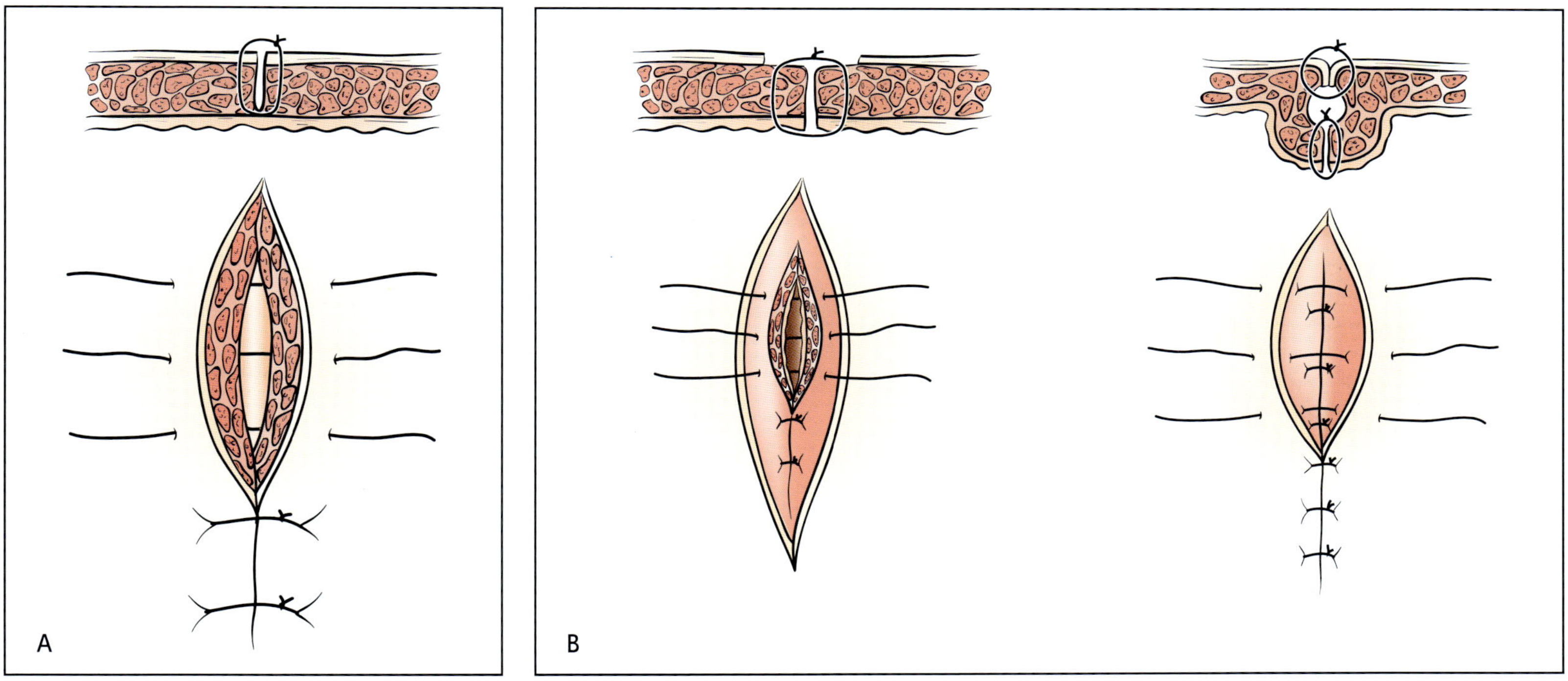

FIGURE 12-25.

Repair of bladder injuries. Partial-thickness bladder injuries are repaired by placing a single layer of 3-0 absorbable or delayed-absorbable sutures through the muscular and serosal layers (**A**). Full-thickness injuries are repaired in two layers with the first layer incorporating the muscular and mucosal layers of the bladder wall and the second layer imbricating the deeper layer by the placement of Lembert sutures through the serosal and muscular layers of the bladder (**B**).

POSTOPERATIVE URINARY DRAINAGE

Ureteral Catheter

- Ureteral damage may require 5 to 7 days of urinary diversion with an excretory urogram and possible cystogram prior to catheter removal.
- Ureteral transections or resections may require 6 to 8 weeks of urinary diversion with an excretory urogram and possible cystogram before catheter removal.

Bladder Catheter

- Period of continuous catheter drainage has to be individualized.
- Consider transurethral catheters for < 24 to 48 hours of continuous drainage.
- Consider suprapubic catheters for > 24 to 48 hours of continuous drainage.
- Intermittent clean self-catheterization may be used instead of continuous drainage as a means of bladder drainage.

FIGURE 12-26.

Postoperative urinary drainage. Ureteral catheters should be positioned to drain urine from the renal pelvis into the bladder or out of the body. Double-J catheters will maintain their position as a result of their coiled tips. Straight catheters must be anchored to a bladder drainage catheter or to the skin to prevent dislodgment. The bladder may be drained by a transurethral or a suprapubic catheter. Balloon transurethral catheters of 14 F or 16 F size are usually adequate. A large number of pericutaneously inserted suprapubic catheters are available. The size of their drainage tube varies from 7 F to 16 F. When hematuria is present, it is better to use a catheter that is 14 F or larger to allow for the possible passage of clots and to facilitate bladder irrigation. In every case, the duration of urinary drainage must be individualized.

REFERENCES

1. Symmonds RE: Ureteral injuries associated with gynecologic surgery: prevention and management. *Clin Obstet Gynecol* 1976, 19:623–643.
2. Hurt WG, Segreti EM: Intraoperative ureteral injuries and urinary diversion. In *Gynecologic and Obstetric Surgery*, edn 2. Edited by Nichols DH, Clarke-Pearson D. St. Louis: Mosby Year Book; 1999.
3. Goodno JA Jr, Powers TW, Harris VD: Ureteral injury in gynecology surgery: a ten-year review in a community hospital. *Am J Obstet Gynecol* 1995, 172:1817–1822.
4. Saidi MH, Sadler RK, Vancaillie TG, *et al.*: Diagnosis and management of serious urinary complications after major operative laparoscopy. *Obstet Gynecol* 1996, 87:272–276.
5. Piscitelli JT, Simel DL, Addison W: Who should have intravenous pyelograms before hysterectomy for benign disease? *Obstet Gynecol* 1987, 69:541–545.
6. Witters S, Cornelissen M, Vereecken R: Iatrogenic ureteral injury: aggressive or conservative treatment, *Am J Obstet Gynecol* 1986, 155:582–584.
7. Manetta A: Surgical maneuver for the prevention of ureteral injuries. *J Gynecol Surg* 1989, 5:291–294.
8. Lee RA: *Atlas of Gynecologic Surgery.* Philadelphia: WB Saunders; 1992.
9. Cruikshank SH: Surgical method of identifying the ureters during total vaginal hysterectomy. *Obstet Gynecol* 1986, 67:277–280.
10. Harris RL, Cundiff GW, Theofrastous JP, *et al.*: The value of intraoperative cystoscopy in urogynecology and reconstructive pelvic surgery. *Am J Obstet Gynecol* 1997, 177:1367–1371.
11. Timmons MC, Addison WA: Suprapubic teloscopy: extraperitoneal intraoperative technique to demonstrate ureteral patency. *Obstet Gynecol* 1990, 75:137–139.
12. Schlossberg SM: Ureteral healing, *Semin Urol* 1987, 5:197–199.
13. Politano VA, Leadbetter WF: An operative technique for correction of vesicoureteral reflux. *J Urol* 1958, 79:932–941.
14. Thompson JD, Benigno BB: Vaginal repair of ureteral injuries. *Am J Obstet Gynecol* 1971, 3:601–610.
15. Boari A: Contributo sperimentale alla plastica dell= uretere. *Atti Acad Sci Med Nat Ferrara* 1894, 68:149–157.
16. Demel R: Ersatz des ureters durch eine Plastik aus der Harnblase (Vorlaufige Mitteilung). *Zentralbl Chir* 1924, 51:2008–2018.

Index

A

B

C

D

E

F

G

H

I

K

L

M

N

O

P

R

S

T

U

V